DIFFERENTIAL DIAGNOSIS IN ULTRASOUND

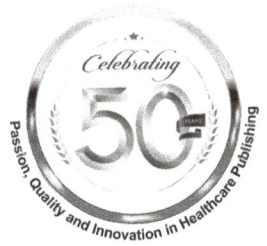

DIFFERENTIAL DIAGNOSIS IN ULTRASOUND

Third Edition

Editors

Sumeet Bhargava
MBBS DNB (Radiodiagnosis) FCGP FIAMS FICRI FIMSA MNAMS

Formerly Associate Professor
Department of Radiology and Imaging
Rama Medical College and Superspecialty Hospital
Ghaziabad, Uttar Pradesh, India

Satish K Bhargava
MBBS MD (Radiodiagnosis)
MD (Radiotherapy) DMRD FICRI FIAMS FCCP FUSI FIMSA FAMS

Formerly Professor and Head
Department of Radiology and Imaging
University College of Medical Sciences (University of Delhi)
Guru Teg Bahadur (GTB) Hospital, New Delhi
Rama Medical College and Superspecialty Hospital, Ghaziabad
and
School of Medical Sciences and Research
Sharda Hospital, Greater Noida, Uttar Pradesh, India

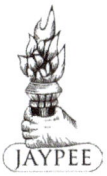

JAYPEE BROTHERS MEDICAL PUBLISHERS
The Health Sciences Publisher
New Delhi | London | Panama

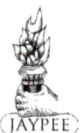 **Jaypee Brothers Medical Publishers (P) Ltd.**

Headquarters
Jaypee Brothers Medical Publishers (P) Ltd
4838/24, Ansari Road, Daryaganj
New Delhi 110 002, India
Phone: +91-11-43574357
Fax: +91-11-43574314
Email: jaypee@jaypeebrothers.com

Overseas Offices
J.P. Medical Ltd
83 Victoria Street, London
SW1H 0HW (UK)
Phone: +44 20 3170 8910
Fax: +44 (0)20 3008 6180
Email: info@jpmedpub.com

Jaypee-Highlights Medical Publishers Inc
City of Knowledge, Bld. 235, 2nd Floor
Clayton, Panama City, Panama
Phone: +1 507-301-0496
Fax: +1 507-301-0499
Email: cservice@jphmedical.com

Jaypee Brothers Medical Publishers (P) Ltd
Bhotahity, Kathmandu, Nepal
Phone: +977-9741283608
Email: kathmandu@jaypeebrothers.com

Website: www.jaypeebrothers.com
Website: www.jaypeedigital.com

© 2019, Jaypee Brothers Medical Publishers

The views and opinions expressed in this book are solely those of the original contributor(s)/author(s) and do not necessarily represent those of editor(s) of the book.

All rights reserved. No part of this publication may be reproduced, stored or transmitted in any form or by any means, electronic, mechanical, photocopying, recording or otherwise, without the prior permission in writing of the publishers.

All brand names and product names used in this book are trade names, service marks, trademarks or registered trademarks of their respective owners. The publisher is not associated with any product or vendor mentioned in this book.

Medical knowledge and practice change constantly. This book is designed to provide accurate, authoritative information about the subject matter in question. However, readers are advised to check the most current information available on procedures included and check information from the manufacturer of each product to be administered, to verify the recommended dose, formula, method and duration of administration, adverse effects and contraindications. It is the responsibility of the practitioner to take all appropriate safety precautions. Neither the publisher nor the author(s)/editor(s) assume any liability for any injury and/or damage to persons or property arising from or related to use of material in this book.

This book is sold on the understanding that the publisher is not engaged in providing professional medical services. If such advice or services are required, the services of a competent medical professional should be sought.

Every effort has been made where necessary to contact holders of copyright to obtain permission to reproduce copyright material. If any have been inadvertently overlooked, the publisher will be pleased to make the necessary arrangements at the first opportunity. The **CD/DVD-ROM** (if any) provided in the sealed envelope with this book is complimentary and free of cost. **Not meant for sale.**

Inquiries for bulk sales may be solicited at: jaypee@jaypeebrothers.com

Differential Diagnosis in Ultrasound

First Edition: 2005
Second Edition: 2013
Third Edition: **2019**
ISBN: 978-93-5270-588-7

Dedicated to
*My late parents Shri Jagannath Bhargava and
Smt Brahama Devi Bhargava
&
My loving late wife Kalpana Bhargava
Whose inspiration and motivation have made
possible to bring out this book*

Satish K Bhargava

Contributors

Amit Sahu DNB (Radiodiagnosis)
Consultant Radiology
Max Superspecialty Hospital
Saket, New Delhi, India

Anoop Kumar Durga Das MD (Radiodiagnosis)
Ex-Resident
Department of Radiology
and Imaging
University College of Medical Sciences (University
of Delhi) and Guru Teg Bahadur (GTB) Hospital
New Delhi, India

Anubhav Sarikwal MD (Radiodiagnosis)
Ex-Senior Resident
Department of Radiology
and Imaging
University College of Medical Sciences (University
of Delhi) and Guru Teg Bahadur Hospital
New Delhi, India

Anupama Tandon MD (Radiodiagnosis)
Associate Professor
Department of Radiology
and Imaging
University College of Medical Sciences (University
of Delhi) and Guru Teg Bahadur Hospital
New Delhi, India

Anurag Agarwal MD (Radiodiagnosis)
Additional Director
National Board of Examinations
New Delhi, India

Ashish Verma DNB (Radiodiagnosis)
Associate Professor
Department of Radiology and Imaging
Institute of Medical Sciences
Banaras Hindu University
Varanasi, Uttar Pradesh, India

Avneesh Kumar Singh DNB (Radiodiagnosis)
Ex-Senior Resident
Department of Radiodiagnosis and Imaging
All India Institute of Medical Sciences
New Delhi, India

Gopesh Mehrotra DNB (Radiodiagnosis)
Professor
Department of Radiology
and Imaging
University College of Medical Sciences (University
of Delhi) and Guru Teg Bahadur Hospital
New Delhi, India

Mamta Motla MD (Radiodiagnosis)
Ex-Senior Resident
Department of Radiology
and Imaging
University College of Medical Sciences (University
of Delhi) and Guru Teg Bahadur Hospital
New Delhi, India

Meenakshi Prakash MD (Radiodiagnosis)
Ex-Resident
Department of Radiology and Imaging
University College of Medical Sciences (University
of Delhi) and Guru Teg Bahadur Hospital
New Delhi, India

Pardeep Kumar MD (Radiodiagnosis)
Senior Resident
Department of Radiology and Imaging
Maulana Azad Medical College and Associated
Govind Ballabh (GB) Pant Hospital
New Delhi, India

Pushpender Gupta MD (Radiodiagnosis)
Department of Radiology
Wake Forest University
Baptist Medical Center
Medical Center Boulevard Winston-Salem
North Carolina, USA

Rajul Rastogi MD (Radiodiagnosis)
Associate Professor
Department of Radiology
and Imaging
Teerthanker Mahaveer University
Moradabad, Uttar Pradesh, India

Satish K Bhargava
MD (Radiodiagnosis) MD (Radiotherapy) DMRD FICRI
FIAMS FCCP FUSI FIMSA FAMS
Formerly Professor and Head
Department of Radiology and Imaging
University College of Medical Sciences (University of
Delhi) Guru Teg Bahadur (GTB) Hospital, New Delhi
Rama Medical College and Superspecialty Hospital
Ghaziabad and School of Medical Sciences and
Research Sharda Hospital
Greater Noida, Uttar Pradesh, India

Shuchi Bhatt MD (Radiodiagnosis)
Associate Professor
Department of Radiology
and Imaging
University College of Medical Sciences (University
of Delhi) and Guru Teg Bahadur Hospital
New Delhi, India

Sumeet Bhargava
MBBS DNB (Radiodiagnosis) FCGP FIAMS FICRI FIMSA
MNAMS
Formerly Associate Professor
Department of Radiology and Imaging
Rama Medical College and Superspecialty Hospital
Ghaziabad, Uttar Pradesh, India

Swati Gupta MD (Radiodiagnosis)
Assistant Professor
Department of Radiology
and Imaging
Maulana Azad Medical College and Associated
LNJP Hospital, New Delhi, India

Thingujam Usha MD (Radiodiagnosis)
Associate Professor
Department of Radiodiagnosis
Jawaharlal Nehru Institute of Medical Sciences
Imphal, Manipur, India

Preface to the Third Edition

With the feedback from the postgraduate students, practicing sonologists and residents, more text and illustrations have been added so as to make this book more handy for better interpretation at bedside. We are sure the book in the present format will be more acceptable and useful to the postgraduate students, residents, and practitioners doing ultrasound in their day-to-day practice.

Sumeet Bhargava
Satish K Bhargava

Preface to the First Edition

Since the introduction of ultrasound (US), this modality has evolved from its primitive nature to its present glamorous status. Its popularity in radiology has always been due to its cost-effectiveness, easy availability and noninvasive nature. Its diagnostic role has been explored in every organ system and its usefulness felt every time. Its support in therapeutic techniques is unparalleled. Radiology without ultrasound is unimaginable.

Almost always real-time US is the initial investigative tool in the radiology department. Many a time, this modality is enough to establish a diagnosis and always provides a direction for further evaluation. Its uniqueness lies in its operator-dependent nature. As the ultrasonologist scans through the region of interest, recognition and interpretation of the important findings are important for establishing and imaging diagnosis. It is also imperative to know the various conditions producing a particular sonographic finding. Only ultrasound can be judiciously used to answer the question posed to the radiologist. This book is a special effort to provide a concise knowledge of the differential diagnosis of a sonographic finding. A list of the various clinical conditions and their short description is the main feature of the text. The information has been kept concise and unnecessary repetition avoided. Line diagrams and illustrations have been added to support the text. The aim of this book is to assist the sonologist with logical interpretation of the scan. We hope this attempt will prove useful to all practicing sonologists.

Sumeet Bhargava
Satish K Bhargava

Acknowledgments

We are grateful to our colleagues and friends who gave timely support and stood solidly behind us in our joint endeavor of bringing out this book which was required keeping in view of wide acceptability of ultrasound in developing countries. We both would like to thank Shri Jitendar P Vij (Group Chairman), Mr Ankit Vij (Managing Director), Ms Chetna Malhotra Vohra (Associate Director–Content Strategy), Ms Madhuri Aggarwal (Development Editor), and all the staff of M/s Jaypee Brothers Medical Publishers (P) Ltd, New Delhi, India, for their efforts and input enabling timely publication of the book.

Contents

1. Chest   1

   1.1 Chest Overview 1
       Satish K Bhargava

   1.2 Pleural Effusion 4
       Sumeet Bhargava, Satish K Bhargava

   1.3 Pleural Plaque 8
       Sumeet Bhargava, Satish K Bhargava

   1.4 Pleural Masses 8
       Satish K Bhargava, Sumeet Bhargava

   1.5 Mediastinal Lymphadenopathy 9
       Pushpender Gupta, Satish K Bhargava

   1.6 Vascular Lesions of Mediastinum 10
       Sumeet Bhargava, Amit Sahu, Satish K Bhargava

   1.7 Cystic Masses of Mediastinum 10
       Sumeet Bhargava, Satish K Bhargava

   1.8 Diaphragm 10
       Satish K Bhargava, Pushpender Gupta

2. Neck Lesions   14

   2.1 Thyroid 14

       2.1.1 Solitary Thyroid Nodule 14
            Satish K Bhargava, Avneesh Kumar Singh, Pushpender Gupta

       2.1.2 Carcinomas 19
            Sumeet Bhargava, Satish K Bhargava, Avneesh Kumar Singh

       2.1.3 Thyroid Calcification 22
            Sumeet Bhargava, Satish K Bhargava, Amit Sahu, Pushpender Gupta

       2.1.4 Differential Diagnosis on the Basis of Echogenicity of Thyroid Nodules 22
            Sumeet Bhargava, Satish K Bhargava, Avneesh Kumar Singh

       2.1.5 Cystic Thyroid Nodule 23
            Satish K Bhargava, Sumeet Bhargava, Pushpender Gupta

   2.2 Salivary Gland 25
       Pushpender Gupta, Satish K Bhargava

       2.2.1 Enlargement of Salivary Gland 25
            Satish K Bhargava, Pushpender Gupta, Gopesh Mehrotra

   2.3 Neck Masses 28
       Satish K Bhargava, Sumeet Bhargava

   2.4 Cervical Lymphadenopathy 33
       Satish K Bhargava, Rajul Rastogi

3. Hepatobiliary System and Abdomen 37
Differential Diagnosis of Liver Lesions 37

- 3.1 Generalized increase in Liver Echogenicity 37
  Satish K Bhargava, Sumeet Bhargava
- 3.2 Generalized Decrease in Echogenicity of Liver 40
  Sumeet Bhargava, Satish K Bhargava, Swati Gupta
- 3.3 Solitary Echogenic Liver Mass 41
  Satish K Bhargava, Sumeet Bhargava
- 3.4 Shadowing Lesions of Liver 43
  Sumeet Bhargava, Satish K Bhargava
- 3.5 Hepatoma, Bull's Eye or Target Lesion of Liver 45
  Sumeet Bhargava, Satish K Bhargava
- 3.6 Periportal Hyperechogenicity of Liver 45
  Sumeet Bhargava, Satish K Bhargava

Noncirrhotic Portal Hypertension 46

- 3.7 Periportal Hypoechogenicity 46
  Sumeet Bhargava, Satish K Bhargava

Liver 47

- 3.8 Focal Hypoechoic Lesions 47
  Pardeep Kumar, Satish K Bhargava
- 3.9 Cystic Lesions of Liver 49
  Amit Sahu, Satish K Bhargava
- 3.10 Mixed Cystic and Solid Lesions 56
  Satish K Bhargava, Pardeep Kumar
- 3.11 Patterns of Hepatic Metastasis 58
  Satish K Bhargava, Pardeep Kumar
- 3.12 Nonvisualization of Gallbladder on Ultrasound 60
  Sumeet Bhargava, Satish K Bhargava
- 3.13 Diffuse Gallbladder Thickening 62
  Sumeet Bhargava, Satish K Bhargava
- 3.14 Focal Gallbladder Thickening 63
  Sumeet Bhargava, Satish K Bhargava
- 3.15 Echogenic Fat in Hepatoduodenal Ligament 66
  Sumeet Bhargava, Satish K Bhargava
- 3.16 Congenital Biliary Cyst 66
  Sumeet Bhargava, Satish K Bhargava
- 3.17 Differential Diagnosis of Pericholecystic Fluid 68
  Ashish Verma, Satish K Bhargava, Sumeet Bhargava
- 3.18 Differential Diagnosis of Intrahepatic Biliary Dilatation 68
  Ashish Verma, Satish K Bhargava, Sumeet Bhargava
- 3.19 Differential Diagnosis of EHBR Dilatation 69
  Satish K Bhargava, Ashish Verma, Sumeet Bhargava
- 3.20 Abdominal Wall Masses 70
  Satish K Bhargava, Ashish Verma, Sumeet Bhargava

3.21 Acute Abdomen 74
Satish K Bhargava, Ashish Verma, Sumeet Bhargava

3.22 Abdominal Lymphadenopathy 81
Satish K Bhargava, Sumeet Bhargava, Ashish Verma

4. Spleen 83

4.1 Nonvisualization of Spleen on Ultrasound 83
Sumeet Bhargava, Satish K Bhargava

4.2 Cystic Lesion of Spleen 83
Sumeet Bhargava, Satish K Bhargava

4.3 Solid Splenic Lesion 86
Sumeet Bhargava, Satish K Bhargava

4.4 Hyperechoic Splenic Lesion 89
Sumeet Bhargava, Satish K Bhargava

5. Pancreas 91

5.1 Differential Diagnosis of Cystic Pancreatic Masses 91
Sumeet Bhargava, Satish K Bhargava, Ashish Verma, Rajul Rastogi

5.2 Differential Diagnosis of Solid/Complex Lesion 93
Satish K Bhargava, Sumeet Bhargava, Ashish Verma

6. Gastrointestinal Tract 97

6.1 Ultrasound Differential Diagnosis of Gastrointestinal Tract 97
Sumeet Bhargava, Gopesh Mehrotra, Rajul Rastogi

6.2 Stomach 98
Sumeet Bhargava, Shuchi Bhatt, Rajul Rastogi

6.3 Gastric Dilatation 99
Sumeet Bhargava, Rajul Rastogi

6.4 Duodenum 101
Satish K Bhargava, Sumeet Bhargava

6.5 Small Bowel and Colon 102
Sumeet Bhargava, Satish K Bhargava, Rajul Rastogi

6.6 Differential Diagnosis of Acute Appendicitis (Appendiceal Lesions) 108
Sumeet Bhargava, Satish K Bhargava, Anoop Kumar Durga Das

6.7 Role of Rectal Endosonography 111
Satish K Bhargava, Sumeet Bhargava, Meenakshi Prakash, Anoop Kumar Durga Das

7. Retroperitoneum 112

7.1 Differential Diagnosis of Solid Masses 112
Ashish Verma, Amit Sahu, Satish K Bhargava, Sumeet Bhargava

7.2 Differential Diagnosis of Pseudomasses 116
Ashish Verma, Sumeet Bhargava, Satish K Bhargava

7.3 Differential Diagnosis of Cystic Lesions and Fluid Collection 116
Sumeet Bhargava, Satish K Bhargava, Ashish Verma

8. Renal — 117

- 8.1 Differential Diagnosis of Renal Pseudotumor 117
  Satish K Bhargava, Rajul Rastogi, Ashish Verma
- 8.2 Differential Diagnosis of Cystic Renal Disease 118
  Sumeet Bhargava, Satish K Bhargava, Ashish Verma
- 8.3 Differential Diagnosis of Complex/Solid Renal Masses 120
  Satish K Bhargava, Ashish Verma, Rajul Rastogi
- 8.4 Differential Diagnosis of Hypoechoic Renal Sinus 123
  Ashish Verma, Satish K Bhargava, Rajul Rastogi
- 8.5 Differential Diagnosis of Hyperechoic Renal Nodules 123
  Amit Sahu, Satish K Bhargava, Shuchi Bhatt
- 8.6 Differential Diagnosis of Dilated Pelvicalyceal System and Ureter 124
  Sumeet Bhargava, Ashish Verma, Satish K Bhargava, Rajul Rastogi

9. Urinary Bladder — 130

- 9.1 Differential Diagnosis of Bladder Wall Thickening 130
  Sumeet Bhargava, Satish K Bhargava, Ashish Verma
- 9.2 Differential Diagnosis of Bladder Contour and Caliber Abnormality 133
  Satish K Bhargava, Sumeet Bhargava, Ashish Verma

10. Adrenal Gland — 136

- 10.1 Bilateral Large Adrenal Gland 136
  Satish K Bhargava, Sumeet Bhargava
- 10.2 Unilateral Adrenal Masses 137
  Satish K Bhargava, Sumeet Bhargava
- 10.3 Large Solid Adrenal Masses 139
  Sumeet Bhargava, Satish K Bhargava
- 10.4 Cystic Adrenal Masses 140
  Sumeet Bhargava, Satish K Bhargava
- 10.5 Adrenal Pseudomasses 140
  Sumeet Bhargava, Satish K Bhargava
- 10.6 Adrenal Calcifications 140
  Sumeet Bhargava, Satish K Bhargava

11. Peritoneal and Mesenteric Masses — 141

- 11.1 Round Solid Masses in Mesentery 141
  Satish K Bhargava, Sumeet Bhargava
- 11.2 Ill-Defined Mass 141
  Satish K Bhargava, Sumeet Bhargava
- 11.3 Loculated Cystic Peritoneal Masses 144
  Satish K Bhargava, Sumeet Bhargava
- 11.4 Solid Peritoneal Lesions 145
  Satish K Bhargava, Sumeet Bhargava

12. Scrotum — 149

- 12.1 Differential Diagnosis of Acute Scrotum 149
  Sumeet Bhargava, Satish K Bhargava, Ashish Verma

12.2 Differential Diagnosis of Scrotal Calcification   151
Satish K Bhargava, Sumeet Bhargava, Ashish Verma

12.3 Differential Diagnosis of Scrotal Gas   152
Satish K Bhargava, Rajul Rastogi, Ashish Verma

12.4 Differential Diagnosis of Scrotal Masses   153
Sumeet Bhargava, Satish K Bhargava, Rajul Rastogi, Ashish Verma

13. Testis and Epididymis   156

13.1 Differential Diagnosis of Cystic Testicular Lesions   156
Ashish Verma, Sumeet Bhargava, Satish K Bhargava

13.2 Pediatric Testicular Masses   157
Sumeet Bhargava, Ashish Verma, Satish K Bhargava
Germ Cell Tumors   158
Stromal Tumors   159
Occult Primary Tumors   159
Testicular Metastasis   159

13.3 Differential Diagnosis of Epididymal Lesions   160
Ashish Verma, Sumeet Bhargava, Satish K Bhargava

14. Prostate   162

14.1 Differential Diagnosis of Prostatic Cyst   162
Amit Sahu, Satish K Bhargava, Sumeet Bhargava, Rajul Rastogi

14.2 Müllerian Cyst   162
Satish K Bhargava, Sumeet Bhargava, Rajul Rastogi

14.3 Ejaculatory Duct Cyst   163
Rajul Rastogi, Sumeet Bhargava, Satish K Bhargava

14.4 Seminal Vesicle Cyst   163
Satish K Bhargava, Ashish Verma, Sumeet Bhargava, Rajul Rastogi

14.5 Hypoechoic Lesions   163
Rajul Rastogi, Anubhav Sarikwal, Sumeet Bhargava

14.6 Prostatic Calcification   165
Sumeet Bhargava, Rajul Rastogi

15. Breast   166

15.1 Cystic Lesions   167
Satish K Bhargava, Rajul Rastogi

15.2 Hyperechoic Lesions   168
Satish K Bhargava

15.3 Hypoechoic Lesions   169
Satish K Bhargava, Mamta Motla

15.4 Ductal Dilatation   170
Anupama Tandon, Satish K Bhargava

15.5 Benign Vs Malignant   170
Anupama Tandon, Satish K Bhargava

15.6 Mastitis   171
Satish K Bhargava, Anurag Agarwal

15.7 Benign Lesions 172
Anurag Agarwal, Satish K Bhargava

15.8 Malignant Lesions 173
Sumeet Bhargava, Rajul Rastogi, Satish K Bhargava

16. Musculoskeletal System 176

16.1 Hyperechoic Foci within the Synovium 176
Rajul Rastogi, Satish K Bhargava

16.2 Cystic Mass in Popliteal Fossa 176
Amit Sahu, Rajul Rastogi, Satish K Bhargava

16.3 Hip Joint Effusion in Adults 176
Sumeet Bhargava, Satish K Bhargava

16.4 Proliferative Synovitis 177
Rajul Rastogi, Satish K Bhargava

16.5 Tendon Tears 177
Rajul Rastogi, Satish K Bhargava

16.6 Pediatric Hip Joint: An Overview 178
Satish K Bhargava, Sumeet Bhargava

16.7 Causes of Articular Cartilage Calcification 188
Amit Sahu, Sumeet Bhargava

Causes of Soft Tissue Nodule Associated Arthritis 188

17. Orbit 189

17.1 Anatomy 189
Satish K Bhargava, Sumeet Bhargava

17.2 Orbital Sonoanatomy and Technique 190
Satish K Bhargava, Sumeet Bhargava

17.3 Sonopathology 192
Satish K Bhargava, Sumeet Bhargava

17.4 Sonological Features of Orbital Diseases 193
Satish K Bhargava, Sumeet Bhargava

17.5 Disease of Retina 198
Satish K Bhargava, Sumeet Bhargava

17.6 Orbital Pathologies 200
Satish K Bhargava, Sumeet Bhargava

18. Neonatal and Infant Brain 208

18.1 Cystic Lesions 208
Shuchi Bhatt, Satish K Bhargava

18.2 Solid Lesions 209
Shuchi Bhatt, Satish K Bhargava

18.3 Prominent Choroid Plexus 209
Shuchi Bhatt, Satish K Bhargava

18.4 Destructive Lesions of Brain 210
Shuchi Bhatt, Satish K Bhargava

18.5 Ventriculomegaly 211
Shuchi Bhatt, Satish K Bhargava

18.6 Congenital and Developmental Malformations 214
Amit Sahu, Shuchi Bhatt, Satish K Bhargava

18.7 Infective Cystic Lesions 216
Shuchi Bhatt, Satish K Bhargava

18.8 Vascular Lesions 217
Sumeet Bhargava, Satish K Bhargava, Anubhav Sarikwal

18.9 Traumatic Cystic Lesions 218
Sumeet Bhargava, Satish K Bhargava, Anubhav Sarikwal

18.10 Intracranial Hemorrhage 218
Sumeet Bhargava, Satish K Bhargava

18.11 Asphyxia 219
Sumeet Bhargava, Satish K Bhargava

18.12 Solid Infective Lesions 220
Sumeet Bhargava, Satish K Bhargava

18.13 Tumors 220
Sumeet Bhargava, Satish K Bhargava

18.14 Congenital Intracranial Infection of Infant and Children 220
Sumeet Bhargava, Satish K Bhargava

18.15 Meningitis 222
Sumeet Bhargava, Satish K Bhargava

18.16 Enlarged Choroid Plexus 222
Sumeet Bhargava, Satish K Bhargava

19. Neonatal and Infant Spine 223

19.1 Spinal Dysraphism 223
Shuchi Bhatt

19.2 Spina Bifida Aperta 224
Shuchi Bhatt

19.3 Spina Bifida Cystica 224
Shuchi Bhatt

19.4 Occult Spinal Dysraphism 225
Shuchi Bhatt

19.5 Tethered Cord 228
Shuchi Bhatt

19.6 Spinal Trauma 229
Shuchi Bhatt

19.7 Tumors 229
Shuchi Bhatt

20. Gynecology and Obstetrics 230

20.1 Free Fluid in Cul-de-Sac 230
Satish K Bhargava, Shuchi Bhatt

20.2 Cystic Pelvic Masses 232
Satish K Bhargava, Shuchi Bhatt, Meenakshi Prakash

20.3 Complex Pelvic Mass 234
Satish K Bhargava, Shuchi Bhatt, Thingujam Usha

20.4 Solid Pelvic Masses 236
Satish K Bhargava, Shuchi Bhatt

20.5 Adnexal Masses 236
Satish K Bhargava, Shuchi Bhatt, Anoop Kumar Durga Das, Swati Gupta

20.6 Ovarian Tumors 241
Satish K Bhargava, Shuchi Bhatt, Meenakshi Prakash
Benign Tumors 241
Malignant Ovarian Neoplasm 242
Ultrasound Features of Malignant Ovarian Lesions 242

20.7 Uterine Masses 243
Shuchi Bhatt, Thingujam Usha, Sumeet Bhargava

20.8 Diffuse Uterine Enlargement 246
Shuchi Bhatt, Anoop Kumar Durga Das

20.9 Thickened Endometrium 247
Amit Sahu, Shuchi Bhatt, Sumeet Bhargava, Swati Gupta

20.10 Differential Diagnosis of Thickened Placenta 255
Satish K Bhargava, Ashish Verma

20.11 Ultrasound Signs of Chromosomal Abnormality 256
Satish K Bhargava, Ashish Verma

20.12 Absent Pregnancy Test with Absent Intrauterine Pregnancy 258
Satish K Bhargava, Ashish Verma

20.13 Fetal Causes of Abnormalities In Liquor Volume 258
Ashish Verma, Satish K Bhargava

20.14 Intra-abdominal Fetal Calcification 260
Satish K Bhargava, Ashish Verma

20.15 Differential Diagnosis of Fetal Thoracic Abnormalities 262
Satish K Bhargava, Ashish Verma

20.16 Unsuccessful First Trimester Pregnancy 264
Satish K Bhargava, Amit Sahu, Ashish Verma

20.17 First Trimester Bleeding 265
Satish K Bhargava, Ashish Verma, Shuchi Bhatt

20.18 Fetal Hydrops 267
Satish K Bhargava, Ashish Verma, Shuchi Bhatt

20.19 Twin Pregnancy/Multifetal Pregnancy 269
Satish K Bhargava, Ashish Verma, Shuchi Bhatt

20.20 Differential Diagnosis of Echogenic Fetal Kidneys 271
Satish K Bhargava, Ashish Verma, Shuchi Bhatt

20.21 Differential Diagnosis of Syndromes Associated with Renal Malformations 272
Satish K Bhargava, Ashish Verma, Shuchi Bhatt

20.22 Differential Diagnosis of Fetal Hydronephrosis 272
Satish K Bhargava, Ashish Verma, Rajul Rastogi

20.23 Fetal Head, Neck and Face 275
Satish K Bhargava, Ashish Verma, Rajul Rastogi

20.24 Differential Diagnosis of Micrognathia 275
Satish K Bhargava, Ashish Verma, Rajul Rastogi

20.25 Differential Diagnosis of Syndromes Associated with Hypertelorism 276
Satish K Bhargava, Ashish Verma, Rajul Rastogi

20.26 Differential Diagnosis of Syndromes Associated with Frontal Bossing 276
Satish K Bhargava, Ashish Verma, Rajul Rastogi
20.27 Differential Diagnosis of Syndromes Associated with
Craniosynostosis and Other Causes 276
Satish K Bhargava, Ashish Verma, Rajul Rastogi
20.28 Differential Diagnosis of Cleft Lip with/without Cleft Palate 277
Satish K Bhargava, Ashish Verma
20.29 Differential Diagnosis of Conditions Associated with Facial Clefting 278
Satish K Bhargava, Ashish Verma
20.30 Fetal Central Nervous System 279
Satish K Bhargava, Ashish Verma
20.31 Fetal Abdominal Wall Defects 283
Satish K Bhargava, Ashish Verma
20.32 Nuchal Fold and Translucency 285
Satish K Bhargava, Ashish Verma
20.33 Prenatal Sonographic Diagnosis of Cardiac Anomalies 285
Satish K Bhargava, Amit Sahu, Ashish Verma
Structural Defects 286

Index *289*

CHAPTER 1

Chest

1.1 CHEST OVERVIEW

Ultrasound (US) is a noninvasive, relatively inexpensive and most rewarding imaging modality, carries no radiation burden, but not much exploited for evaluation of chest disease because of basic (inherent) properties of US waves not to pass through bony cage and air-filled lungs. However, over a couple of years, US has emerged as a useful tool in evaluating wide range of perplexing clinical problems of chest due to presence of fluid in pleural space, consolidating or atelectatic lung or even tumor, provide window for US to penetrate and this has helped in diagnosis of certain conditions or limit the differential diagnosis (DD) of conditions under consideration.

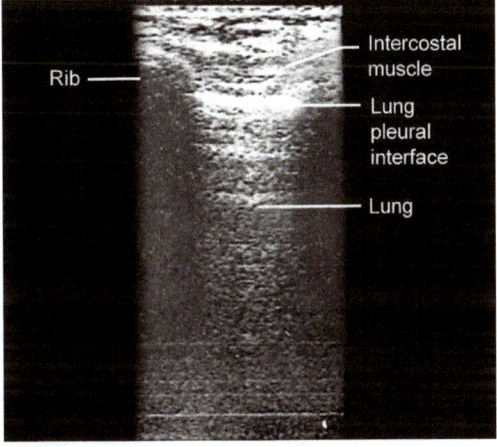

Fig. 1.1.1: Normal lung as seen in transverse section. Ribs with distal shadowing are shown with intercostal muscles. The lung pleural interface is seen as an echogenic line.

1. *Chest wall* **(Fig. 1.1.1)**: It has helped in diagnosing soft tissue abscesses, masses, osteomyelitis, rib tumors and even fracture where plain X-ray gives only soft tissue swelling or obliteration of costophrenic angle (may be due to pleural fluid or sometimes by rib tumor) and also where rib erosion is due to underlying carcinoma. Sometimes, when clinically mass is suspected with fractures, US can be used as a first modality particularly in children to avoid radiation by getting an X-ray chest.

2. *Mediastinum*: Anterior mediastinum can be very well-evaluated by US through suprasternal route by elevating shoulders and extending the neck. This will avoid structures particularly thymus in children. Even paratracheal and hilar adenopathy can be diagnosed especially in tubercular patients where it is not only helpful in diagnosis but also in follow-up when child is on antitubercular therapy, thus avoiding unnecessary radiation and getting repeated X-rays.

3. *Lung parenchyma*: It is also helpful in differentiating cystic lesions of the lung parenchyma like hydatid cyst **(Fig. 1.1.2)** consolidation **(Figs. 1.1.3 to 1.1.5)**, collapse and tumor of lung. Also differentiates a tumor and pleural fluid/consolidation above the diaphragm from (subpulmonic effusion) below the diaphragm.

4. *Pleura*: US is a good modality to differentiate pleural lesions from parenchymal ones.

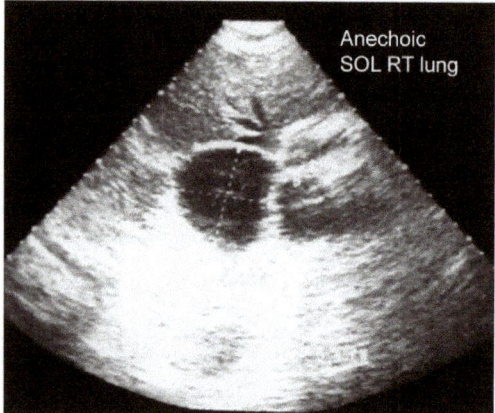

Fig. 1.1.2: Lung hydatid seen as anechoic cystic lesion in transverse scan of lung. (SOL: space occupying lesion; RT: right)

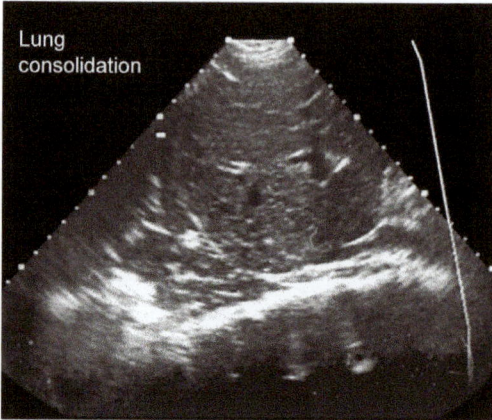

Fig. 1.1.3: Consolidation—seen as a homogeneous hypoechoic lesion with air bronchogram in right lower lobe of lung.

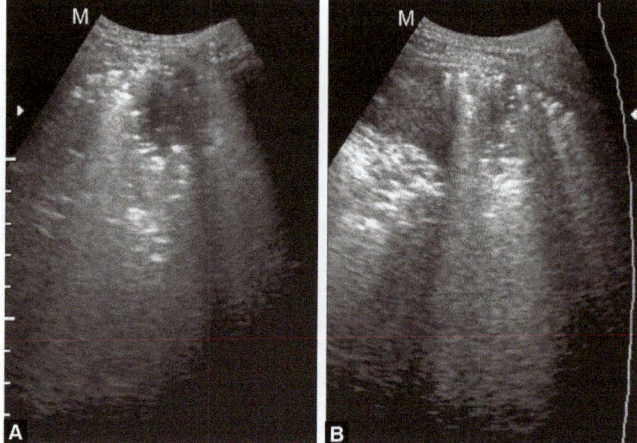

Figs. 1.1.4A and B: US scans showing consolidation with cavitation in lower lobe. (M: mass)

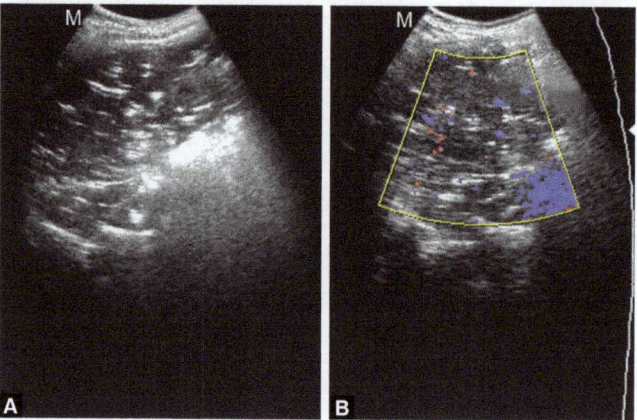

Figs. 1.1.5A and B: US scans show lobar consolidation with presence of color flow on color Doppler flow imaging (CDFI). (M: mass)

It is also helpful in diagnosing minimal amount of fluid in pleural cavity, even 5–10 mL of fluid, thus avoiding need of lateral decubitus film/lateral chest film.

i. It also gives the etiology of pleural fluid due to its appearance as anechoic, hypoechoic, echogenic, presence of debris, nodules and types of septa.
ii. Anechoic—all transudates are anechoic, however, all anechoic collections are not transudates. About one-third of exudative collection tends to be anechoic in the beginning.
iii. Hypoechoic—Usually exudative effusions, empyema and later stages of hemothorax.
iv. Echogenic—Hemothorax or empyema.
v. Debris—Represents settled down pus cell, blood cells, etc.
vi. Septations—Usually represent process of loculation and fibrosis occurring in pleural effusion. Thin clean septa with no or very minimal debris—tubercular pleural effusion. However, thick, shaggy irregular septations with debris—pyogenic effusion.
vii. Pleural nodule/masses **(Figs. 1.1.6A to C)**, represent meso-thelioma, metastatic nodule and tuberculomata.

In addition to characteristics septations the thickness of parietal pleura and combined (parietal + visceral) also give etiological diagnosis. As tubercular pleural effusion-parietal pleural thickness varies 2–8 mm and combined pleural varies from 4–10 mm. In pyogenic pleural effusion, parietal pleural thickness varies from 5–22 mm and combined 8–27 mm. In hemothoraces (post-traumatic) thick irregular mantle of pleura around hypoechoic pleural collection is seen, pleural thickness varies from 12–18 mm.

Pleural effusion v/s ascites: Bare area sign—if fluid interface is abutting the bare area of liver than it is pleural effusion and if it is not than it is ascites.

Diaphragmatic crus sign—pleural effusion is posterolateral and superior to crus of diaphragm while ascites is anteromedial and inferior to crus of diaphragm.

5. *Intervention*: US is very helpful in fine needle aspiration biopsy, pleural tapping, guided pleural aspiration and tube placement.
6. *ICU*: US is very helpful in critically ill-patients that is trauma and ICU-needs serial X-rays to see day-to-day changes in lesions like consolidation and lung abscess

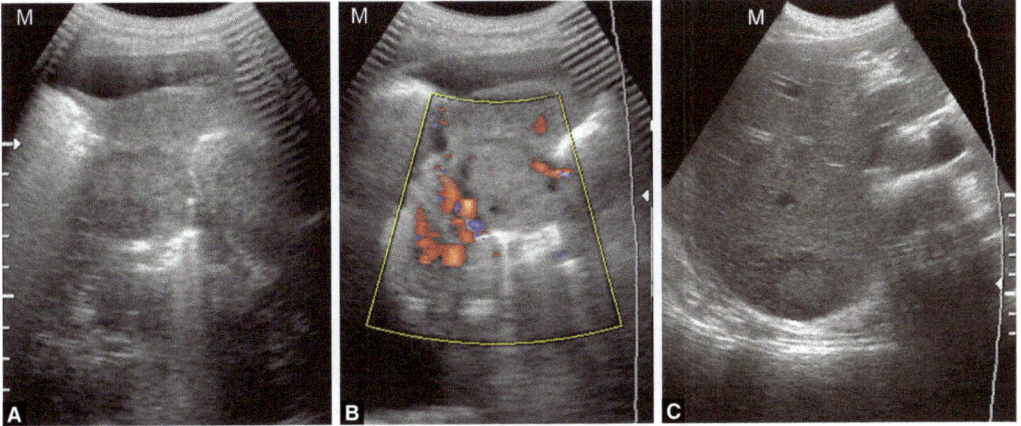

Figs. 1.1.6A to C: US scans show pulmonary mass with color flow associated with mild pleural effusion causing compression atelectasis of underlying parenchyma and hepatic metastases. (M: mass)

(**Fig. 1.1.7**), particularly when there is inability to position the patient as required and usually substandard quality of X-rays.

Limitations

- Pneumothoraces/hydropneumothorax
- Limited information about mediastinum, hilar and proximal airways
  - Limited information of the underlying lung parenchyma in the setting of complex pleural and lung parenchymal disease.
  - No preferred for complicated interventional procedures, such as empyema drainage with a pigtail catheter or biopsy of pleural masses.
- Restricted field of view
- Familiarity of clinician
- Operator dependent.

Other Advantages

- Lower cost
- Increase flexibility
- No radiation
- Good guidance tool

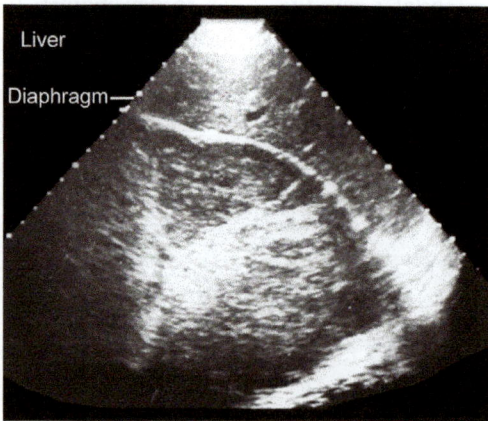

Fig. 1.1.7: Lung abscess—a large predominantly hypoechoic space-occupying lesion (SOL) with internal septae and posterior enhancement is seen in lower lobe of right lung. Aspiration revealed pus Inversion of diaphragm is seen.

- Repeated evaluation with no radiation cost
  - Portability in ICU settings
  - Better in differentiating pleural effusion from pleural thickening
  - More sensitive than X-ray in differentiating pleural fluid from consolidation
  - Ultrasound guidance is associated with a reduced risk of pneumothorax during thoracentesis.

Ability to detect abdominal lesions associated with causative of chest lesion as liver abscesses leading to pleural effusion.

1.2 PLEURAL EFFUSION

Pleural effusion can be transudative or exudative.

Signs of pleural fluid on USG:

Transudative effusion: Pleural (fluid) that changes shape with respiration.

Exudative effusion:
- Fluid with floating echodensities
- Septations—thick and shaggy (**Figs. 1.2.1A to C**)
- Fibrin strands
- May be anechoic fluid
- Echogenic fluid (**Fig. 1.2.2**)
- Pleural nodules
- Thickened pleura.

Causes of Transudative Pleural Effusion

1. Increased hydrostatic pressure
   - Congestive heart failure
   - Superior vena cava (SVC) obstruction
   - Constrictive pericarditis.
2. Decreased osmotic pressure
   - Cirrhosis with ascites
   - Peritoneal dialysis
   - Acute glomerulonephritis
   - Nephrotic syndrome
   - Urinary tract obstruction

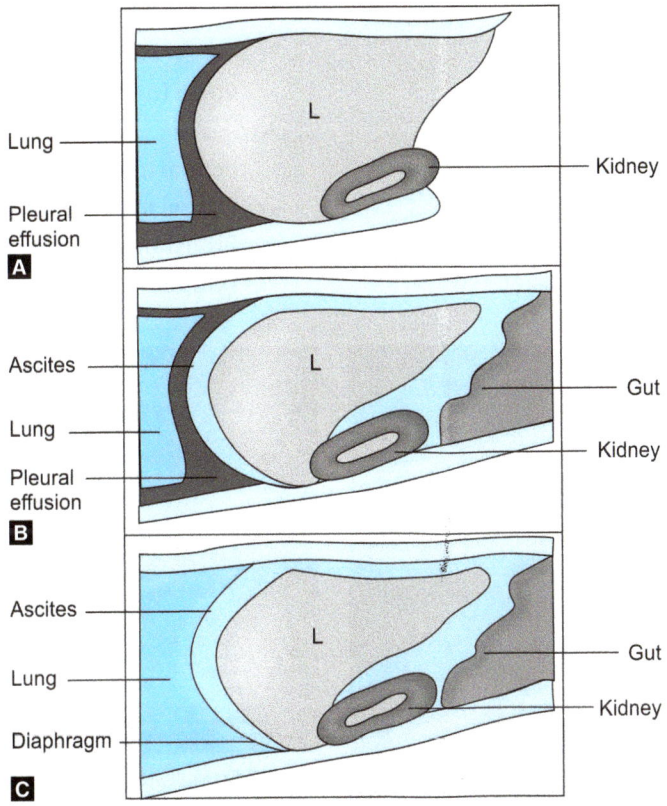

Figs. 1.2.1A to C: (A) Pleural effusion superior to the diaphragm; (B) Pleural effusion and ascites outlining the diaphragm; (C) Ascites only. Irregular outline of the gut is seen due to ascites. (L: liver)

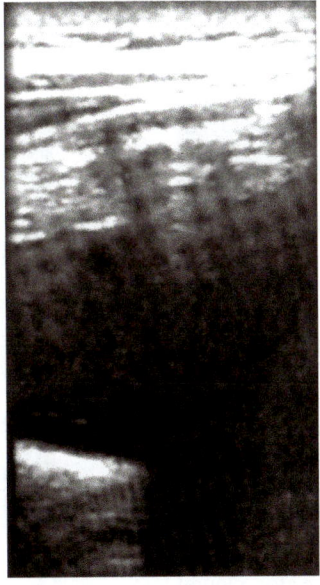

Fig. 1.2.2: Longitudinal intercostal view in a patient with pleural effusion showing echogenic surface of visceral and parietal pleura.

- Hypoalbuminemia
- Overhydration
- Hypothyroidism.

Causes of Exudative Pleural Effusion (Figs. 1.2.3 to 1.2.10)

1. Infection
   - Parapneumonic effusion
   - Empyema (see **Fig. 1.1.7**)
   - Tuberculosis
   - Fungi (nocardia, actinomycosis).
2. Neoplasm
   - Pleural metastasis
   - Pleural mesothelioma
   - Bronchogenic carcinoma
   - Lymphoma.

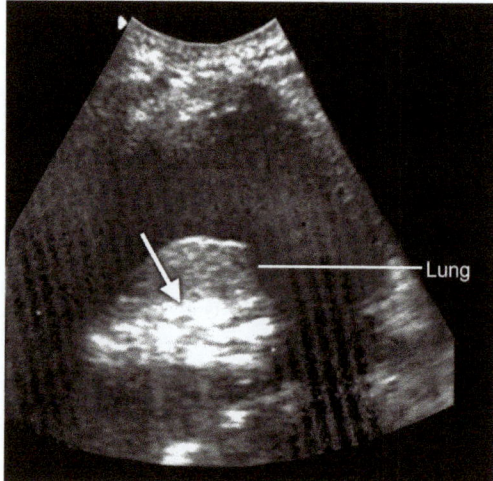

Fig. 1.2.3: Longitudinal intercostal view—pleural effusion and collapsed lung showing echogenic gas-filled bronchus (arrow) within the collapsed lung.

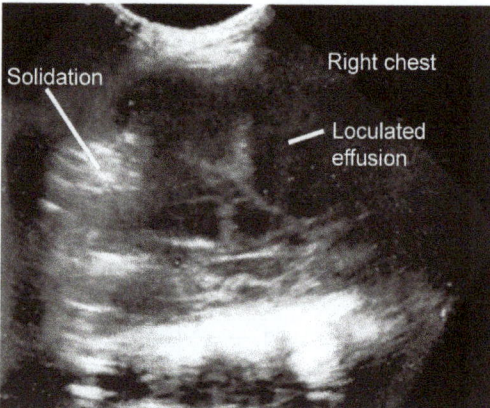

Fig. 1.2.5: Multiseptated fluid collection seen in right pleural cavity in the case of infected pleural effusion.

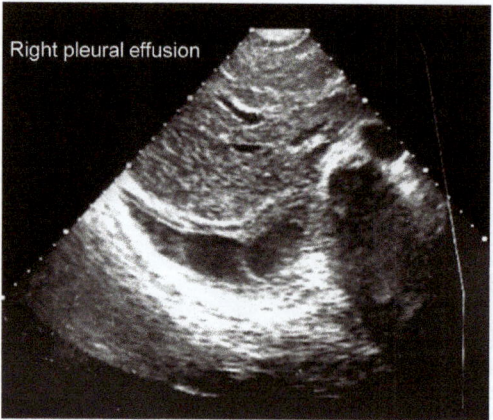

Fig. 1.2.4: Loculated multiseptated fluid collection seen in the pleural cavity with associated pleural thickening.

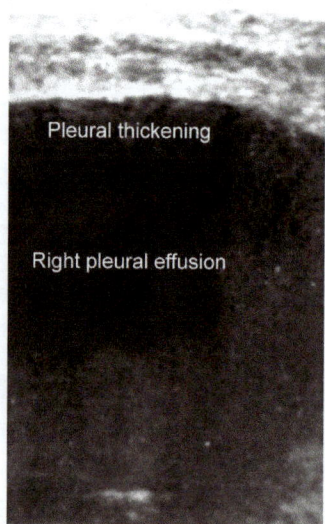

Fig. 1.2.6: Thickened pleura seen along with pleural effusion.

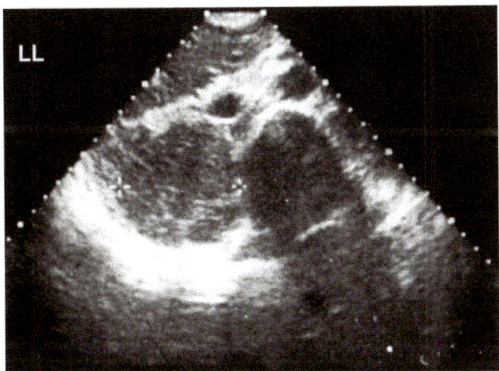

Fig. 1.2.7: A predominantly hypoechoic solid mass lesion seen in right lower lobe (LL) of lung.

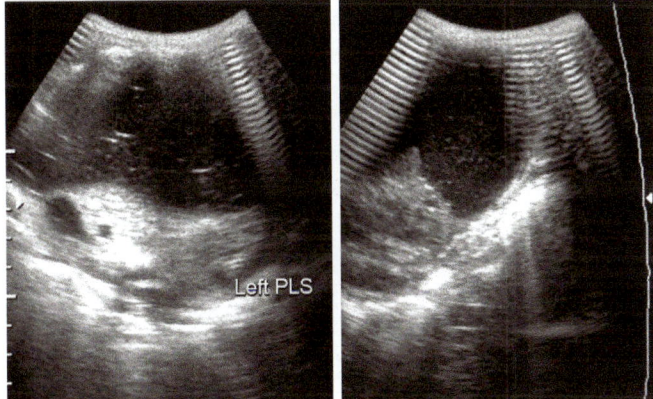

Fig. 1.2.8: US scans show hydropneumothorax with compression atelectasis of underlying pulmonary parenchyma. (PLS: pleural lung scan)

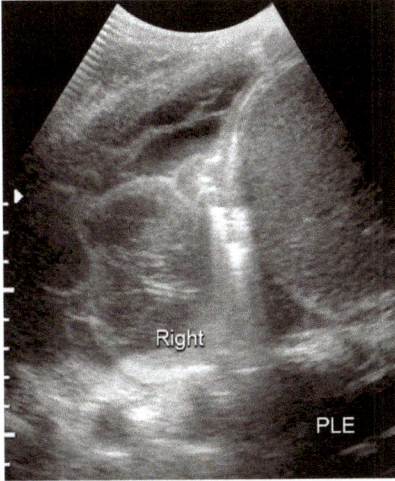

Fig. 1.2.9: US scan shows tuberculous pleural effusion with pleural thickening. (PLE: pleural effusion)

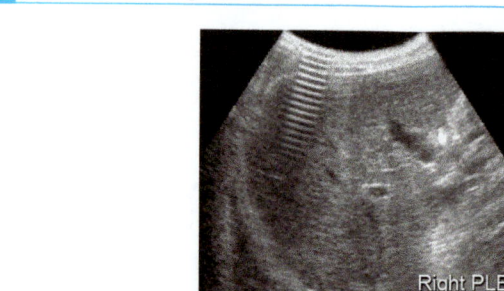

Fig. 1.2.10: US scans show presence of organizing pleural effusion (PLE).

3. Vascular
   - Pulmonary emboli.
4. Collagen vascular disease
   - Systemic lupus erythematosus (SLE)
   - Rheumatoid arthritis.
5. Abdominal disease
   - Subphrenic abscess
   - Pancreatitis.
6. Trauma
   - Hydrothorax.
7. Miscellaneous
   - Drug induced effusion
     - Uremia
     - Hypothyroidism
     - Acute respiratory distress syndrome (ARDS).

1.3 PLEURAL PLAQUE

Common causes of pleural plaque includes:
- Pneumonia
- Asbestos exposure
- Pulmonary infarction
- Trauma
- Chemical pleurodesis
- Drug-related pleural disease.

Plaques resulting from asbestos exposure are usually confined to the parietal pleura. Ultrasound demonstrates pleural plaques as smooth, elliptical, hypoechoic pleural thickening.

Visceral pleural plaques are differentiated from parietal pleura by observing the 'gliding sign' during respiration.

Calcified pleural plaques are irregular, echogenic and produce acoustic shadowing and comet tail artifact.

Differential diagnosis to be considered while diagnosing pleural plaques:
- Diffuse pleural thickening
- Extrapleural fat
- Pleural tumors
- Pleural pseudotumors
- Rib fracture.

1.4 PLEURAL MASSES

1. Loculated pleural effusion
2. Metastasis
3. Malignant mesothelioma
4. Pleural fibroma
5. Fibrin balls.

Loculated Pleural Effusion

Anechoic collection seen within the pleural cavity.

Metastasis

Pleural effusion associated with malignant disease may result from:

- Malignant cell implantation on the pleura (common causes: lung, breast and GIT cancers)
- Obstruction of pleura or pulmonary lymphatics (common causes: lymphoma, breast cancer)
- Obstruction of pulmonary veins usually by lung cancers
- Malignant cells shed freely into pleural space
- Obstruction of thoracic ducts, resulting in chylous effusion (usually due to lymphoma).

Sonographic findings favoring malignant etiology.
- Solid nodules in the pleural space
- Circumferential pleural thickening
- Nodular pleural thickening or >1 cm pleural thickening
- Pleural thickening involving the mediastinal pleura.

Pleural Mesothelioma

Malignant mesothelioma is a rare and usually fatal pleural tumors associated with asbestos exposure.

Imaging Findings

Diffuse pleural thickening, often nodular and irregular (86%).
- Calcification in pleura (74%)
- Focal pleural mass (25%).

Rib destruction occurs with advanced disease.

Pleural Fibroma (Local Benign Mesothelioma)

A smooth lobular mass, 2–15 cm diameter arising more frequently from the visceral pleura.
- Pedunculated mass changes shape with respiration (30–50%)
- Forms an obtuse angle with the chest wall.

Fibrin Balls

These develop in serofibrinous pleural effusion and become visible following absorption of fluid.
- Small and tend to be situated near the lung base.
- May disappear spontaneously or remain unchanged for many years.

1.5 MEDIASTINAL LYMPHADENOPATHY

Tuberculosis	Sarcoidosis	Lymphoma
Unilateral	Bilateral	Bilateral
—	Symmetric	Asymmetric
Right paratracheal and tracheobronchial nodes are most commonly involved	Bilateral hilar with or without right paratracheal, aortopulmonary window lymphadenopathy	Superior mediastinum most common site with or without unilateral or bilateral hilar nodes
—	• Mediastinal lymph node (LN) with or without hilar LN-unusual • Characteristic involvement of bronchopulmonary nodes, than hilar nodes	In non-Hodgkin lymphoma (NHL) involvement of other nodal groups (cardiophrenic, posterior media stinal) also seen more commonly
Low attenuation	Isodense	Isodense
Mild homogeneous enhancement to rim enhancement	Homogeneous mild to moderate enhancement	Mild homogeneous enhancement
May show calcification	May show rim calcification	Calcification unusual without treatment
More likely to be confluent	Discrete May be confluent with large nodal masses	Usually discrete

1.6 VASCULAR LESIONS OF MEDIASTINUM

Ultrasound is an excellent, noninvasive method of diagnosing masses of vascular origin in the mediastinum.

Vascular nature of a suspected mass can be confirmed by ultrasound using imaging supplemented by color flow and spectral Doppler effect:
- Tortuous brachiocephalic artery
- Aneurysm of the aorta
- Aneurysm of the sinus of Valsalva
- Right-sided aortic arch
- Double aortic arch
- Dilated superior vena cava.

1.7 CYSTIC MASSES OF MEDIASTINUM

1. Congenital cyst (Benign)
   - Bronchogenic cyst
   - Pericardial cyst
   - Esophageal duplication cyst
   - Neuroenteric cyst
   - Thymic cyst.
2. Mature cystic teratoma
3. Meningocele (Lateral)
4. Lymphangioma
5. Cystic degeneration
   - Hodgkin's disease
   - Metastasis to lymph nodes
   - Nerve root tumors
6. Mediastinal abscess
7. Pancreatic pseudocyst.

Ultrasonography can be useful in evaluating a mass adjacent to pleural surface or cardiophrenic angle. At US, the benign cysts typically appear as anechoic thin-walled masses with increased through transmission.
- Ultrasound is used to characterize wall thickness, septations, vascularity, appearance of internal fluid, location and relationship to adjacent structures.

Pericardial cyst-results from aberrations in the formation of celomic cavities. Pericardial cysts are invariably connected to the pericardium but only a few cases unable to show communication with the pericardial sac. Thus ultrasound can help in detecting the pericardial involvement.

The majority of pericardial cysts arise in anterior cardiophrenic, more commonly on the right side. Occasionally cysts are pedunculated.

Mature Cystic Teratoma

These are cystic tumors composed of well-differentiated derivations from at least two of the three germ layers.

Majority of dermoid cysts are in the anterior mediastinum.

Most cystic teratoma are multilocular but unilocular cystic lesions also occur.

They may contain four types of tissues- including fluid, fat, soft tissues, calcium but fluid containing cystic component are usually prominent.

A fat fluid level within the mass is highly specific finding but is seen less frequently.

Cystic Degeneration

Many tumors and lymph nodes can undergo cystic degeneration and demonstrate mixed solid and cystic elements. If degeneration is extensive, the appearance of the lesion is indistinguishable from those of a congenital cyst. Cystic degeneration of a solid mass is more likely to occur after radiation therapy or chemotherapy but may be seen prior to treatment.
- A mediastinal abscess or pancreatic pseudocyst appears as a fluid containing mediastinal cystic mass, but clinical features usually permit differentiation from true cysts or neoplasms.

1.8 DIAPHRAGM

Bilateral diaphragmatic elevation
a. Shallow inspiration (most common).

b. Abdominal cause (USG useful by showing fluid, fetus or an abdominal mass as the cause)
   1. Obesity
   2. Pregnancy
   3. Ascites
   4. Any large abdominal mass.
c. Pulmonary causes—USG little use
   1. Chext X-ray/CT required making the diagnosis.
d. Neuromuscular disorders
   1. Myasthenia gravis—chest CT may show thymoma.
   2. Amyotropic lateral sclerosis—USG is of little use.
   - MRI required for diagnosis.

Unilateral Diaphragmatic Elevation

Subpulmonic Pleural Effusion

- Ultrasound confirmatory
- Shows the presence of fluid is pleural cavity with normal relative position of both domes of diaphragm.

Pulmonary Causes

- USG may show the presence of elevation of one dome of diaphragm may be due to liver lesions also (**Figs. 1.8.1 and 1.8.2**) as compared to other dome. However, underlying lung is usually not evaluated by ultrasound
- Chest X-ray/CT will confirm the cause for diaphragmatic elevation and relation to diaphragm with other structures.

Phrenic Nerve Paralysis (Diaphragmatic Paralysis)

- May occur due to:
  - Primary lung tumor
  - Malignant mediastinal
  - Iatrogenic
  - Idiopathic.
- Diagnosis is made on USG by observing the absent or paradoxical movement on

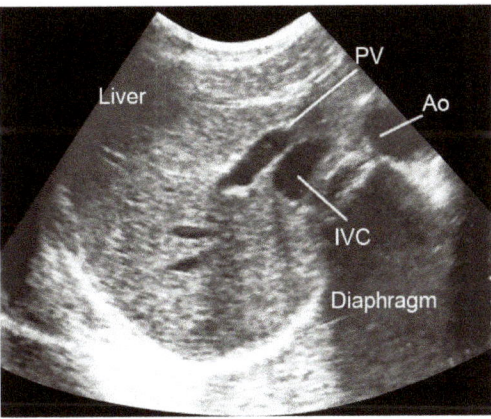

Fig. 1.8.1: Liver in transverse scan—right lobe of liver. (Ao: aorta; IVC: inferior vena cava; PV: portal vein)

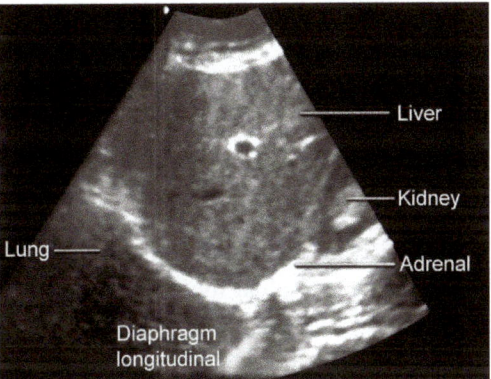

Fig. 1.8.2: Longitudinal image showing the various relation along the anteroposterior extent of the diaphragm on right side.

the affected side with usual or exaggerated excursion on the opposite side. Paradoxical movement can be elicited by the coughing or sniffing tests.

Abdominal Causes

- Subphrenic abscesses
  - In appropriate clinical setting usually history of surgery
  - USG shows—elevated hemidiaphragm
- Reduced or absent movement of the ipsilateral diaphragm
  - Subdiaphragmatic anechoic or hypoechoic collection

- Usually ipsilateral pleural effusion present
- *Liver mass:* Tumor, echinococcal cyst, abscess
- Distended stomach or colon
- Interposition of colon.

Diaphragmatic Hernia (Fig. 1.8.3)
- USG may show the discontinuity of the dome of diaphragm
- Bowel, spleen, kidney may be visualized inside thorax above dome of diaphragm
- Contralateral displacement of heart is visualized
- In congenital diaphragmatic hernia, polyhydramnios may be associated after 25 weeks.

Eventration of Diaphragm
- Complete—more commonly on left
- Partial—more commonly on right
- Complete eventration of diaphragm can be diagnosed by ultrasound
- Ultrasound in focal eventration shows evidence of typical focal diaphragmatic bulge filled by liver **(Figs. 1.8.4 and 1.8.5)**.

Diaphragmatic Rupture
- Traumatic—blunt or penetrating trauma
- Infection—ruptured amebic liver abscess
- In post-traumatic rupture in large, usually over 10 cm, defects ultrasound may detect—disruption of diaphragmatic echoes. Herniation of abdominal viscera into thorax-associated pleural effusion. Sometimes, small diaphragmatic rents may be difficult to detect, but due to availability of high frequency transducers, it is now possible to detect small disruption of diaphragmatic contour.

Neoplasms
- Very rarely diaphragmatic neoplasms
- Primary—various types of sarcomas

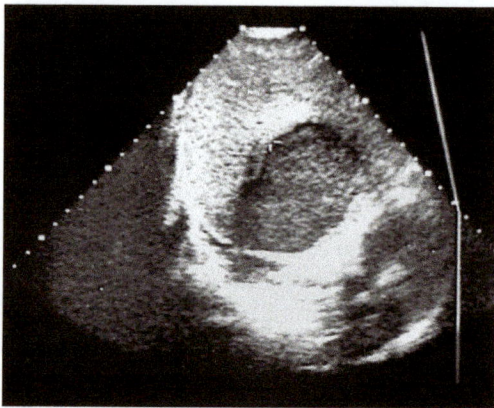

Fig. 1.8.4: Amebic liver abscess—a hypoechoic space-occupying lesion (SOL) is seen in the posterosuperior aspect of liver with evidence of posterior enhancement. It is extending into subdiaphragmatic space.

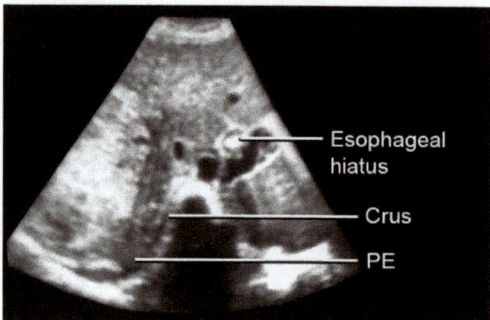

Fig. 1.8.3: Diaphragmatic hiatus for inferior vena cava (IVC), esophagus and aorta. (PE: pleural effusion)

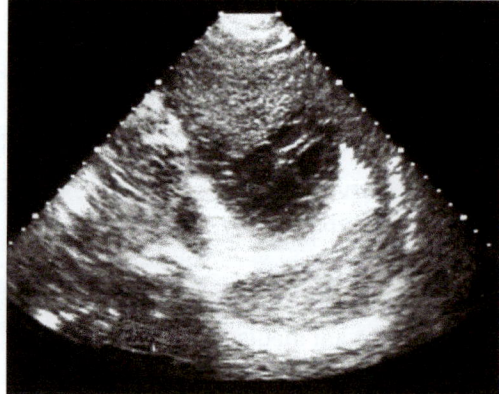

Fig. 1.8.5: Subdiaphragmatic collection—fluid collections with multiple internal septae is seen below the diaphragm.

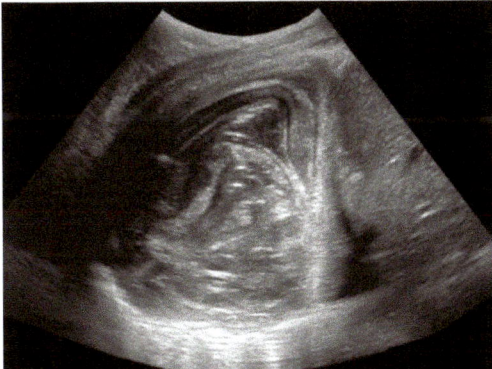

Fig. 1.8.6: Cystic lesion with internal membrane and daughter cyst in the lower lobe of right lung.

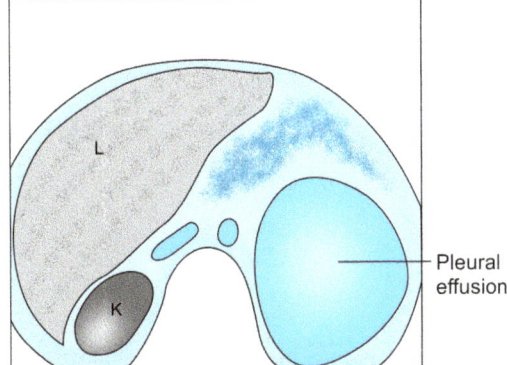

Fig. 1.8.8: Transverse view—a large pleural effusion inverting the diaphragm can look like a large cyst. (L: liver; K: kidney)

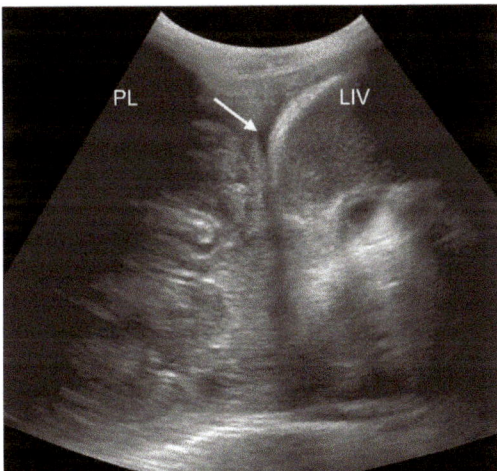

Fig. 1.8.7: Cystic lesion with internal membranes in the lower lobe of right lung with minimal subdiaphragmatic fluid. (PL: pleura; LIV: liver)

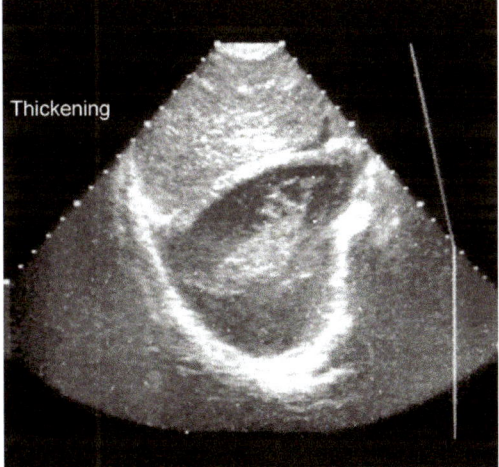

Fig. 1.8.9: Free-fluid seen in right pleural cavity with collapsed lung inside—note the inverted diaphragm.

- Various lung lesions like hydatid (**Figs. 1.8.6 and 1.8.7**)
- Fibroma
- Secondary—local invasion by adjacent pleural, peritoneal, thoracic and abdominal wall malignancies
- Distant metastasis from bronchogenic or ovarian carcinoma
- Wilms' tumor and osteogenic sarcoma are less
- More common on left side, due to protective effect of liver on right side

- Part of diaphragm or entire diaphragm may be affected
- May occur due to large pleural effusion or neoplasm, pushing the diaphragm downwards (**Figs. 1.8.8 and 1.8.9**)
- May show little or asynchronous motion with respiration.

Ultrasound should be the primary imaging modality to see for the cause of elevated diaphragm. In helps to give an etiology at many instances and could narrow down the differential diagnosis in others.

CHAPTER 2

Neck Lesions

2.1 THYROID

2.1.1 Solitary Thyroid Nodule

- Hyperplastic adenomatous nodule
- Adenoma
- Lymphoma
- Carcinoma
- *USG features of benign goitrous nodules*:
  - A thoroughly cystic appearance
  - Moving comet tail artefacts
  - Fluid-fluid level
  - Widespread cystic changes in isoechoic or highly reflective nodules
  - Highly reflective nodules
  - A perilesional thin, uniform thickness echo-poor halo
  - Well-defined and regular margins
  - Peripheral egg shell-like or large coarse calcification
  - A perilesional blood flow pattern (Basket pattern).
- *USG signs for malignancy are*:
  - Low reflectivity
  - Irregular margins
  - Thick irregular halo
  - Microcalcification
  - Intranodal blood flow pattern
  - Hypervascularity
  - Vessel encasement
  - Invasion of vessels and adjacent structures.
- *Hyperplastic or adenomatous nodule*:
  - Isoechoic, if large, may be hyperechoic. Less commonly hypoechoic
  - Thin peripheral hyperechoic halo, complete
  - Perinodal blood flow. However, hyperfunctioning (Basket pattern)
  - Adenomatous nodules frequently show both perinodal and intranodal vascularity
  - *May show degenerative changes*:
    - Purely an echoic—due to serous or colloid fluid.
    - If hemorrhage occurs—echogenic fluid or fluid-fluid level may be present.
    - If dense colloid material is present—comet tail artefact may be seen.
    - Thin intracystic septation—which are avascular on Doppler study.
    - Peripheral (eggshell-like) or large and coarse calcification may be seen.
- *Adenomas*:
  - Solid, may be hyper-iso-or hypoechoic
  - Thick and smooth peripheral hypoechoic halo (**Figs. 2.1.1.1 and 2.1.1.2**)
  - Spoke- and wheel-like arrangement of vessels on Doppler study
  - Sometimes adenomatous nodules are hyperplastic and multiple (**Figs. 2.1.1.3 to 2.1.1.6**).
- *Lymphoma*:
  - Large hypoechoic lobulated mass which is nearly avascular
  - May show large cystic areas due to necrosis
  - May show encasement of neck vessels
  - Heterogeneous echotexture of remaining thyroid parenchyma due to associated chronic thyroiditis.

Neck Lesions

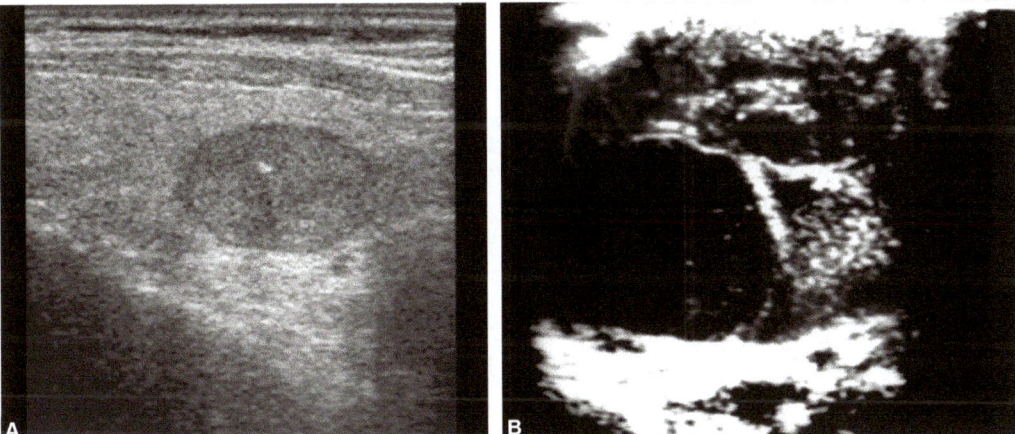

Figs. 2.1.1.1A and B: A solitary thyroid nodule with homogeneous parenchyma in a euthyroid patient. Hypoechoic halo is visible around space occupying lesions.

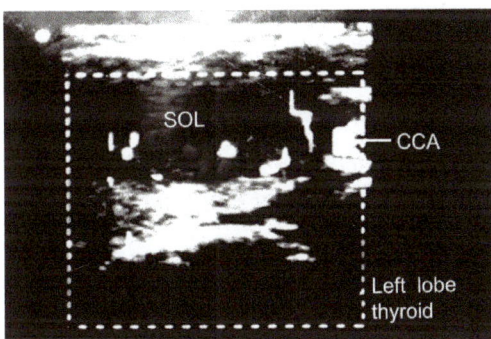

Fig. 2.1.1.2: Doppler images of above lesion reveals no vascularity in the mass but color flow corresponding to the halo is seen. (SOL: space-occupying lesion; CCA: common carotid artery)

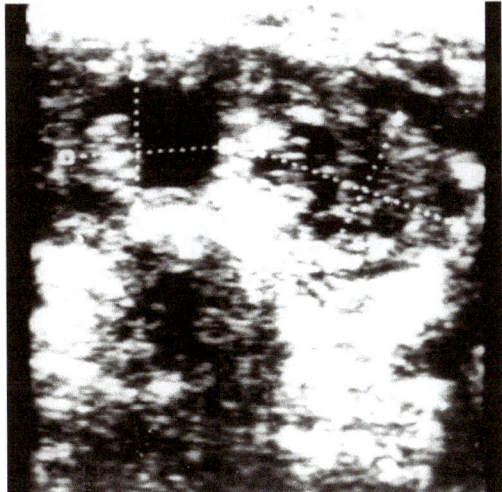

Fig. 2.1.1.3: Transverse scan neck showing multiple space-occupying lesions involving left lobe and isthmus of thyroid. Cystic areas seen in nodules without calcification—multinodular goiter.

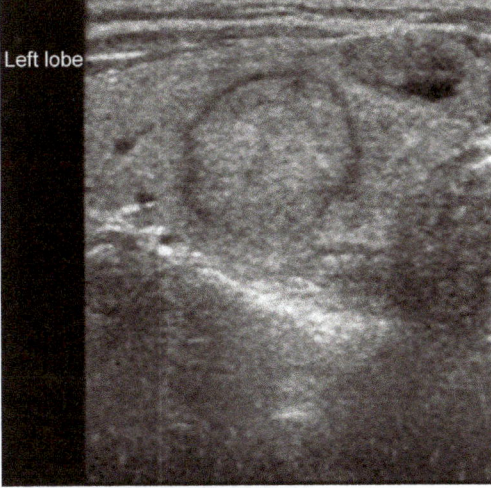

Fig. 2.1.1.4: US scan shows a hyperplastic nodule.

Ultrasound Differentiation of Benign and Malignant Thyroid Nodule

Ultrasound criteria predictive of malignant thyroid nodules are:
- Taller than wide shape
- Spiculated/irregular margin
- Markedly hypoechogenic nodule
- Predominantly solid compression
- Presence of microcalcification in a solid nodule (3-fold risk)
- Macrocalcification in a solid nodule (2-fold risk)
- Absence of halo
- Intranodular vascularity.

Thyroid nodules which necessitates biopsy are four classic patterns (Reading et al. 2005).
1. A hypoechoic nodule with microcalcifications
2. Coarse calcifications in a hypoechoic nodule
3. Well-marginated ovoid solid nodules with a thin hypoechoic halo
4. A solid mass with refractive shadowing from the edges, which is believed to occur as a result of fibrosis.

Thyroid nodules which do not necessitates biopsy. The four classic patterns are:
1. Small (<1 cm) colloid-filled cystic nodules
2. A small with a honeycomb appearance consisting of internal cystic spaces with thin echogenic walls
3. Diffuse multiple small hypoechoic nodules with intervening echogenic bands, indicating of Hashimoto's thyroiditis
4. A homogeneously hyperechoic nodule.

Four Specific Morphological Patterns Highly Predictive of Benignity (Bonavita et al. 2009)

Type 1: Spongiform or honeycomb pattern is characteristic of colloid nodules and goiter and consists of diffuse internal cysts without vascularity, i.e. iso or a vascular.

Type 2: This pattern is a cystic nodule containing a central plug of a vascular colloid **(Fig. 2.1.1.7)**.

Type 3: Giraffe pattern is typical of Hashimoto's thyroiditis and is a nodule with appearance of

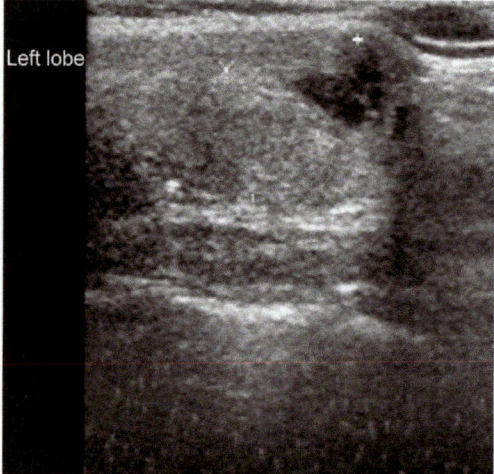

Fig. 2.1.1.5: US scan shows adenomatous nodule with cystic degeneration.

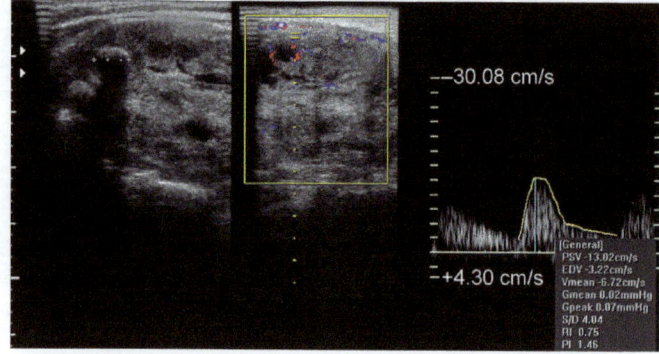

Fig. 2.1.1.6: US and color Doppler scans show adenomatous nodule with internal calcification and cystic degeneration and internal vascularity of moderate resistance.

Neck Lesions

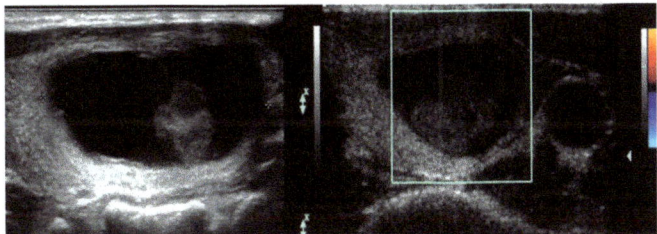

Fig. 2.1.1.7: USG images showing well-defined anechoic nodule with central colloid plug with no vascularity "pattern 2" in left lobe of thyroid gland suggestive of colloid goiter.

hide of a giraffe, i.e. light blocks separated by a black bands.

Type 4: White knight or hyperechoic nodule (**Fig. 2.1.1.8**) is a variation of type 3 which was found commonly to be a regenerative nodule of Hashimoto's thyroiditis.

US Elastography—Importance in Differentiating Benign versus Malignant Thyroid Nodule

Ultrasound elastography (**Figs. 2.1.1.9A and B**) is a noninvasive device developed to obtain information on tissue stiffness. The technique can evaluate the degree of distortion of tissues under application of an external force and is based on the principle that the softer parts of the tissue deform easily than the harder parts under compression, thus allowing an objective determination of tissue stiffness. The 4-point scale characterized by a different pattern in the color scale, depending upon the magnitude of the strain: Red (Soft tissue), Green (Intermediate degree of stiffness), and Blue (Anaplastic tissue).

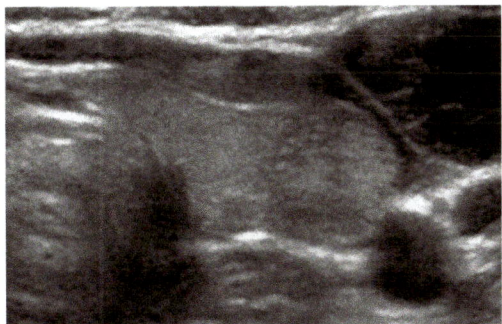

Fig. 2.1.1.8: USG image showing well-defined hyperechoic nodule "white knight" in left lobe of thyroid gland suggestive of benign nodule.

	ES	Elastogram pattern
ES 1	Elasticity in the whole area examined	Homogeneously green inside the nodule
ES 2	Elasticity in a large portion of the examined area	Almost the whole tumor is displayed in light green with some peripheral and/or central blue area (Figs. 2.1.1.10A and B)
ES 3	No elasticity/stiffness in a large portion of the examined area	Almost the whole tumor is displayed in a dark blue with some green and red areas
ES 4	No elasticity in the whole examined area	Homogeneously dark blue

Differential Diagnosis of Diffuse Thyroid Disease

- *Diffuse nontoxic goiter* (**Fig. 2.1.1.11**):
  - Diffuse glandular enlargement with uniform or irregular echogenicity that may be increased or decreased
  - Diffuse in homogeneous echogenicity or multiple focal hypoechoic nodules in a relatively normal thyroid gland.

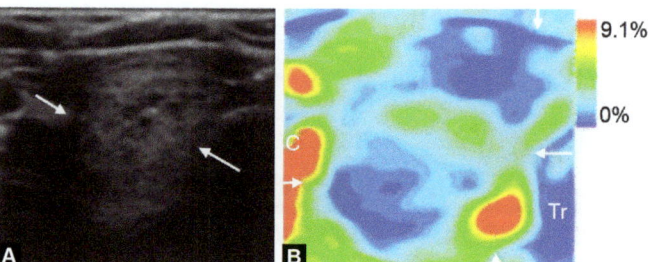

Figs. 2.1.1.9A and B: (A) Transverse US image shows a predominantly solid nodule with small cystic areas (arrows); (B) Elastogram shows the heterogeneous appearance within nodule. This was diagnosed as a nodular goiter at fine-needle aspiration cytology (FNAC).

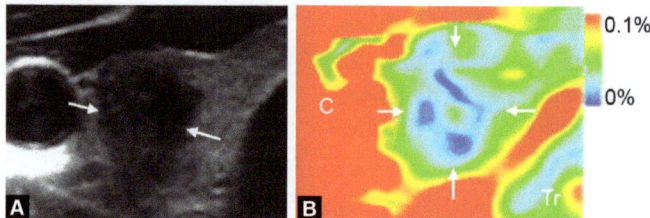

Figs. 2.1.1.10A and B: (A) Transverse US image shows a hypoechoic nodule (arrows) with irregular borders and tiny punctate calcifications in it; (B) Elastogram at same level shows stiff areas within lesion (blue region). This was diagnosed as papillary carcinoma at fine-needle aspiration cytology (FNAC).

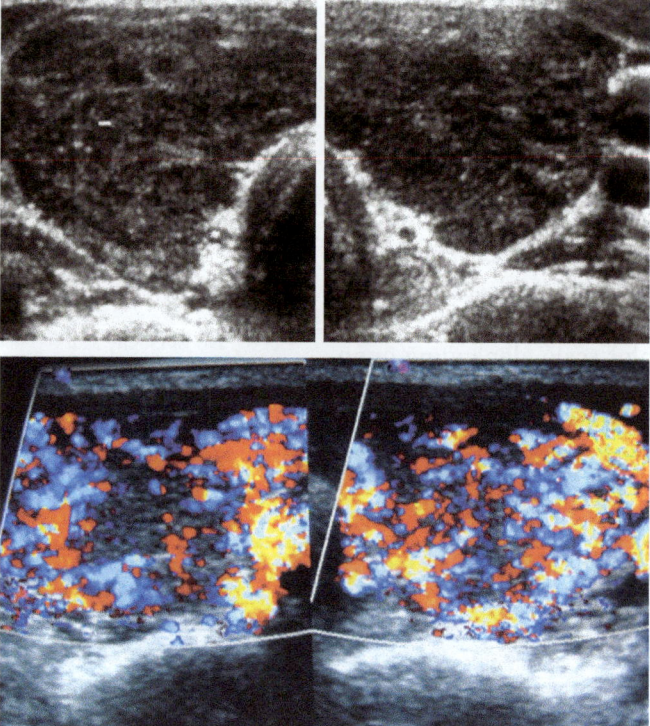

Fig. 2.1.1.11: USG images showing enlarged heteroechoic thyroid gland with hypoechoic areas with increased vascularity in a case of diffuse toxic goiter.

Neck Lesions

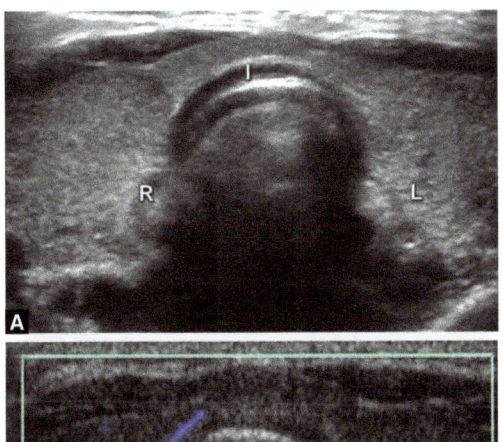

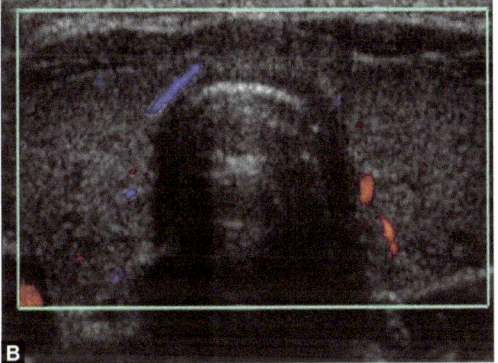

Figs. 2.1.1.12A and B: USG images showing hypoechoic areas in both thyroid lobes with decreased vascularity in a case of Hashimoto's thyroiditis. (I: isthmus; R: right; L: left)

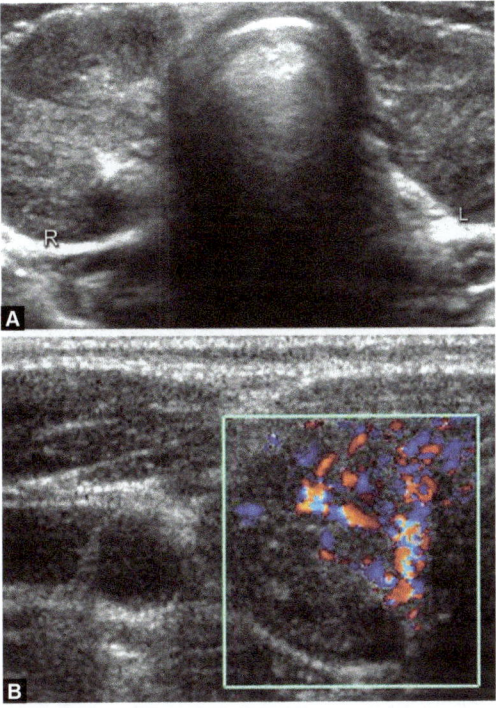

Figs. 2.1.1.13A and B: USG thyroid images showing heteroechoic enlarged thyroid gland with nodular change and increased vascularity in a case of de Quervain's thyroiditis.

- *Diffuse toxic goiter—Graves' disease*:
  - Inhomogeneous echotexture with diffusely hypoechoic parenchyma due to extensive lymphocytic infiltration.
  - Color Doppler-hypervascular pattern as "thyroid inferno"
  - Peak systolic velocities exceeds 70 cm/sec.
- Chronic autoimmune lymphocytic (Hashimoto's thyroiditis) **(Figs. 2.1.1.12 and 2.1.1.13)**
  - May be normal or more often enlarged in size
  - Coarse heterogeneous echogenicity of the parenchyma, generally more hypoechoic than normal thyroid
  - The vascularity on color Doppler is normal or decreased.

2.1.2 Carcinomas

Papillary Carcinoma (Figs. 2.1.2.1A and B)
- About 90% hypoechoic
- Microcalcifications may be present
- Hypervascularity, both intranodal and perinodal with disorganized arrangement of vessels on Doppler study
- Enlarged cervical lymph nodes due to metastasis, which may also show microcalcifications. Occasionally on USG cervical lymph node metastasis may be cystic.

Follicular Carcinoma (Figs. 2.1.2.2A and B)
- Features similar to adenoma, except for:
  - Irregular tumor margins
  - Thick irregular hypoechoic halo

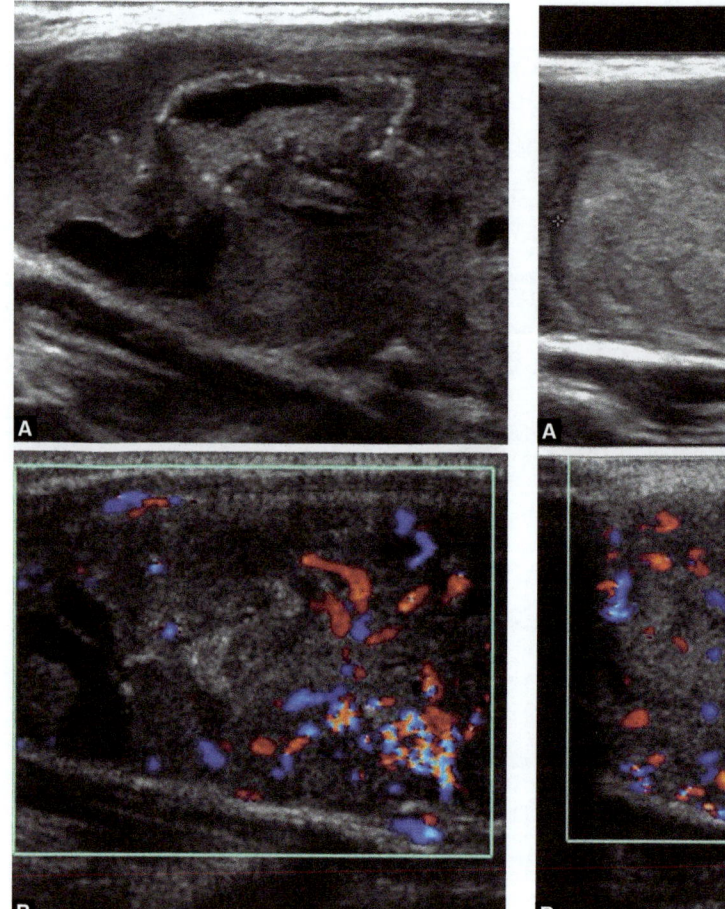
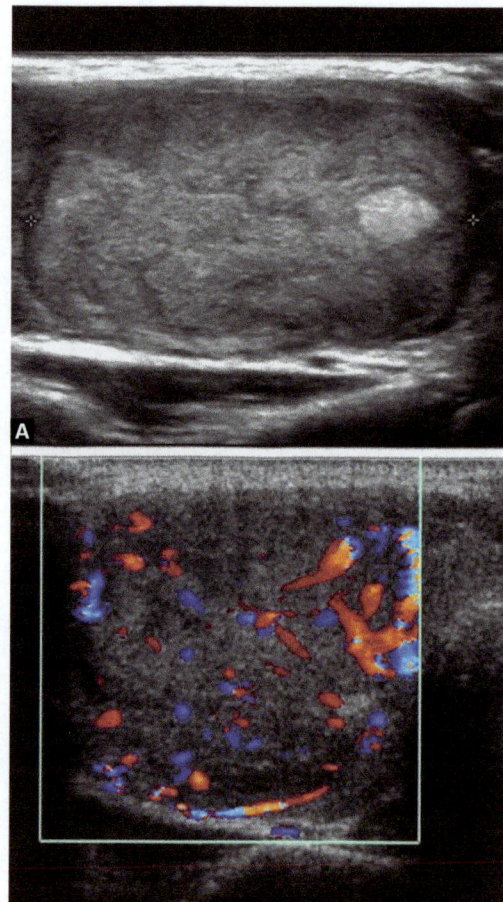

Figs. 2.1.2.1A and B: Ultrasound images of thyroid showing well-defined nodule with clustered microcalcifications well-defined perilesional halo showing increased vascularity in a case of papillary carcinoma of right lobe of thyroid.

Figs. 2.1.2.2A and B: Ultrasound images of thyroid showing well-defined nodule with well-defined perilesional halo showing increased vascularity in a case of follicular adenoma of right lobe of thyroid.

- Both intra- and perinodal vascularity with tortuous and chaotic arrangement of internal blood vessels on color Doppler.

Anaplastic Carcinoma Thyroid (Fig. 2.1.2.3)

- Large, hypoechoic
- Ill-defined margins

- Encase or invade blood vessels and muscles in the neck.

Medullary Carcinoma Thyroid

- Sonographic appearance similar to papillary carcinoma (hypoechoic, irregular margins, hypervascularity) except that the local invasion and metastasis to cervical nodes **(Figs. 2.1.2.4 to 2.1.2.6)** occurs

Neck Lesions

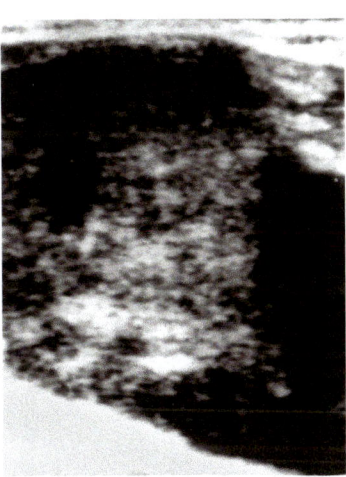

Fig. 2.1.2.3: Anaplastic carcinoma thyroid. Ultrasound image showing a large heteroechoic lesion involving right lobe of thyroid with brightly echogenic focus suggestive of calcification.

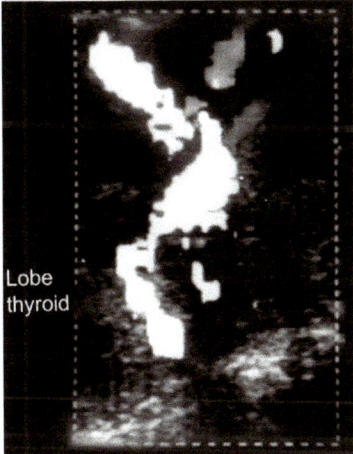

Fig. 2.1.2.5: Color velocity imaging revealed high velocity flow throughout the parenchyma suggestive of malignancy—medullary carcinoma.

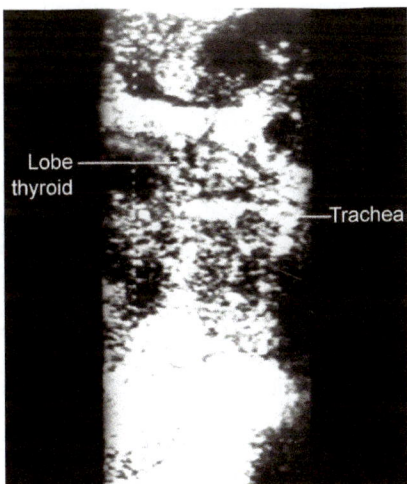

Fig. 2.1.2.4: Heterogeneous multinodular parenchymal pattern of thyroid along with obscuration of anatomical planes seen in elderly patient. Discrete lymph nodes were also seen in posterior triangle.

- more frequently in patients with medullary carcinoma
- May show microcalcifications similar to papillary carcinoma
- Familial in 20% patient and essential component of MEN type II syndrome.

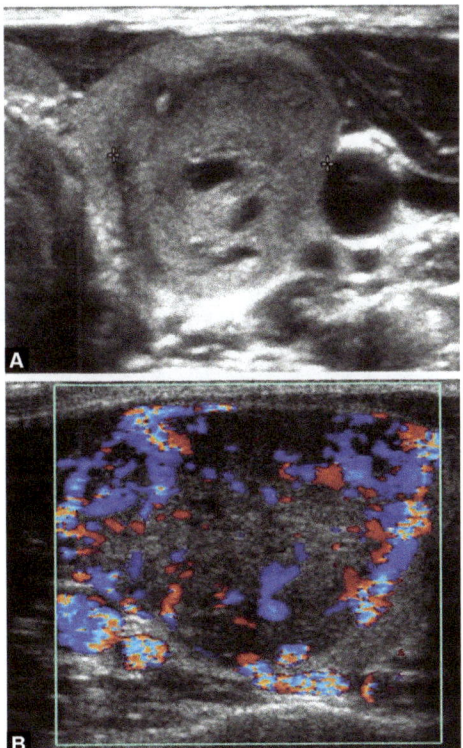

Figs. 2.1.2.6A and B: Ultrasound images of thyroid showing well-defined nodule with coarse calcification with ill-defined perilesional halo posteromedially and showing increased vascularity in a case of medullary carcinoma of left lobe of thyroid.

2.1.3 Thyroid Calcification

- Peripheral or egg shell-like calcification is a feature of benign thyroid nodule
- Scattered large and coarse calcification (**Fig. 2.1.3.1**) is, if seen the nodule is more, likely to be benign
- Scattered fine and punctate calcifications (Microcalcification) are seen in papillary carcinoma of thyroid (psammoma bodies) or medullary carcinoma of thyroid caused by reactive fibrosis and calcification around amyloid deposits.

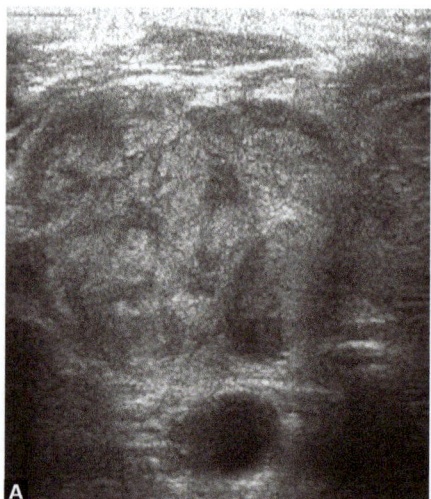

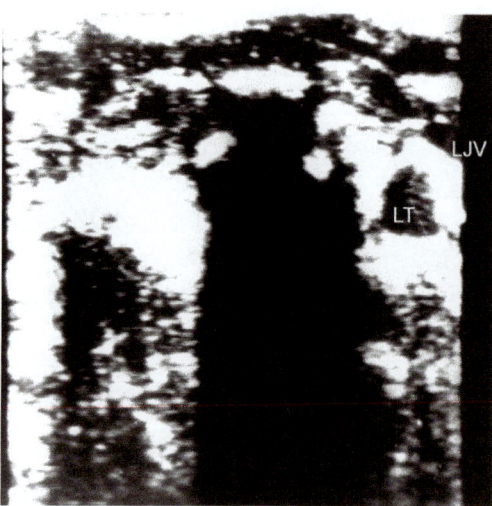

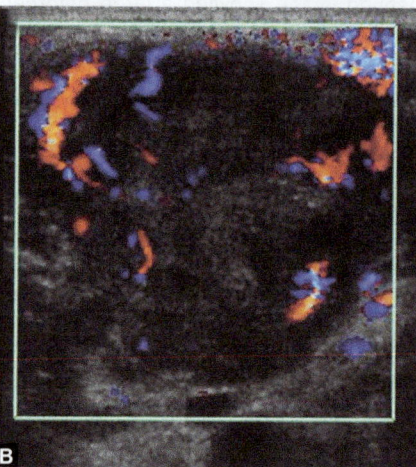

Fig. 2.1.3.1: Multiple coarse calcification seen within well-defined regular isoechoic, nodule in thyroid-multinodular goiter.

Figs. 2.1.4.1A and B: Ultrasound images of thyroid showing well-defined nodule with showing increased vascularity in a known case of carcinoma lung suggestive of metastasis to right lobe of thyroid.

2.1.4 Differential Diagnosis on the Basis of Echogenicity of Thyroid Nodules

- *Hypoechoic nodule*:
  - Can be both benign or malignant
  - Most thyroid cancers are hypoechoic, however, few benign nodules can also be hypoechoic
  - Because of much greater incidence of benign thyroid nodules, as compared to thyroid cancer, in fact most hypoechoic thyroid nodules are thought to be benign unless proved otherwise. However, sonographically strong suspicion of malignancy be kept
  - Look for after features such as margins, halo pattern of calcification, color flow pattern to differentiate benign from malignant nodule (**Figs. 2.1.4.1A and B**).
- *Hyperechoic nodule*: A predominantly hyperechoic nodule is more likely to be benign.

- *Isoechoic nodule*: It (visible because of peripheral sonolucent rim) has an intermediate risk of malignancy (16–84%). Again, look for other sonographic features favoring benign or malignant nodules.

2.1.5 Cystic Thyroid Nodule

Benign

- A nodule that has a significant cystic **(Fig. 2.1.5.1)** component is usually benign adenomatous (colloid) nodule **(Fig. 2.1.5.2)**, that has undergone degeneration **(Fig. 2.1.5.3)** or hemorrhage.

Features favoring are:
- Purely anechoic
- Echogenic fluid or moving fluid-fluid level
- Bright echogenic foci with comet-tail artefact
- Thin septations; avascular on Doppler study
- A true epithelium-lined, simple thyroid cyst is extremely rare.

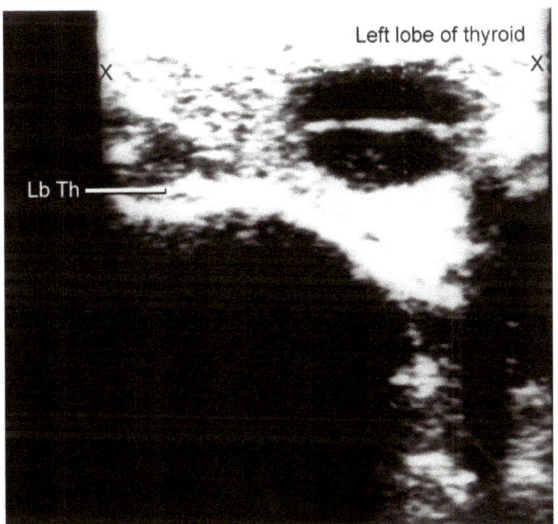

Fig. 2.1.5.1: Well-defined regular predominantly cystic nodule with septation seen within left lobe of thyroid—multinodular goiter. (Lb Th: lobe of thyroid)

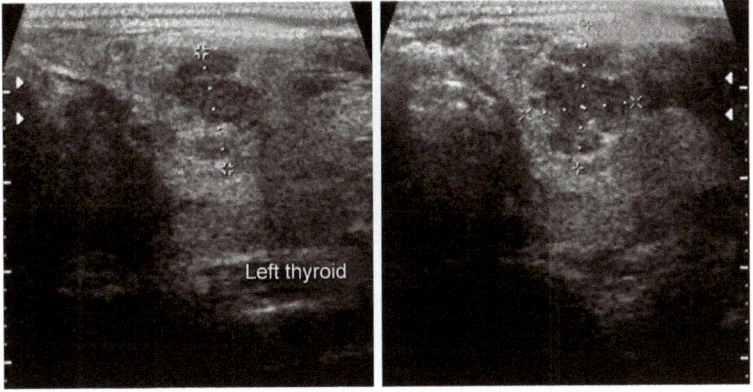

Fig. 2.1.5.2: US scans show colloid nodule of thyroid.

Malignant

Papillary carcinomas may show cystic component, features favoring papillary carcinoma are:

- Solid projection (1 cm or more) with blood flow on color Doppler
- Presence of microcalcification **(Figs. 2.1.5.4A and B)**.

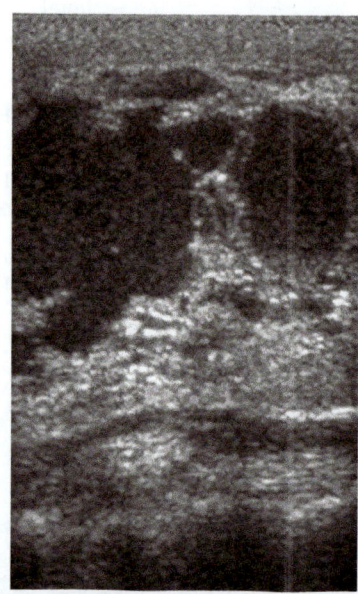

Fig. 2.1.5.3: US scan shows cystic degeneration in thyroid nodule.

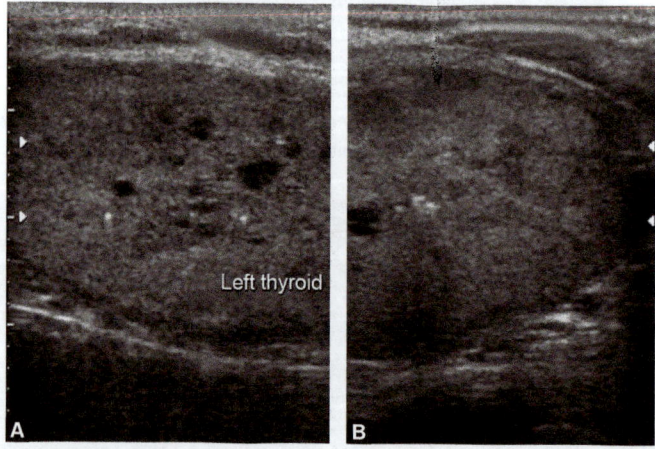

Figs. 2.1.5.4A and B: US scans show follicular adenoma of thyroid with internal calcification and cystic changes.

2.2 SALIVARY GLAND

2.2.1 Enlargement of Salivary Gland

Hypertrophy

- Enlarged gland with normal size, shape and echotexture
- *May be due to:*
  - Obesity
  - Diabetes
  - Liver cirrhosis
  - Uremia.
- Racial (Egyptians–North Africans).

Acute Sialadenitis

- Probe tenderness
- Enlarged gland
- Hypoechoic slightly heterogeneous echotexture
- Small echo poor areas may be observed inside the gland due to microabscesses
- Large abscesses **(Fig. 2.2.1.1)** may develop which are seen as fluid-filled areas with irregular borders and internal debris.

Chronic Sialadenitis (Fig. 2.2.1.2)

- Commonly due to Sjögren's syndrome
- *Classical triad of:*
  - Keratoconjunctivitis sicca
  - Xerostomia
  - Autoimmune disorders most commonly rheumatoid arthritis.
- Typical USG features of multiple cystic areas scattered throughout the salivary glands as a result of peripheral nonobstructive sialectasis. These cystic areas has well-defined but irregular margins **(Fig. 2.2.1.3)**.
- Four point USG scale:
  Grade 0: No parenchymal changes
  1. Occasional microcysts (< 2 mm in diameter) and minimal heterogeneity.
  2. Diffuse cysts (> 2 mm).

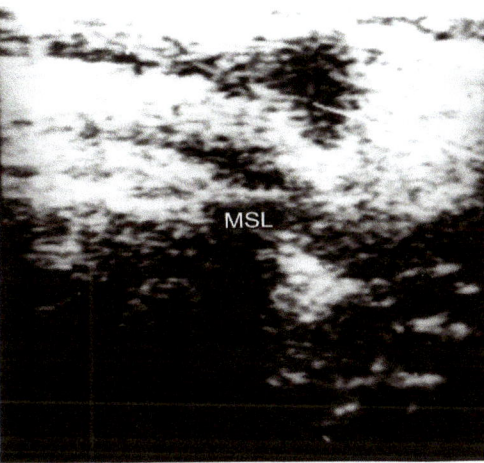

Figs. 2.2.1.1: Longitudinal scan—parotid gland of the patient shows hypoechoic abscess with a track seen anterior of muscle plane. (MSL: muscular layer)

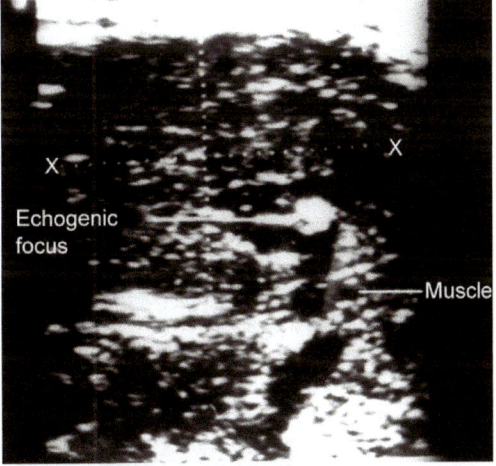

Fig. 2.2.1.2: Transverse scan of the submandibular gland shows diffusely hypoechoic and coarse echo texture of the gland parenchyma with irregularity of the margins. The finding suggestive of sialadenitis. An echogenic focus (calcification) was seen within glandular parenchyma.

3. Large confluent cysts with septations (confluent masses) and a highly heterogeneous structure.
4. Disappearance of parenchymal texture in atrophic glands with undefined margins and reduced volume.

- On Doppler—a diffuse increase in parenchymal blood flow signals and decrease in arteriolar resistance.
- *Sialolithiasis*:
  - Most common in submandibular gland
  - Seen as highly echogenic foci with posterior acoustic shadowing **(Fig. 2.2.1.4)**
  - Associated ductal dilatation may be seen.

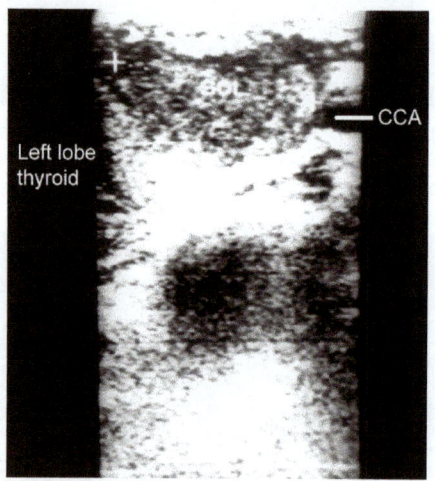

Fig. 2.2.1.3: Ultrasound showing a well-defined hypoechoic lesion with mixed solid and cystic areas in right submandibular region. Benign submandibular tumor. (CCA: common carotid artery)

- *Tumors*
  - Most common tumor of salivary glands is pleomorphic adenoma (mixed tumor—60-70%) **(Figs. 2.2.1.5 to 2.2.1.8)**
  - On USG—homogeneous, solid, echo poor structure, sharp margins with discrete posterior acoustic enhancement
  - Surface may be lobulated
  - Peripheral echo poor areas may be observed due to hemorrhage or cystic degeneration
  - On color Doppler peripheral "basket pattern" of flow seen
  - Most common salivary gland tumor to have calcifications and ossifications within the tumor matrix.

Adenolymphoma (Warthin's Tumor)

- Most common lesion to occur as multifocal unilateral and bilateral disease
- On USG—echo poor with sharp margins, but appear less homogeneous than pleomorphic adenoma
- One or more cystic areas that produce a well-defined posterior acoustic enhancement.

Tumors >5 cm have higher proportion of cystic component than smaller ones.

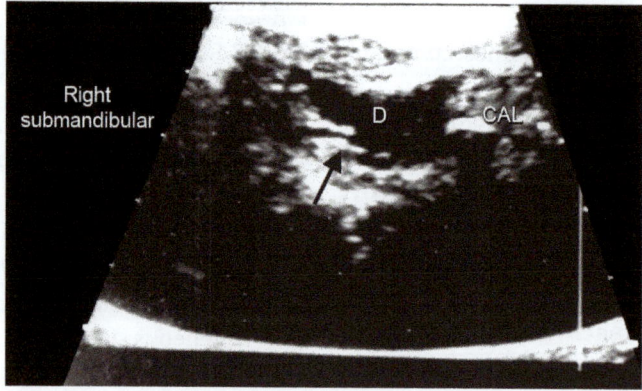

Fig. 2.2.1.4: US (sagittal scan) showing an echogenic focus with distal shadowing in Wharton's duct which is dilated. Dilated ductal system within gland can be seen very well (arrow). (D: dilated; CAL: calculus)

Neck Lesions

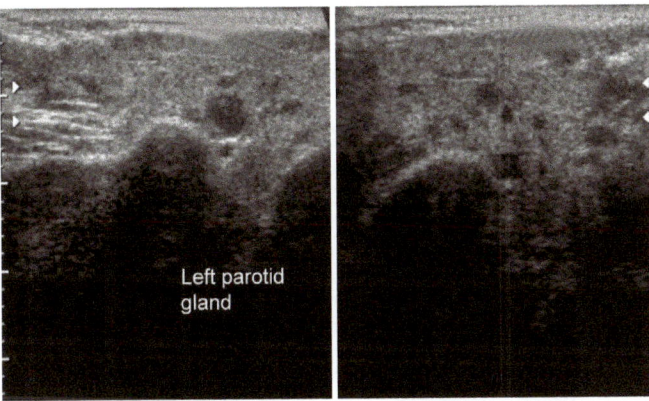

Fig. 2.2.1.5: US scans show granulomatous parotitis.

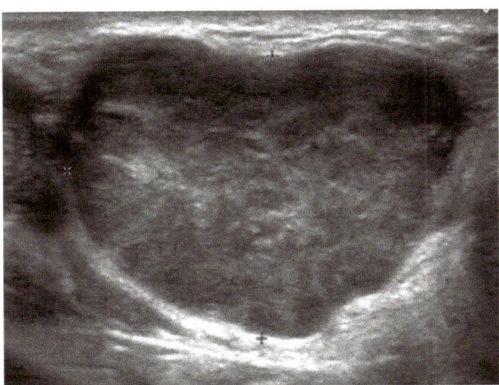

Fig. 2.2.1.6: Pleomorphic adenoma involving the superficial lobe of parotid gland.

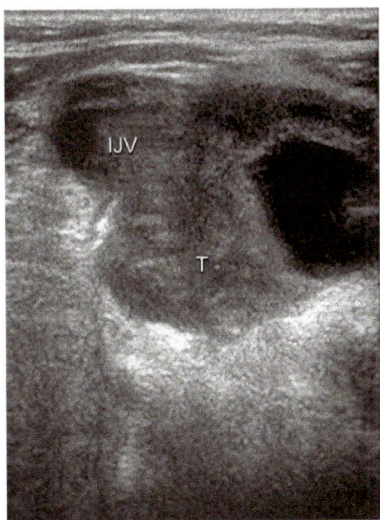

Fig. 2.2.1.7: Lymph nodal mass (marked as T) invading into the internal jugular vein (IJV).

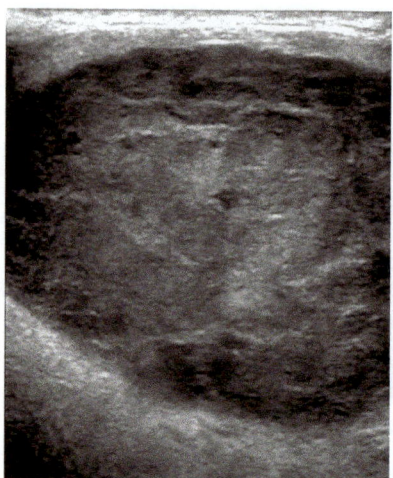

Fig. 2.2.1.8: Pleomorphic adenoma in the parotid gland.

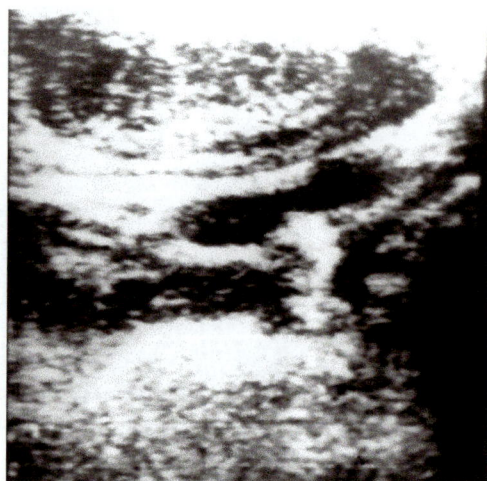

Fig. 2.3.1: Well-defined, encapsulated thick-walled space occupying lesion seen in anterior triangle of neck in lower half. The contents of the lesion were hyperechoic along with debris—brachial cyst.

Mucoepidermoid Carcinoma

- Most common salivary gland malignancy
- Heterogeneously hypoechoic with well-defined margins which stand out distinctly from the normal hyperechoeic gland parenchyma
- Marked tendency to spread into adjacent structures
- Cystic areas may be present and rarely focal calcification may be seen.

2.3 NECK MASSES

Congenital Lesions

Branchial Cyst (Fig. 2.3.1)

- Not generally evident at birth, but during childhood
- In anterior triangle of neck along the anterior margin of sternocleidomastoid muscle
- Round or oval, usually echofree masses with thin regular walls, clearly demarcated from the sternoclei domastoid muscle
- If infected—low level, then internal echos may be seen.

Thyroglossal Cyst

- Usually present in childhood
- Characteristic medial location
- May be anterior or posterior to hyoid bone or within the bone itself
- Movement towards the oral cavity during swallowing or tongue protrusion
- USG appearance is similar to bronchial cyst except for midline location anywhere between the thyroid isthmus and the blind foramen of the tongue.

Cystic Hygroma

- Usually located in posterior triangle of neck
- Present at birth
  - Usually can be detected on antenatal ultrasound
  - On USG—multilocular, thin septa, thin regular margins, clear demarcation from surrounding structures
- Fine low to medium level internal echos are present
  - Presence of septations and larger volume indicate poor fetal outcome.

Neck Lesions

Inflammatory Lesions (Cervical Phlegmon)

- Usually located in posterior triangle of neck **(Fig. 2.3.2)**
- Present at birth
    - On USG—multilocular, thin septa, thin regular margins, clear demarcation from surrounding structures
- Fine low to medium level internal echos are present
- Sometimes well-defined multiloculated lesions are seen with posterior acoustic enhancement **(Fig. 2.3.3)**.

Abscess (Figs. 2.3.4 to 2.3.6)

- Usually involve the subcutaneous and subfascial planes but may extend into deeper structures
- On USG—echofree or echo poor fluid collection with thick irregular wall with

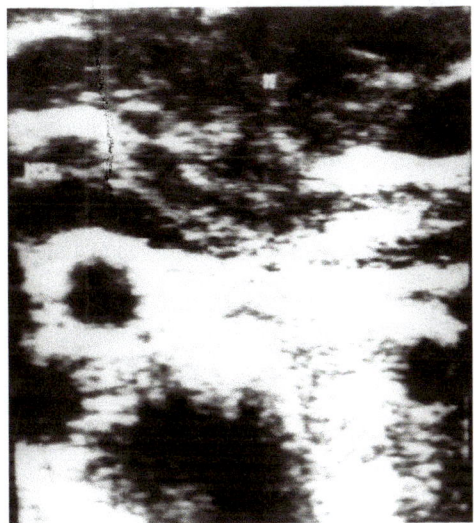

Fig. 2.3.4: Multiple tubercular abscess—a transverse sonogram in a patient of hypoechoic ill-defined mass within the strap muscles—tubercular etiology.

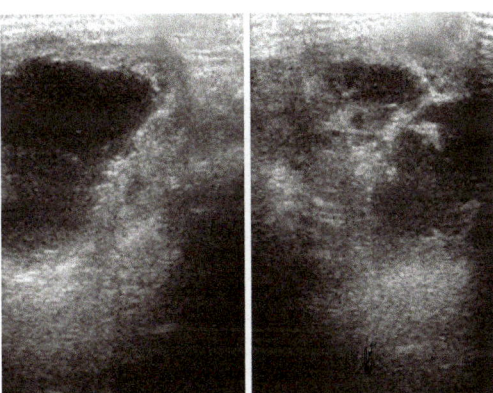

Fig. 2.3.2: US scans show inflammatory necrotic mass in neck.

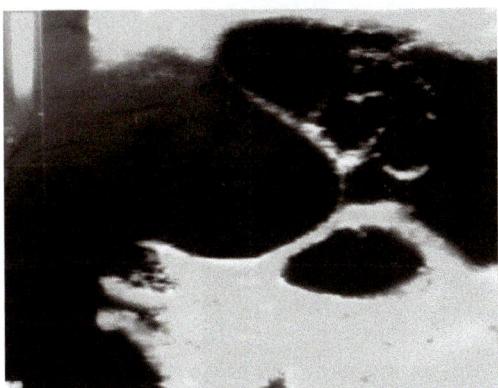

Fig. 2.3.3: Cystic lymphangioma: Ultrasound of left side of neck showing a well-defined multiloculated lesion with posterior acoustic enhancement.

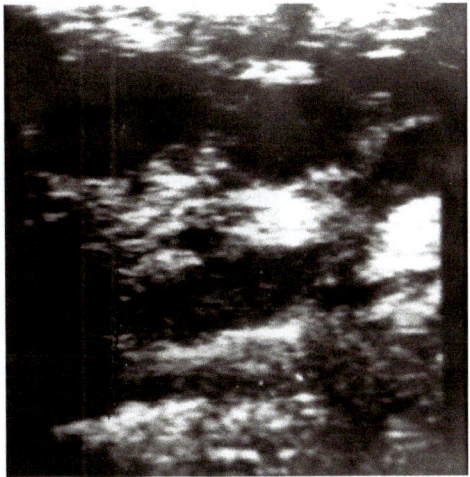

Fig. 2.3.5: Multiple matted lymph nodes seen. All multiple abscesses regressed on ATT.

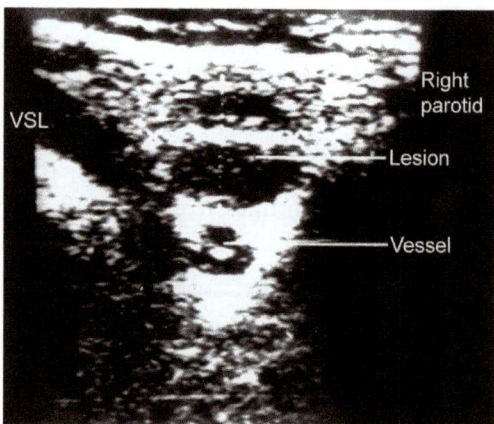

Fig. 2.3.6: Hypoechoic lesion seem to be arising from parotid and reaching up to submandibular gland. Vessels were seen reaching up to margin of the lesions. (VSL: vessel)

irregular margins extending through fascial and muscular planes
- Always associated with local adenopathy
- May cause thrombosis of the internal jugular chain.

Benign Tumors

Hemangioma (Figs. 2.3.7 and 2.3.8)

- It can be either cutaneous or deeply located
- Soft, relatively mobile, sometimes pulsatile masses
  - USG—mass of low reflectivity with irregular margins
- It may show tubular hypoechoic areas or sponge-like pattern due to tiny vessels and/or small blood pools

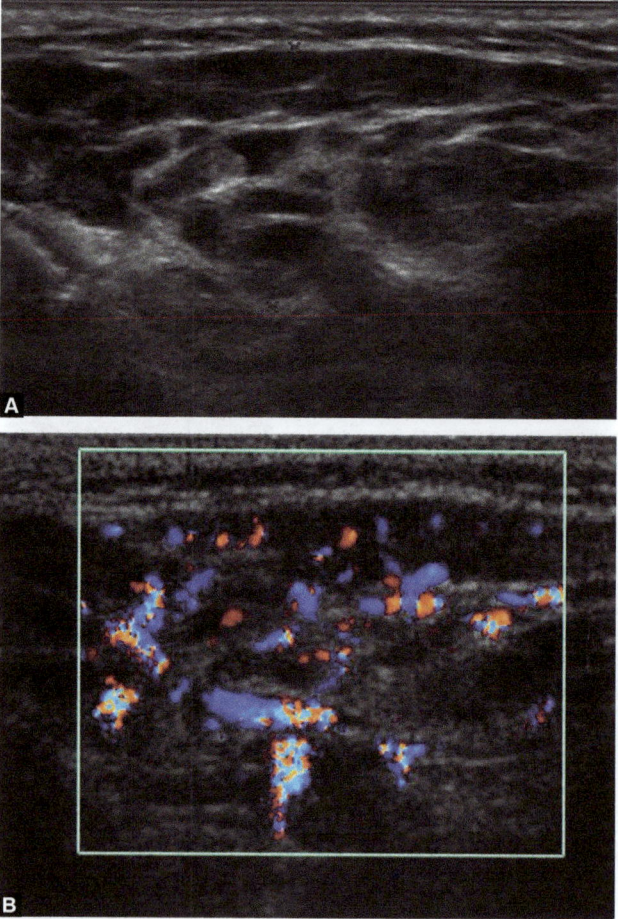

Figs. 2.3.7A and B: Multiple small hypoechoic lesions in the enlarged parotid gland with increased vascularity.

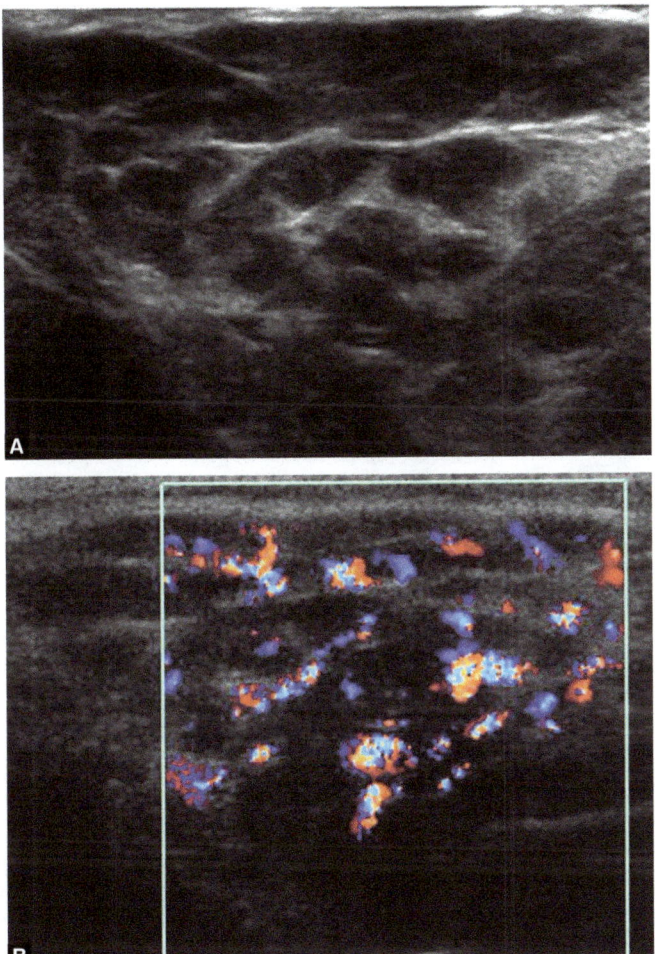

Figs. 2.3.8A and B: Ultrasound images of parotid showing multiple hypoechoic lesion with increased vascularity in a child suggestive of hemangiothelioma.

- Phleboliths may be seen as echogenic foci with posterior acoustic shadowing
- Internal flow may be seen on Doppler.

Lipoma (Fig. 2.3.9)

- Either subcutaneous or in deep tissue spaces
- May be well—circumscribed or diffuse
  - USG—moderately or highly reflective encapsulated masses with fibrous strands
- No signs of local invasion, with well-defined margins
- No flow signals on Doppler studies.

Nerve Tumors (Ganglioneuromas, Neurinomas, Schwannomas and Neurofibromas)

- Their typical site along the nerve paths and atrophy of the adjacent muscular structures supplied by them
  - USG—homogeneous masses of low reflectivity with regular margins, often surrounded by highly reflective rim
- Adjacent structures are generally displaced and compressed, but are never invaded by the mass

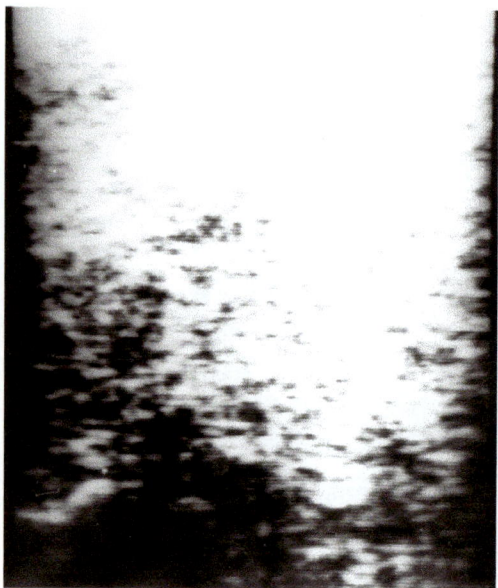

Fig. 2.3.9: Ultrasound, neck showing homogeneously hyperechoic lesion containing linear echogenic lines parallel to skin surface—lipoma.

- Show little or no internal flow, except for carotid body tumors (chemodectomas) which have characteristic location at cervical vessels and are highly vascular **(Figs. 2.3.10 and 2.3.11)**.

Malignant Tumors

- *Except for thyroid cancer, malignant cervical neoplasms are rare—can be:*
    - Bronchial epithelioma
    - Malignant chemodectoma
    - Liposarcoma
    - Rhabdomyosarcoma—tumors of cervical esophagus.
- *USG—Signs of malignancy are:*
    - Lobulated, irregular, ill-defined margins
    - Invasion or infiltration of adjacent muscles or blood vessels
    - No distinguishing feature for individual malignancy.

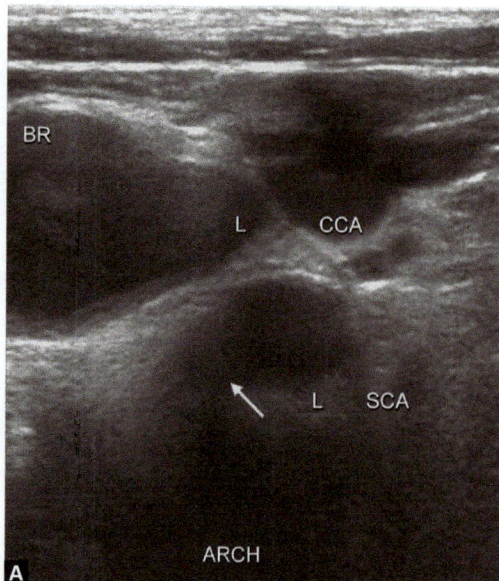
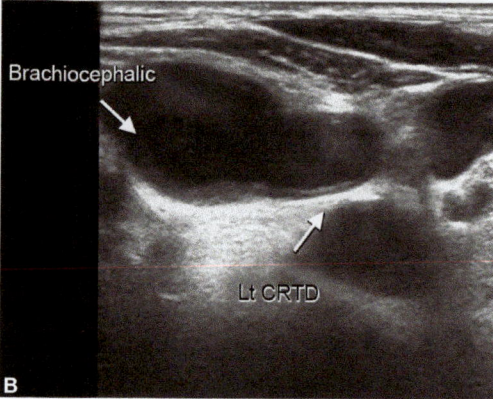

Figs. 2.3.10A and B: Anomalous origin of left CCA from right brachiocephalic trunk. (CCA: common carotid artery; SCA: subclavian artery; BR: brachiocephalic; ARCH: arch of aorta; Lt CRTD: left common carotid artery).

- Tumors arising from pharynx or esophagus can be shown to have relationship with digestive tract on ultrasound or barium studies.

Neck Lesions

2.4 CERVICAL LYMPHADENOPATHY

Cervical Lymph Nodes Levels

- Level IA submental lymph nodes
- Level IB submandibular lymph nodes
- Level II internal jugular (deep cervical) chain from the base of the skull to the inferior border of the hyoid bone
- Level III internal jugular (deep cervical) chain from the hyoid bone to the inferior border of the cricoid arch
- Level IV internal jugular (deep cervical) chain between the inferior border of the cricoid arch and the supraclavicular fossa
- Level V posterior triangle or spinal accessory nodes
- Level VI central compartment nodes from the hyoid bone to the suprasternal notch
- Level VII nodes inferior to the suprasternal notch in the upper mediastinum.

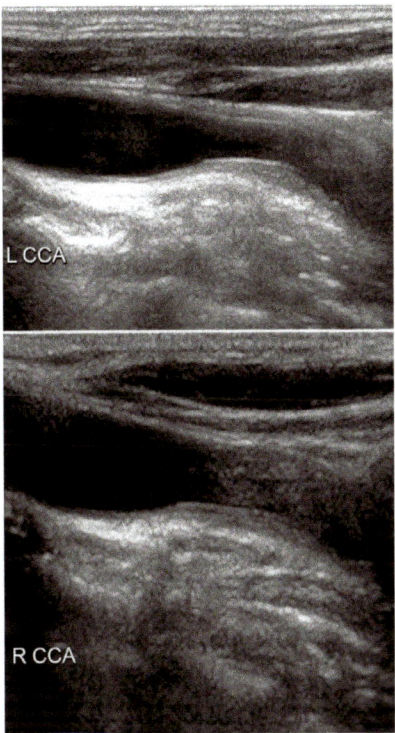

Fig. 2.3.11: Narrowing of the lumen of the left CCA due to atherosclerotic plaque. (L CCA: left common carotid artery; R CCA: right common carotid artery)

Features of cervical lymphadenopathy.

	Features	Benign	Malignant
1.	Roundness index (L > S) Long/short axis diameter	>2	<2
2.	Hilum present	Echogenic hilum (slit-like) or eccentric hilum or completely absent	Thin hilum
3.	Eccentric cortical widening	Less common	More common
4.	Pattern of involvement	Usually diffuse cortical involvement	Usually multifocal
5.	Flow pattern	Completely absent limited to hilar region	Diffuse increase in vascularity, with a wide range of velocities and uneven distribution mainly concentrated in the cortex
6.	Extracapsular nodal spread	Usually absent	Present more often

Some Characteristic Ultrasound Appearances (Figs. 2.4.1 to 2.4.6)

- In lymphomas (untreated), the node is usually markedly echo poor (pseudocystic) owing to the homogeneous arrangement of cellular sheets
- Cystic cervical nodes may be seen in metastatic deposits from squamous cell

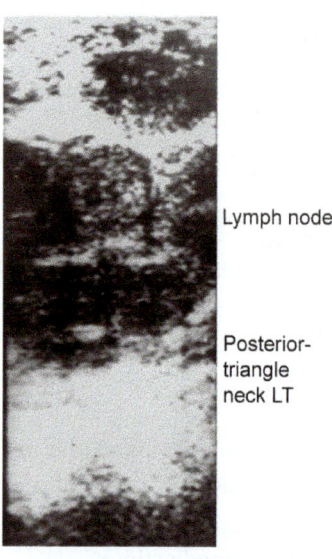

Fig. 2.4.1: Posterior cervical lymph nodes were also enlarged and showed evidence of cavitation, matting and distal enhancement suggestive of tubercular etiology.

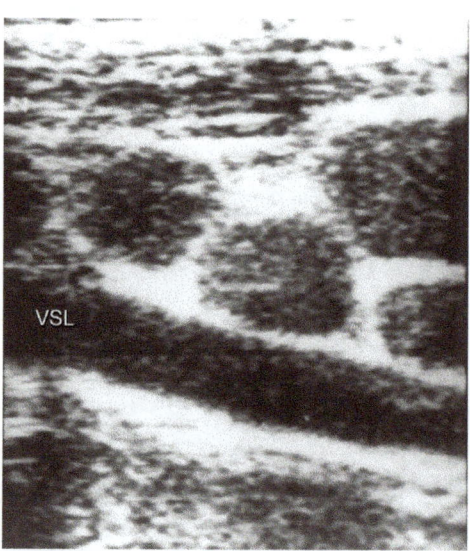

Fig. 2.4.2: Multiple large size, discrete, hypoechoic, supraclavicular (Region-7) nodes seen. No distal enhancement, matting, and involvement of surrounding soft tissues—Metastatic lymph nodes—abdominal scanning revealed gallbladder malignancy. (VSL: vessel)

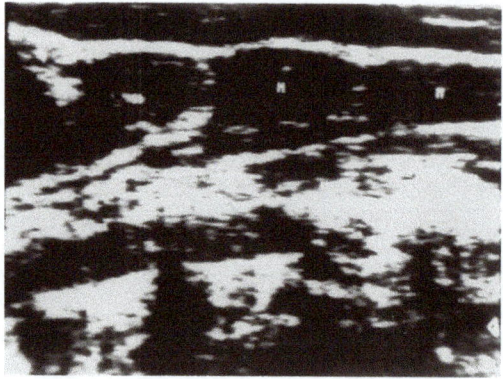

Fig. 2.4.3: Multiple hypoechoic discrete lymph nodes in submandibular region (Region-2), without matting of involvement of surrounding tissues along with distal enhancement. FNAC-lymphomatous changes.

Neck Lesions

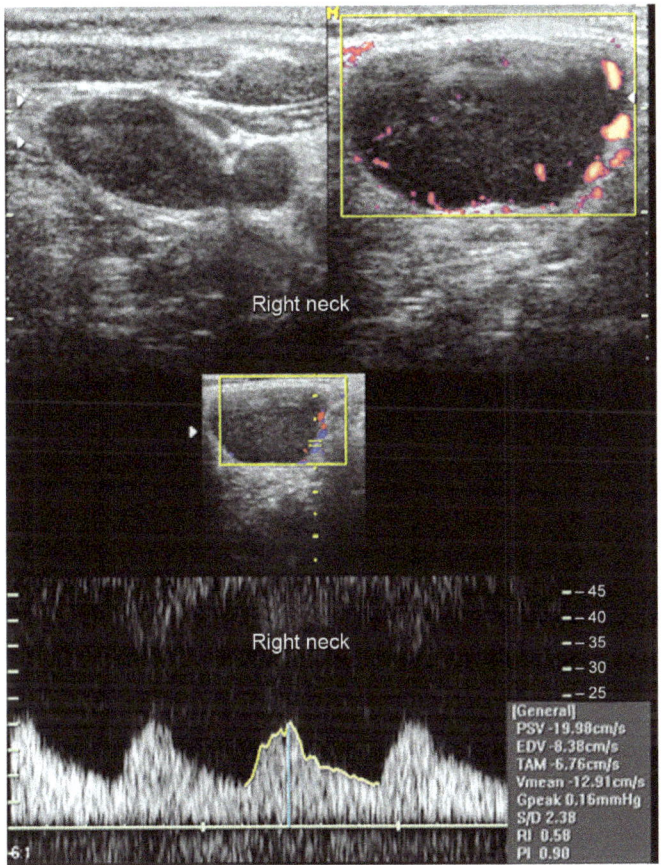

Fig. 2.4.4: US and color Doppler scans show inflammatory adenopathy of neck.

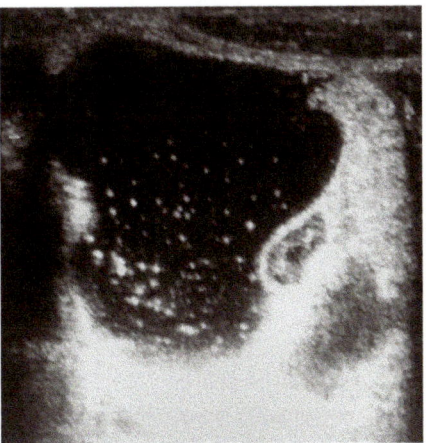

Fig. 2.4.5: Colloid goiter.

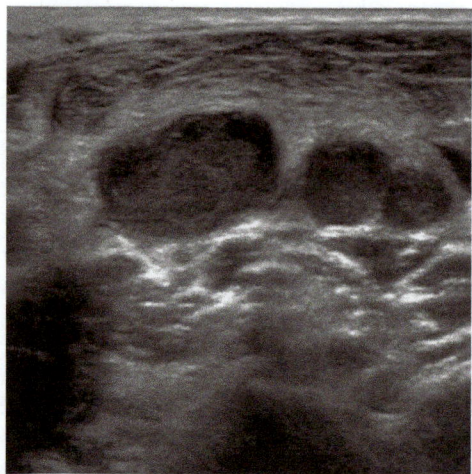

Fig. 2.4.6: Multiple enlarged cervical lymph nodes.

carcinoma or cystic papillary carcinoma of the thyroid gland
- Large cortical calcification may occur in granulomatous diseases or in metastatic muscles following radiotherapy or chemotherapy
- Microcalcification may occurs in nodes, following metastasis from papillary or medullary carcinomas of the thyroid gland.

CHAPTER 3

Hepatobiliary System and Abdomen

DIFFERENTIAL DIAGNOSIS OF LIVER LESIONS

3.1 GENERALIZED INCREASE IN LIVER ECHOGENICITY

- Fatty infiltration
- Cirrhosis
- *Hepatitis:*
  - Acute alcoholic hepatitis
  - Chronic hepatitis
  - Granulomatous hepatitis.

During examination of liver, it is must to examine all surfaces of liver including Riedel's lobe **(Fig. 3.1.1)**.

Fatty Infiltration

Fatty infiltration is an acquired, reversible disorder of metabolism resulting in an accumulation of triglycerides within the hepatocytes.

The most common cause of fatty liver is obesity. Other causes of fatty liver are:
- Excessive alcohol intake
- Hyperlipidemia
- Diabetes
- Excessive exo or endogenous corticosteroids
- Pregnancy
- Glycogen storage disease, etc.

Sonographically liver shows, increased echogenicity **(Fig. 3.1.2)** with a normal smooth echotexture giving the typical appearance of a 'bright liver' increased attenuation of sound beam is also a feature here. Fatty infiltration can be divided into three categories **(Fig. 3.1.3)**:

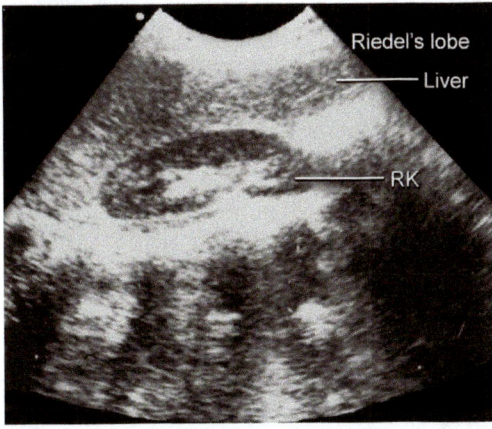

Fig. 3.1.1: Riedel's lobe—it is an extension (inferior) of the right lobe which often overlies the kidney. (RK: right kidney)

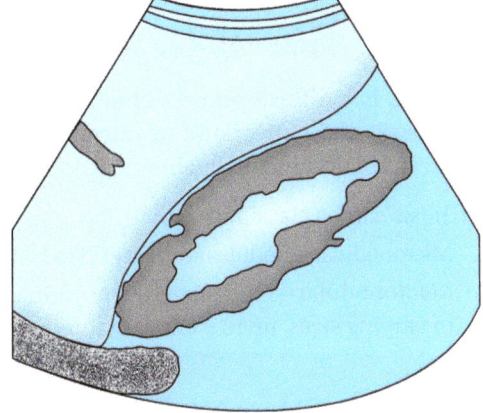

Fig. 3.1.2: Diffuse increase in echogenicity of liver—to be compared with renal echogenicity.

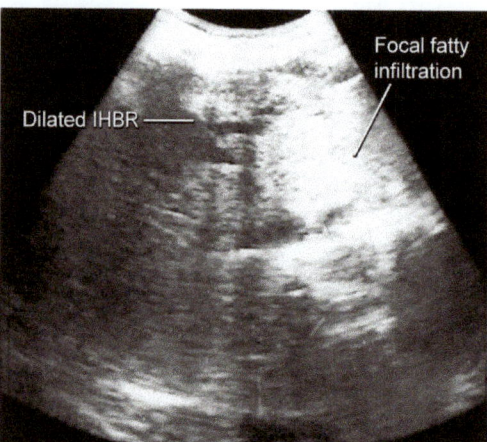

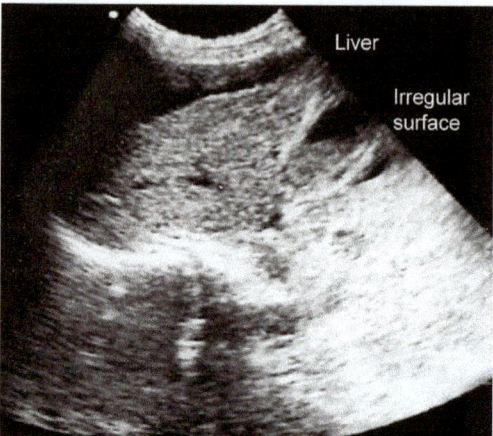

Fig. 3.1.3: Focal fatty infiltration in transverse scan of liver showing focal fatty change as hyperechoic well-defined lesion with no distortion of normal vascular architecture. (IHBR: intrahepatic biliary radicals)

Fig. 3.1.4: Irregular liver surface is seen clearly due to ascites in a case of cirrhosis.

1. Mild—minimal diffuse increase in echogenicity, normal visualization of diaphragm and intrahepatic vessel border.
2. Moderate—diffuse increase in echogenicity of liver, slightly impaired visualization of intrahepatic vessel border and diaphragm.
3. Severe—marked increase in echogenicity, poor penetration of posterior segment of right lobe of liver, poor or nonvisualization of hepatic vessels and diaphragm.

Cirrhosis (Figs. 3.1.4 to 3.1.7)

Cirrhosis is a diffuse process characterized by fibrosis and conversion of normal liver architecture into structurally abnormal nodules.

Cirrhosis can be classified into:
1. Micronodular—nodules are of size 0.1 to 1 cm.
2. Macronodular—characterized by nodules of varying sizes, up to 5 cm in diameter.

Etiology

- Alcohol consumption—most common cause of micronodular cirrhosis

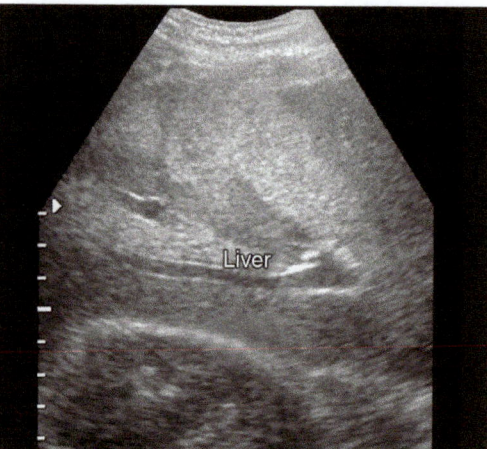

Fig. 3.1.5: US scan shows area of fat sparing in hepatic parenchyma. (US: ultrasound)

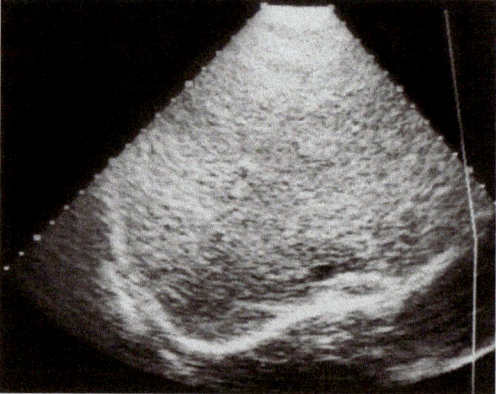

Fig. 3.1.6: Coarse and increased echotexture of liver with loss of definition of portal vein wall—cirrhosis.

Hepatobiliary System and Abdomen

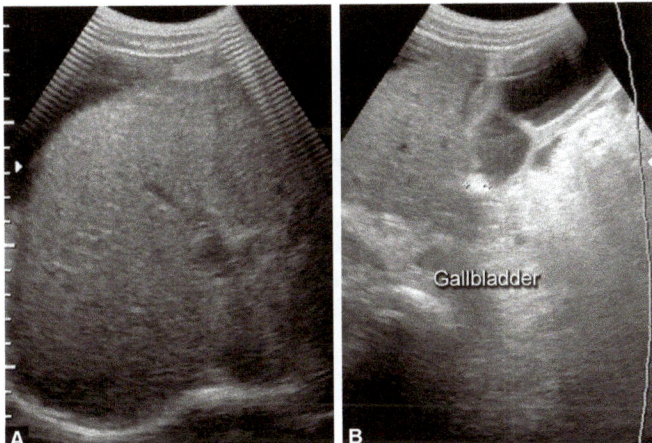

Figs. 3.1.7A and B: US scans show nodular surface of liver in a patient of cirrhosis associated with ascites and mural thickening of gallbladder (GB).

- Chronic viral hepatitis—most common cause of macronodular cirrhosis
- Biliary cirrhosis
- Wilson's disease
- Primary sclerosing cholangitis
- Hemochromatosis.

Sonographic Findings of Cirrhosis

- Volume redistribution—in early stage liver may enlarge while in advanced stage it may shrunken with relative enlargement of caudate or left or both lobes of liver. The ratio of width of caudate and right lobe of liver of more than 0.65 is considered indicative of cirrhosis
- Increased echogenicity with no significant increased attenuation of sound beam
- Coarse and heterogeneous echotexture—loss of definition of the portal vein walls
- Nodular surface—irregularity of the liver surface as seen in micronodular disease is a definitive sign of cirrhosis.

Hepatitis

- Acute alcoholic hepatitis—an enlarged 'right' liver showing increased attenuation of sound beam as evident on ultrasonography. Clinical history is required to distinguish it from other causes of fatty infiltration
- Regenerative nodules—represents regenerating hepatocytes surrounded by a fibrous septa. On ultrasound they appear as iso- or hypoechoic with a thin echogenic border
- Dysplastic nodules—larger than regenerating nodules, and premalignant.

Chronic Hepatitis

The sonographic features are:
- Diffusely increased echogenicity and altered echotexture
- Increased attenuation may be seen depending upon the amount of fatty change
- Periportal cuffing
- Hepatomegaly
- Thickening of gallbladder wall.

Granulomatous hepatitis (**Figs. 3.1.8A and B**) occurs in tuberculosis, sarcoidosis and brucellosis and may appear as a bright liver indistinguishable from other causes of increased echogenicity.

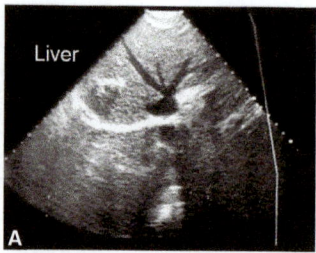
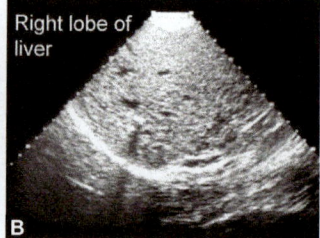

Figs. 3.1.8A and B: Healed granuloma seen in right lobe of liver as hyperechoic focus with distal acoustic shadowing.

3.2 GENERALIZED DECREASE IN ECHOGENICITY OF LIVER

- Acute hepatitis **(Figs. 3.2.1 and 3.2.2)**—in this condition, there is diffuse swelling of the hepatocytes, proliferation of the Kupffer cells lining. On ultrasound, the liver appears diffusely hypoechoic and is referred is as 'dark liver'.
  Other features are:
  - Accentuated brightness of the portal triads
  - Periportal cuffing
  - Hepatomegaly and
  - Thickening of gallbladder wall.
- Diffuse malignant infiltration—homogeneous hypoechoic appearance is not very common. However, diffuse disorganization

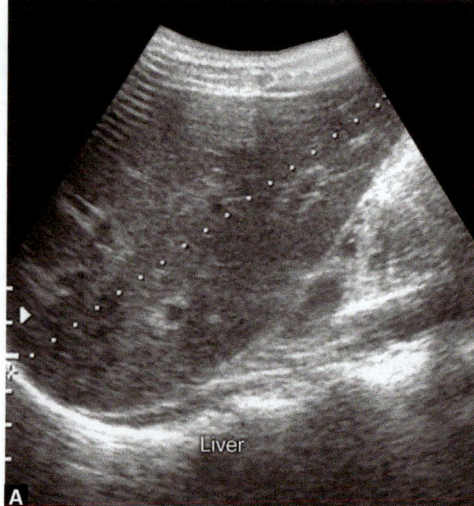

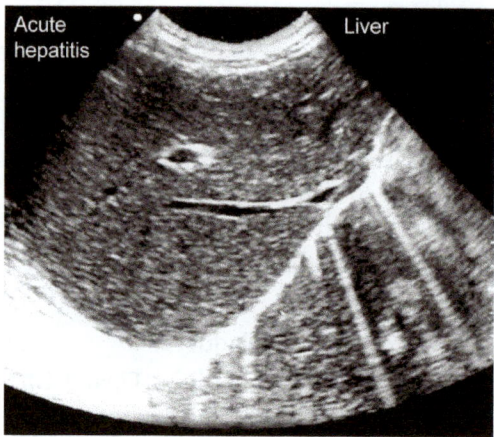

Fig. 3.2.1: Acute hepatitis.

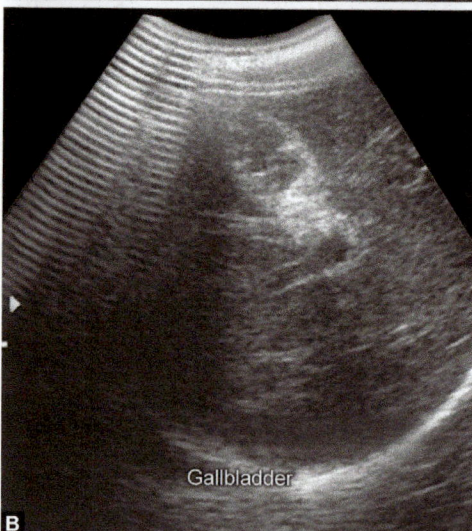

Figs. 3.2.2A and B: US scans show acute hepatitis with associated mural thickening of gallbladder.

Hepatobiliary System and Abdomen

of the hepatic parenchyma is common from. Breast, lung and malignant melanoma are the most common primary tumors to give this type of pattern. Leukemic or lymphomatous infiltration also gives this sonographic appearance
- Candidiasis—most common appearance. This corresponds to progressive fibrosis
- Congestive cardiac failure
- Acquired immunodeficiency syndrome (AIDS)
- Radiation injury.

3.3 SOLITARY ECHOGENIC LIVER MASS

- Focal fatty infiltration
- Fibrosis
- Adenoma
- Lipoma
- Focal nodular hyperplasia (**Fig. 3.3.1**)
- Hemangioma
- Hepatoma
- Metastasis
- Hematoma
- Focal fatty infiltration—regions of increased echogenicity are present within a background of normal liver parenchyma.

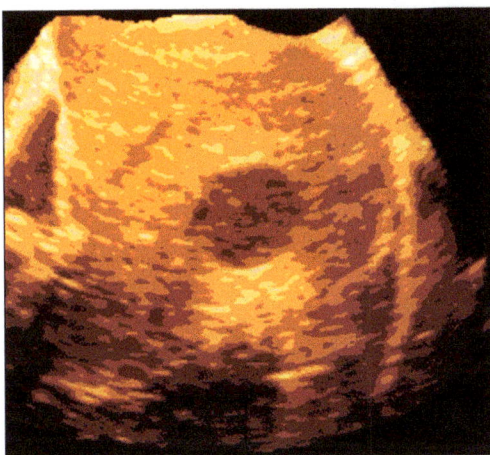

Fig. 3.3.1: 3D US scan shows focal nodular hyperplasia (FNH) lesion in liver.

Most common seen in the periportal region of medial segment of left lobe of liver.
  - Lack of mass effect
  - No displacement of hepatic vessels
  - Geographic margin
  - Rapid change with time.
- Adenoma—usually smooth solitary masses which are well-encapsulated. Microscopically tumor consists of normal hepatocytes but bile ducts and Kupffer cells are absent. It is much common in women and has an association with the use of oral contraceptives. They usually presents with a palpable mass in right hypochondrium, pain or hemorrhage.

  Sonographically it may be hyper, hypo- or isoechoic to liver parenchyma and indistinguishable from paroxysmal nocturnal hemoglobinuria (PNH).

  With hemorrhage a fluid component may be seen within or around the mass.
- Lipoma are extremely rare. An association between the hepatic lipoma, renal angiomyolipoma and tuberous sclerosis.

  On ultrasound appears as an echogenic mass, indistinguishable from a hemangioma, echogenic mets, or focal fat, unless the mass is large and near the diaphragm in which case differential sound transmission through the fatty mass will produce a discontinuous or broken diaphragm sign.
- Focal nodular hyperplasia (FNH) (**Fig. 3.3.1**) is the second most common benign liver mass and formed from proliferation of normal non-neoplastic hepatocytes related to an area of vascular malformation. This lesion is more common in women of childbearing age and are clinically silent on sonography. FNH appears as a subtle liver mass which is difficult to differentiate in echogenicity from the adjacent normal liver parenchyma.

  Subtle contour abnormality and displacement of vascular structures raises

the possibility of FNH, the central scar appears as a hypoechoic linear or stellate area within the central portion of the mass.
- Hemangioma (**Fig. 3.3.2**)—cavernous hemangioma is the most common variety of benign liver tumor. Woman to man ratio is approximately 5:1.

On sonography the lesion appears homogeneously hyperechoic. The increased echogenicity is due to numerous interfaces between the walls of the cavernous sinuses and the blood within them. Few cases also show posterior acoustic enhancement.

Few atypical features can also be seen:
- A nonhomogeneous central area containing hypoechoic portion
- An echogenic border either a thin rim or thick rind
- Scalloping of the margin of the lesion.
- Hepatoma (**Figs. 3.3.3 and 3.3.4**)—the masses may be hyperechoic, complex or echogenic. Most small (<5 cm) hepatocellular carcinoma (HCC) are hypoechoic.

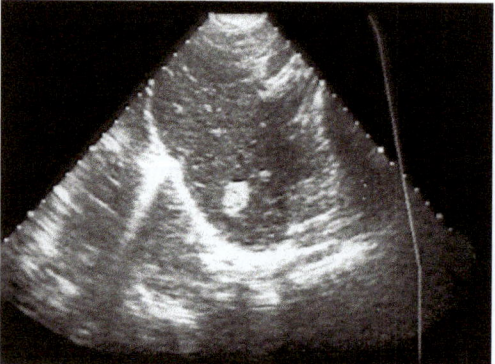

Fig. 3.3.2: Right lobe of liver shows a tiny highly reflective cavernous hepatic hemangioma.

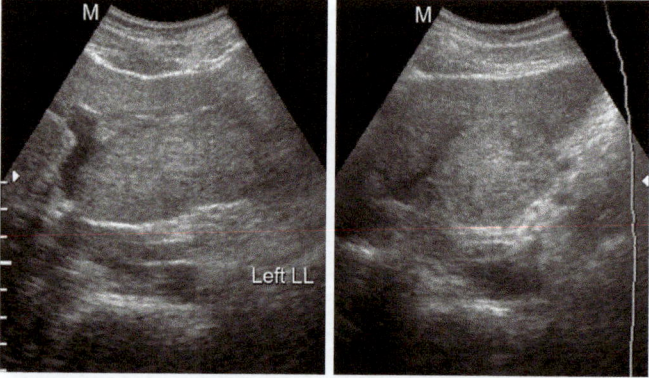

Fig. 3.3.3: US scans show presence of hepatic adenoma in left hepatic lobe. (LL: lower lobe; M: mass)

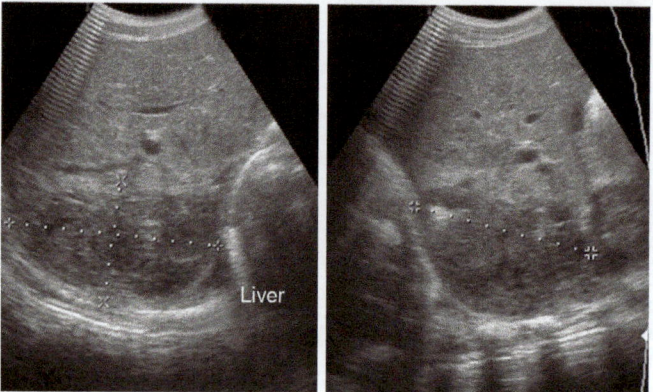

Fig. 3.3.4: US scans show evidence of resolving hepatic hematoma.

A thin peripheral hypoechoic halo which corresponds to fibrous capsule is seen most often in small HCC.

With time as the size increases, masses tend to become more complex and inhomogeneous as a result of necrosis and hemorrhage.

Small tumors may appear diffusely hyperechoic secondary to fatty metamorphosis or sinusoidal dilatation.

Metastasis (Figs. 3.3.5 and 3.3.6)

It may present as a single focal lesion, although multiple lesions are more commonly encountered. Patterns of hepatic metastases:

- *Hypoechoic (most common):*
  - Lung carcinoma
  - Breast carcinoma
  - Pancreatic adenocarcinoma
  - Lymphoma
- *Hyperechoic:*
  - Colorectal carcinoma
  - Renal cell carcinoma
  - Kaposi sarcoma
  - Neuroendocrine tumors
  - Choriocarcinoma
- *Calcified:* Mucinous adenocarcinoma (gastrointestinal tract and ovary)
- *Peripheral hypoechoic halo:* Lung carcinoma
- *Cystic:*
  - Ovarian carcinoma
  - Pancreatic adenocarcinoma
  - Colorectal carcinoma
  - Ovarian carcinoma
- *Infiltrative:*
  - Lung carcinoma
  - Breast carcinoma
  - Melanoma.

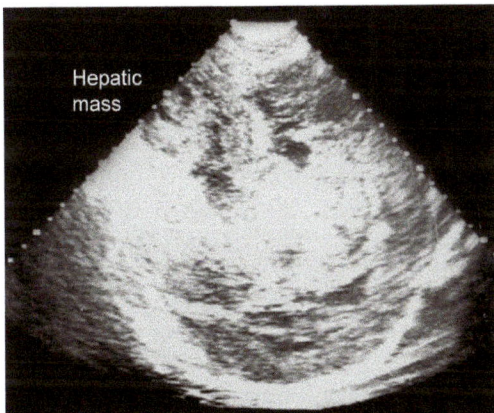

Fig. 3.3.5: A large space occupying lesion of heterogeneous echotexture is seen occupying almost whole of the right lobe of liver. A rim of normal liver tissue is seen on the posteromedial aspect of the mass.

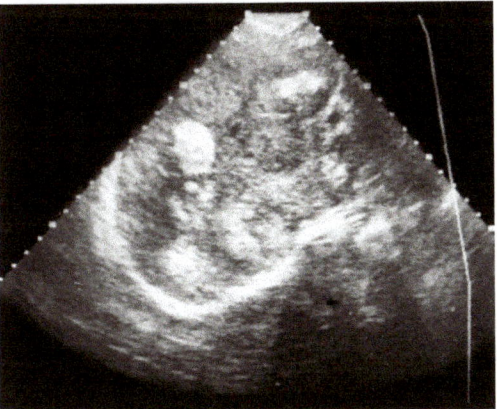

Fig. 3.3.6: The liver is studded with hyperechoic metastases from carcinoma stomach.

3.4 SHADOWING LESIONS OF LIVER

- *Multiple and small*
  - Healed granuloma **(Fig. 3.4.1)**—tuberculosis, histoplasmosis, and less commonly brucellosis and coccidioidomycosis.
- *Curvilinear*
  - Hydatid **(Fig. 3.4.2)**—liver is the most common site of hydatid diseases. The most common cause of hydatid in human is *Echinococcus granulosus*. Most cysts are in the right lobe and are clinically silent.

    Calcification seen in 20–30% of cases. Calcification does not indicate death of the parasite but extensive calcification indicates inactive cyst.

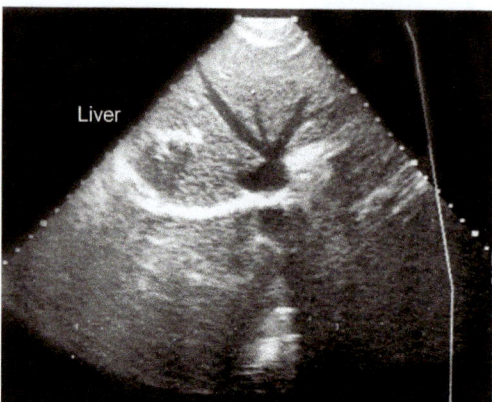

Fig. 3.4.1: Healed granuloma seen in right lobe of liver as hyperechoic focus with distal acoustic shadowing.

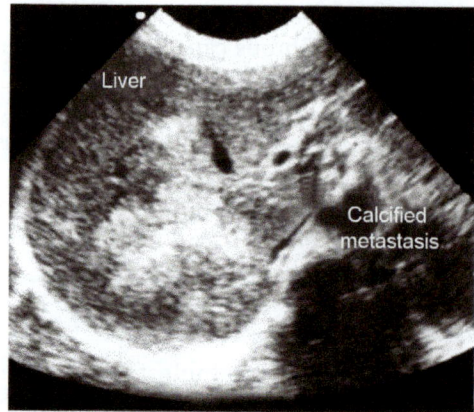

Fig. 3.4.3: Calcified metastases—multiple well-defined hyperechoic lesion with evidence of calcification within it. Patient was a case of adenocarcinoma stomach.

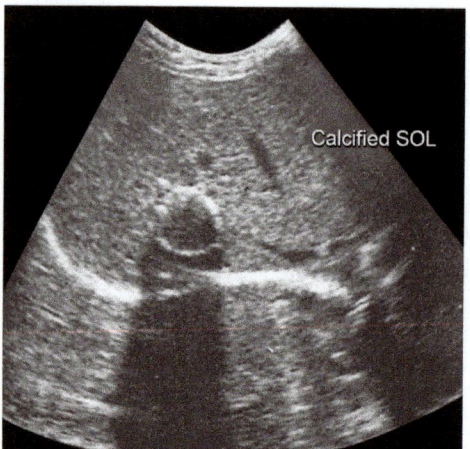

Fig. 3.4.2: Calcified hydatid—transverse scan of liver showing a well-defined rounded SOL with a hyperechoic wall and distal acoustic shadowing. (SOL: space occupying lesion)

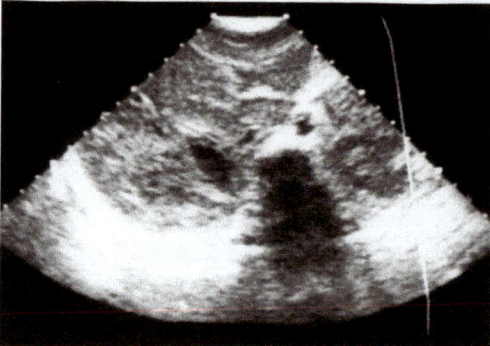

Fig. 3.4.4: An ill-defined lesion is seen in right lobe with multiple areas of hypo- and hyperechogenicity suggestive of resolving hematoma in a patient of blunt abdominal trauma.

　　Calcification of the daughter cysts produces several rings of the calcification.
- Abscess—especially amebic abscess when the right lobe is most frequently affected.
• *Localized*
  - Metastasis **(Figs. 3.4.3 and 3.4.4)**—calcification in metastasis is uncommon but colloid carcinoma of the rectum, colon or stomach calcify most frequently. It may be amorphous, flaky, stippled or granular and solitary or multiple. Calcification may follow radiotherapy or chemotherapy.
  - Hepatoma (rare)—calcification may be punctate, stiffened or granular.
  - Hematoma—previous history of significant liver trauma may give a clue to the diagnosis.
• *Sunray spiculation:*
  - Hemangioma—phleboliths may also occur but are uncommon

- Metastasis—infrequently in metastasis from colloid carcinoma.

3.5 HEPATOMA, BULL'S EYE OR TARGET LESION OF LIVER

It appears as echogenic center surrounded by a hypoechoic rim **(Fig. 3.5.1)**.
- Candidiasis
- Metastasis
- Lymphoma, leukemia
- Sarcoidosis, granulomatous—tuberculosis, brucellosis
- Septic emboli
- Other opportunistic infection
- Kaposi's sarcoma.

Candidiasis

The liver is frequently involved secondary to hematogenous spread of mycotic infection in other organs, most commonly lungs. Patients are usually immunocompromised.

1-4 cm lesion having a hyperechoic center and a hypoechoic rim. This appearance is seen when neutrophil counts returns to normal. The echogenic center represents inflammatory cells.

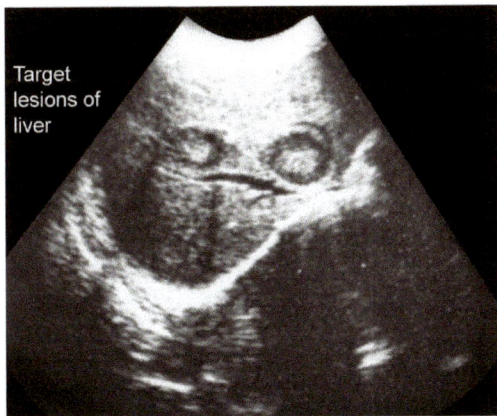

Fig. 3.5.1: Right lobe of liver shows the concentric ring pattern of the "target" or "bull's eye" lesion. This pattern is more often seen with larger lesions.

Metastasis

Bull's eye or target appearance is seen in metastasis from bronchogenic carcinoma. Characterized by a peripheral hypoechoic zone. This pattern is also seen in metastasis from gastrointestinal—colorectal, urogenital—kidney and ovary and pancreatic carcinomas.

Lymphoma and Leukemia

Multiple hypoechoic hepatic masses are more common in primary non-Hodgkin's lymphoma of the liver or lymphoma associated with AIDS.

Kaposi's Sarcoma

Although frequent in patients with AIDS diagnosis at autopsy is rarely diagnosed by imaging.

3.6 PERIPORTAL HYPERECHOGENICITY OF LIVER

- Air in biliary tree
- Schistosomiasis
- Cholecystitis
- Recurrent pyogenic cholangitis.

Air in Biliary Tree (Fig. 3.6.1)

Could be secondarily to following sphincterotomy, following passage of a stone, patulous sphincter in the elderly, postoperative following spontaneous biliary fistula.

Schistosomiasis

Hepatic schistosomiasis is caused by *S. mansoni, S. japonicum, S. mekongi*. Sonographic features of schistosomiasis are widened echogenic portal tracts, sometimes reaching a thickness of 2 cm.

Initially the liver size is enlarged; however, as the periportal fibrosis progresses, the liver becomes contracted and the feature of portal hypertension develops.

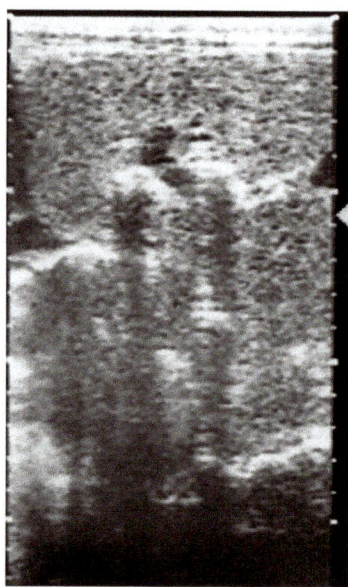

Fig. 3.6.1: Pneumobilia echogenic foci with dirty shadowing is suggestive of gas in the lumen of biliary tree.

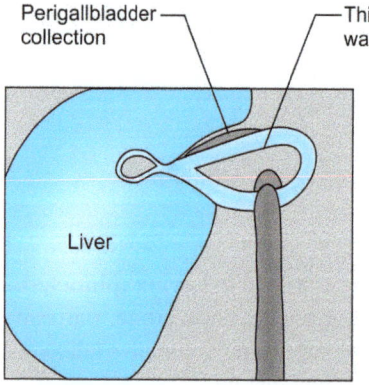

Fig. 3.6.2: Acute cholecystitis. The gallbladder wall is thickened and there is a perigallbladder collection. A gallstone is present. The gallbladder was very tender.

Cholecystitis (Fig. 3.6.2)

Other features of cholecystitis:
- Gallstone
- Focally tender gallbladder
- Impacted gallstone
- Gallbladder (GB) sludge
- Diffuse wall thickening.

Recurrent Pyogenic Cholangitis

The recurrent pyogenic cholangitis (RPC) occurs in any patient with prolonged bile stasis. Intrahepatic biliary calculi are very common in RPC. The stones are usually multiple and develop in the intra- and extrahepatic ductal system.

The lateral segment of the left lobe is the most commonly involved.

Sonography shows these stones to have a dramatic range of appearance. They can be of moderate echogenicity and lack acoustic shadowing. With very large stones acoustic shadowing frequently predominates.

NONCIRRHOTIC PORTAL HYPERTENSION

3.7 PERIPORTAL HYPOECHOGENICITY

- Orthotopic liver transplant rejection particularly seen when central and peripheral parts of the liver are affected.
- May also seen in nonrejecting liver transplants and seen because of tracking of extrahepatic fluid and severed lymphatic channel.
- Congestive hepatomegaly.
- Blunt abdominal trauma seen because of distended periportal lymphatics and lymphedema associated with elevated central venous pressure following vigorous intravenous (IV) fluid replacement.
  Related to severity of injury and associated with a higher mortality.
- Cholangitis—minimal luminal bile duct dilatation smooth or irregular wall thickening of the intrahepatic bile ducts.
- Viral hepatitis.
- Malignant lymphatic obstruction.

LIVER

3.8 FOCAL HYPOECHOIC LESIONS

Benign

- Abscess
- Hydatid cyst
- Hematoma
- Cavernous hemangioma
- Complicated simple cyst
- Hepatic adenoma.

Malignant

- Metastasis
- Hepatocellular carcinoma
- Lymphoma.

Abscess (Fig. 3.8.1)

Candidiasis—liver is frequently involved secondary to hematogenous spreads and patients are generally immunocompromised.

- USG—there are various sonographic appearances but uniformly hypoechoic pattern is most common. Other appearances are:
  - 'Wheel within a wheel'—peripheral hypoechoic zone with an inner echogenic wheel and central hypoechoic nidus
  - Bull's eye—small lesion having a hyperechoic center and a hypoechoic rim
  - Echogenic—due to calcification representing scar formation
  - Pyogenic—regions of early suppuration may appear solid usually hypoechoic related to the presence of necrotic hepatocytes. Frankly purulent abscesses are cystic
  - Amebic abscess—usually seen as oval or round, hypoechoic lesion with a homogeneous pattern of internal echoes.

Complicated Cyst (Hydatid or Simple) (Figs. 3.8.2A and B)

Following hemorrhage or infection, in a hydatid or simple cyst, it may appear sonographically as hypoechoic lesion.

Cavernous Hemangioma

- Most common benign tumor of the liver
- The spectrum of appearances on ultrasound is variable. Majority have a sharply defined, highly reflective solid tumor usually less than 2 cm in diameter and with a homogeneous echopattern
- It may appear as a nonhomogeneous central area containing hypoechoic portions which may appear uniformly granular
- A hemangioma may appear hypoechoic within the background of a fatty infiltrated liver.

Hepatic Adenoma

Usually the patient is asymptomatic but pain may occur in the setting of bleeding or infarction in the lesion.

Usually a capsulated, solitary mass, 8–15 cm in size.

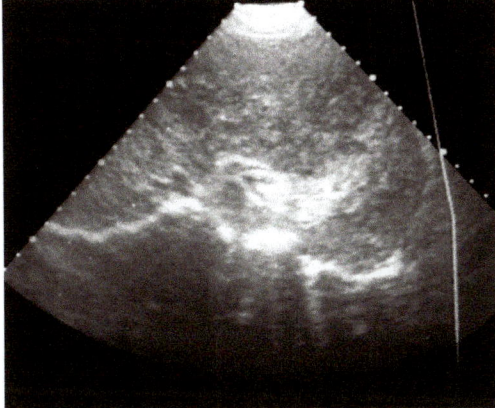

Fig. 3.8.1: Liver abscess information seen as an ill-defined hypoechoic lesion in the left lobe of liver.

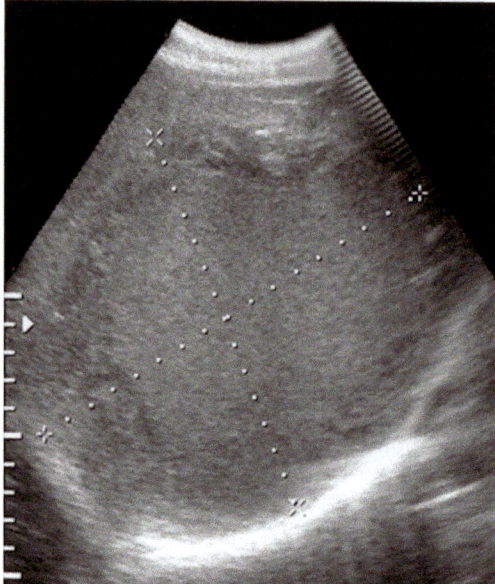

Fig. 3.8.2A: US scan shows complicated hydatid cyst (infected cyst).

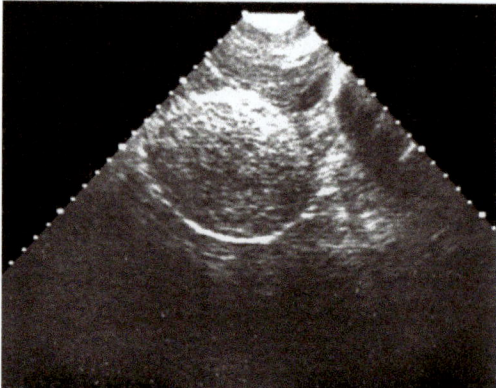

Fig. 3.8.2B: Transverse scan of right lobe of liver showing an infected hydatid cyst.

USG—sonographic appearance of adenoma is nonspecific. It may present as a hypoechoic, hyperechoic or isoechoic mass with hemorrhage, a fluid component may be evident within or around the mass. Hepatic adenomas may regress following cessation of the contraceptive pill.

Metastasis (Figs. 3.8.3 and 3.8.4)

Hypoechoic lesions may be produced by any type of primary tumor but they are the typical pattern seen in untreated metastatic breast or lung cancer.

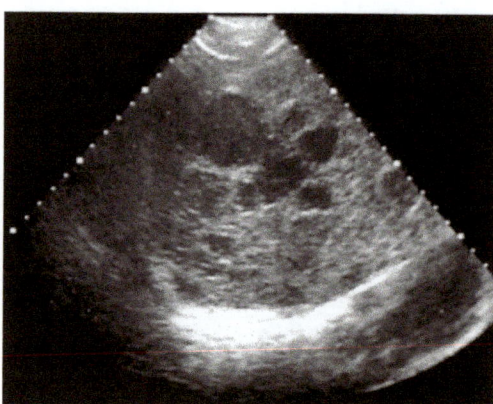

Fig. 3.8.3: Multiple hypoechoic lesions— metastatic breast.

Hepatocellular Carcinoma (Figs. 3.8.5 and 3.8.6)

Three forms of the early disease are described:
1. Nodular—single or multiple
2. Massive—>5 cm
3. Diffuse.
   - It is the small (<5 cm) nodular type HCC which presents usually as a hypoechoic lesion.
   - But as the size enlarges the tumor tends to become more complex

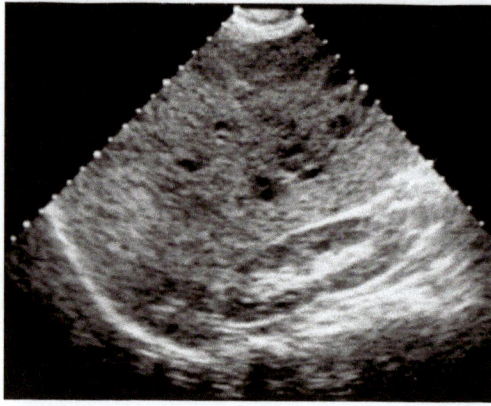

Fig. 3.8.4: An enlarged liver showing multiple hypoechoic deposits.

Hepatobiliary System and Abdomen

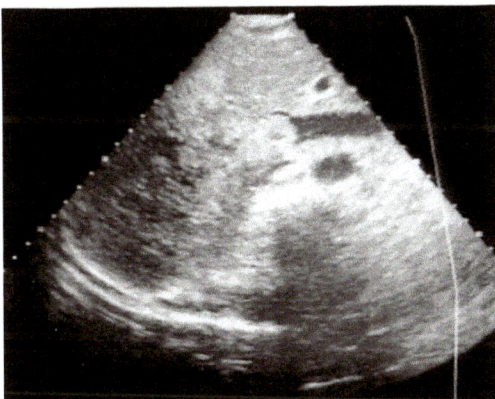

Fig. 3.8.5: An ill-defined predominantly hyperechoic SOL seen in right lobe invading the portal vein suggestive of HCC with tumor thrombus in portal vein.

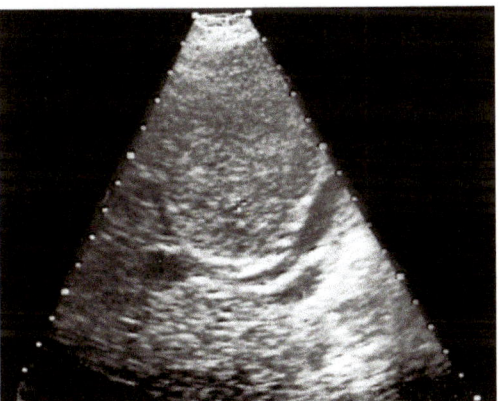

Fig. 3.8.6: Hepatocellular carcinoma: An isoechoic liver mass indenting the portal vein. The margins of the lesion are not apparent.

and inhomogeneous as a result of hemorrhage and necrosis.

Lymphoma

Lymphomatous involvement of the liver may manifest as hypoechoic masses. The difference in the reflectivity of the normal liver and the lesion may be very obvious, as the lymphoma have a very uniform cellular architecture with little stromal tissue, so few interfaces are produced sometimes lesions may even be echo-free.

The pattern of multiple hypoechoic liver masses is more typical of primary non-Hodgkin's lymphoma of liver or lymphoma associated with AIDS.

3.9 CYSTIC LESIONS OF LIVER

Differential Diagnosis

Developmental Lesions

- Hepatic cyst **(Fig. 3.9.1)**
- Peribiliary cysts
- Adult polycystic disease
- Bile duct hamartoma (von Meyenburg complex)
- Caroli disease.

Infectious Causes

- *Abscess:*
  - Pyogenic
  - Amebic
- Hydatid cyst.

Neoplastic

- Biliary cyst adenoma and cystadeno-carcinoma
- Metastasis
- Rarely hepatocellular carcinoma and cavernous hemangioma.

Miscellaneous

- Hematoma
- Biloma.

Hepatic Cyst

The frequent presence of columnar epithelium within simple hepatic cysts suggests they have a ductal origin, although their precise cause is unclear.

- Patient is usually asymptomatic, occasionally may develop pain and fever secondary to cyst hemorrhage or infection.

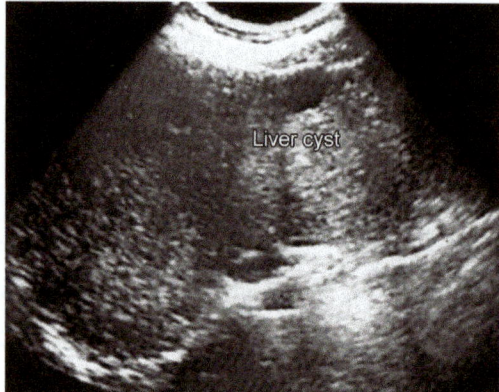

Fig. 3.9.1: Simple liver cyst.

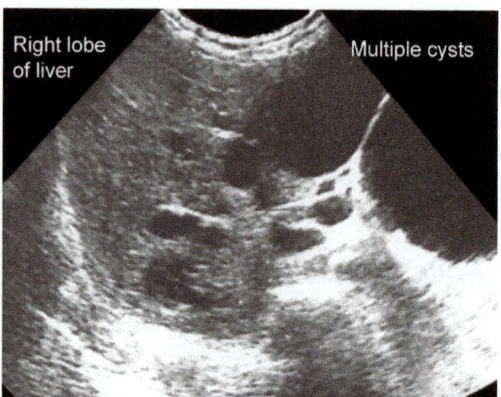

Fig. 3.9.2: Polycystic liver—multiple simple cysts of variable sizes are seen in transverse scan of adult liver in a case of polycystic kidney disease.

USG—benign hepatic cysts are anechoic with a well-defined, thin wall and posterior acoustic enhancement. On hemorrhage or infection, the cyst may contain internal echoes and septations, a thickened wall or may appear solid.

Peribiliary Cysts

These cysts have been described in patients with severe liver disease. Usually range in size from 0.2 cm to 2.5 cm and located centrally within the porta hepatis or at the junction of the main right and left hepatic ducts.

USG—seen as discrete, clustered cysts or as tubular appearing structures having thin septae, paralleling the bile ducts and portal veins.

Adult Polycystic Disease (Fig. 3.9.2)

Polycystic renal disease is a relatively common condition affecting 1 in 500. Approximately one-third of patients with polycystic kidney disease are found to have liver cysts.
- Polycystic liver disease is more likely to be symptomatic than simple cysts.
  USG—multiple cysts may distort the liver architecture or cause hepatomegaly. As with simple cysts hemorrhage or infection may occur.

Bile Duct Hamartoma (von Meyenburg Complexes)

These are small focal developmental lesions of the liver composed of groups of dilated intrahepatic bile ducts with a collagenous stroma.

USG—they are demonstrated as small lesions of low reflectivity or areas of high reflectivity with ring down artifacts related to the cholesterol crystals within the dilated tubules.

von Meyenburg complex (VMC) may occur with other congenital disorders such as congenital hepatic fibrosis or polycystic kidney or liver disease.

Caroli's Disease

It is a congenital abnormality that is most likely inherited in an autosomal recessive fashion. It can occur in focal or diffuse form and is characterized by saccular, communicating intrahepatic bile duct ectasia.

USG—it reveals multiple cystic like spaces throughout the liver substance.

Communication between the cysts and bile ducts is important to distinguish this condition from polycystic liver disease.

Extrahepatic bile ducts are usually unaffected.

Pyogenic Abscess (Fig. 3.9.3)

Most commonly arises as a complication of an intra-abdominal infection with direct portal venous spread to the liver. Clinical presentation may be variable but fever, pain, pleurisy, nausea and vomiting are all common.

USG—frankly purulent abscesses appear cystic, with the fluid ranging from echo-free to highly echogenic.

- Occasionally gas producing organisms give rise to echogenic foci with a posterior reverberation artifact
- The abscess wall can vary from well-defined to irregular and thick.

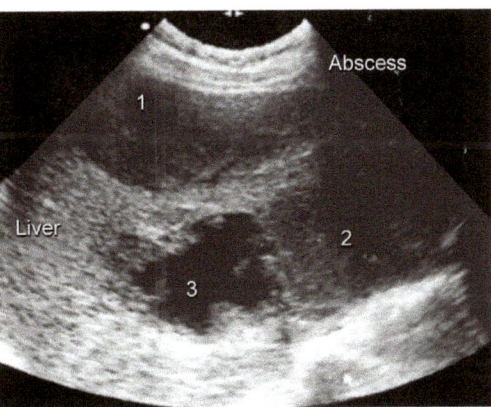

Fig. 3.9.3: Multiple liver abscess seen as large hypoechoic lesions showing internal echoes and posterior acoustic enhancement.

Amebic Abscess (Figs. 3.9.4 to 3.9.6)

Hepatic infection by the parasitic *Entamoeba histolytica* is the most common extraintestinal manifestation of amebiasis.

Most common presenting symptom is pain.

USG—usually a round or oval-shaped lesion, absence of a prominent abscess wall, hypoechogenicity, distal acoustic enhancement, fine low level echoes and contiguity with the diaphragm.

As compared to pyogenic liver abscess two sonographic patterns are significantly more prevalent in amebic abscess-round or oval shape and hypoechoic appearance with fine internal echoes at high gain.

Hydatid Disease (Figs. 3.9.7 to 3.9.13)

The most common cause of hydatid disease in humans is infestation by the parasite *Echinococcus granulosus*. It is most prevalent

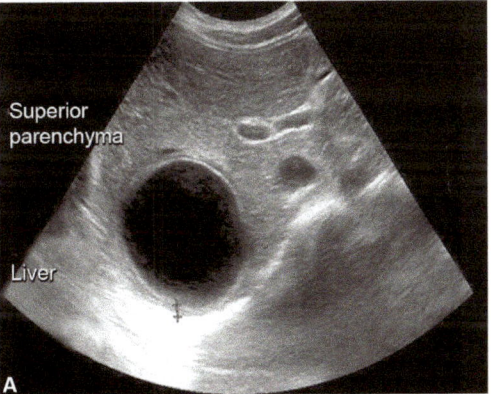

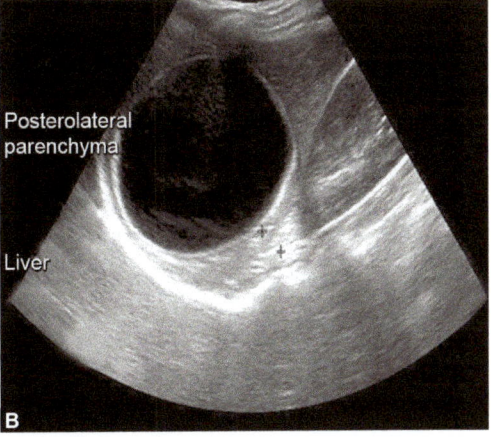

Figs. 3.9.4A and B: Large rounded anechoic cystic lesion with thick wall suggestive of abscess in the right lobe of liver.

52 Differential Diagnosis in Ultrasound

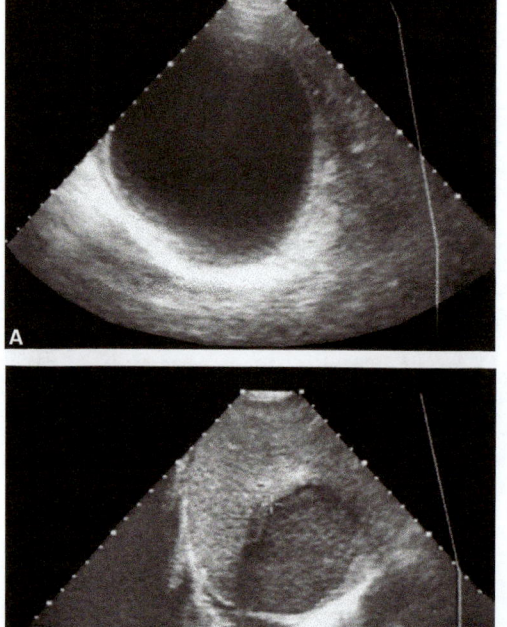

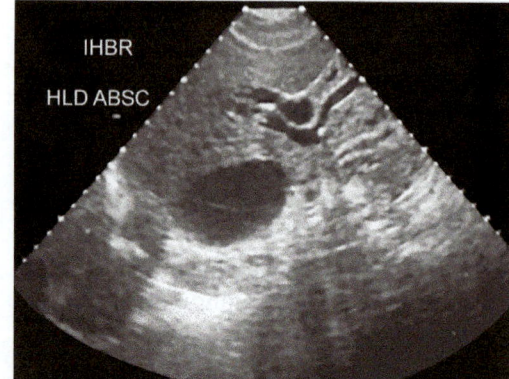

Figs. 3.9.5A and B: (A) A large amebic abscess seen replacing the right of liver. It has well-defined walls and absence of internal echoes, distal acoustic enhancement is present; (B) Amebic liver abscess—a hypoechoic SOL is seen in the posterosuperior aspect of liver with evidence of posterior enhancement. It is extending into subdiaphragmatic space.

in sheep and cattle of developing countries like India. These slow growing cysts have three layers:
1. Pericyst—outermost, formed of hosts dense connective tissue capsule.
2. Ectocyst—external membrane of cyst, approximately 1 mm thick, which may calcify.
3. Endocyst—inner germinal layer gives rise to blood capsules that enlarge to form protoscoliosis.

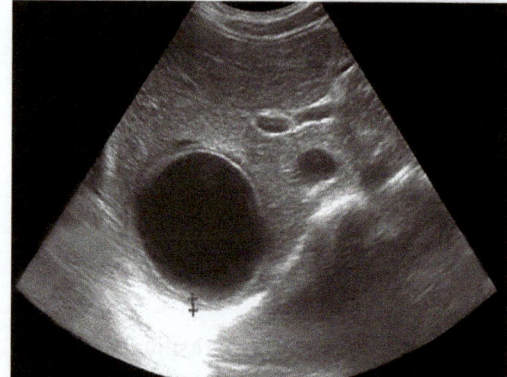

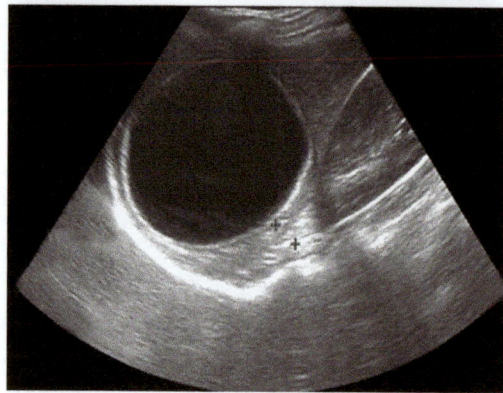

Fig. 3.9.6: An oval well-defined anechoic cystic lesion in posterior aspect of right lobe suggestive of amebic liver abscess. Large rounded anechoic cystic lesion with thick wall suggestive of abscess in the right lobe of liver. (IHBR: intrahepatic biliary radicals; HLD: hepatic liver disease; ABSC: abscess)

Hepatobiliary System and Abdomen

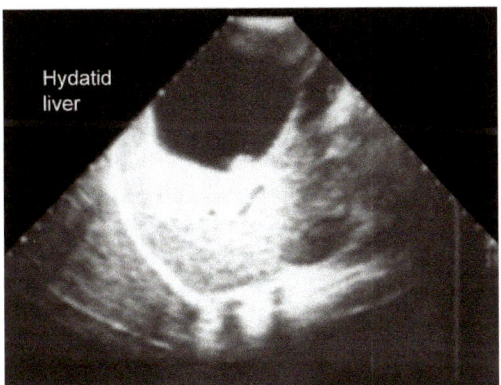

Fig. 3.9.7: Subcostal scan of liver shows a large cyst with a small mural nodule. Complement fixation test revealed hydatid cyst.

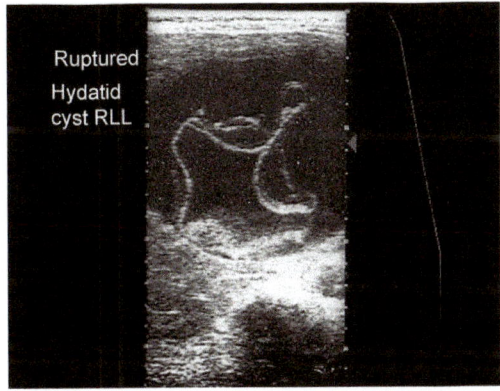

Fig. 3.9.9: Hydatid cyst in a liver showing complete detachment of membranes giving the pathognomonic appearance of ultrasound waterlily sign. Hydatid sand is also seen at the bottom of the cyst.

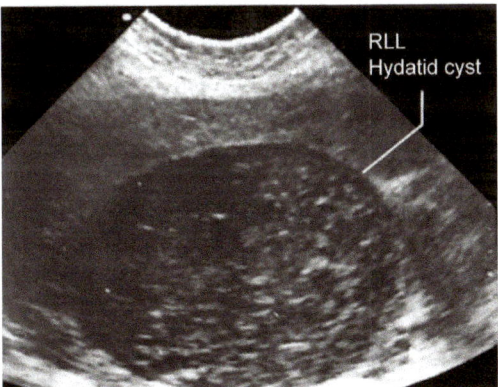

Fig. 3.9.8: Infected hydatid is seen as well-defined hypoechoic SOL—daughter cysts are filled up with debris and margins of cysts are indistinct. (RLL: right lower lobe)

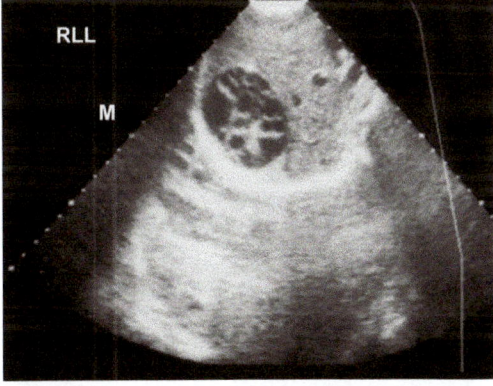

Fig. 3.9.10: Classical hydatid cyst: Pathognomonic appearance of hydatid cyst with multiple daughter cyst producing the characteristic cart wheel or honeycomb appearance. (RLL: right lower lobe; M: mass)

USG—a variety of ultrasound appearances may be demonstrated by hydatid cysts.
- Simple cysts containing no internal architecture except sand, visibility of this can be improved by moving the patient during examination.
- Separation of the membrane producing a pathognomonic 'ultrasound' 'waterlily sign' results from detachment and collapse of the inner germinal layer from the ectocyst.
- Daughter cysts—the development of daughter cysts from the lining germinal membrane produces a characteristic appearance of cysts enclosed with a cyst, described as a cart wheel or honeycomb cyst.
- Multiple cysts—with heavy or continued infestation multiple primary parent cysts may develop within the liver, often producing hepatomegaly with normal liver tissue between the individual cysts.

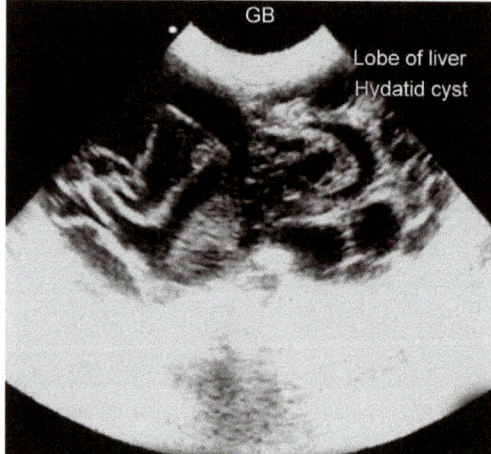

Fig. 3.9.11: Two adjacent hydatid cysts, one showing detachment of germinal layer and the other showing multiple daughter cysts. (GB: gallbladder)

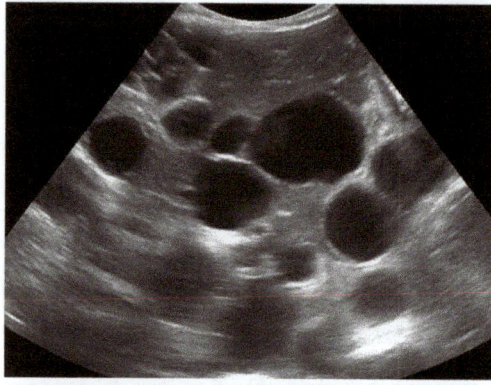

Fig. 3.9.12: Multiple hydatid cysts in liver.

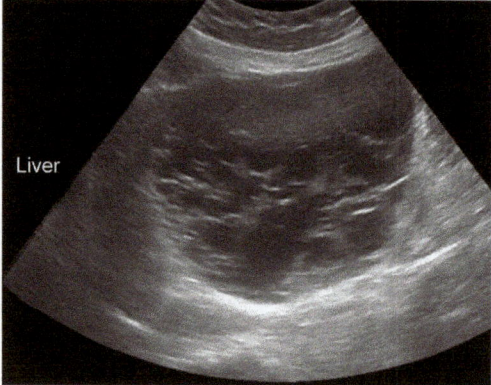

Fig. 3.9.13: Transabdominal image of the liver showing cystic lesion with multiple daughter cysts sonography of hydatid cyst.

Densely calcified masses—the distinction between simple cyst and hydatid disease of simple type may be aided by following features:
- Wall calcification may occur after many years in hydatid after the initial infection. Simple liver cysts rarely calcify
- Debris consisting of sand or scoliosis may be present within hydatid cysts
- It may be possible to discern the two layers of the wall of a hydatid cyst.

Biliary Cystadenoma and Cystadenocarcinoma

Biliary cystadenoma are rare, usually slow growing multilocular cystic masses, more commonly seen in right lobe of liver. They occur predominantly in middle-aged woman and are considered premalignant lesions.

USG—usually seen as a solitary cystic mass with thick septae, mural nodular and rarely capsular calcification. Polypoid, pedunculated excrescences are seen more commonly in biliary cystadenocarcinoma than in cystadenoma.

Metastasis (Fig. 3.9.14)

Mostly the cystic metastasis occurs due to extensive necrosis, seen more commonly in metastatic sarcoma, which typically have low level echoes and a shaggy, thickened wall.

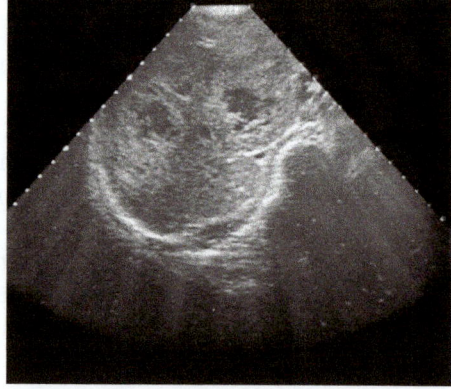

Fig. 3.9.14: Two large metastatic lesions are seen with central hypoechoic areas with irregular margins suggestive of necrosis.

Uncommonly primary neoplasms having a cystic component may produce cystic lesions such as colorectal carcinoma and cystadenocarcinoma of the ovary.

Cystic metastasis can be distinguished from the benign hepatic cyst by features like presence of mural nodules, thick walls, fluid-filled levels and internal septations.

Hepatocellular Carcinoma and Giant Cavernous Hemangioma (Fig. 3.9.15)

These are the two most common primary neoplasms of the liver that rarely manifest as an entirely or partially cystic mass, usually related to internal necrosis.

In about 90% of patients with HCC, complications or signs of underlying liver cirrhosis, such as left hepatic lobe or caudate lobe hypertrophy, regenerating nodules, splenomegaly, etc. may be seen. Tumor characteristics of HCC like biliary or vascular invasion and a capsule should suggest the diagnosis.

Liver Hematoma (Figs. 3.9.16 and 3.9.17)

The etiology of a liver hematoma may be blunt abdominal trauma or rupture of a neoplasm

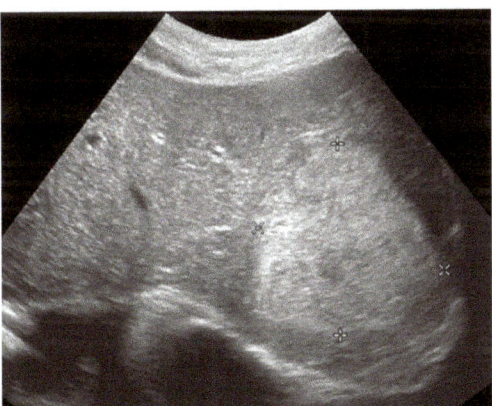

Fig. 3.9.15: Hemangioma (in calipers) in left lobe of liver having hyperechoic appearance.

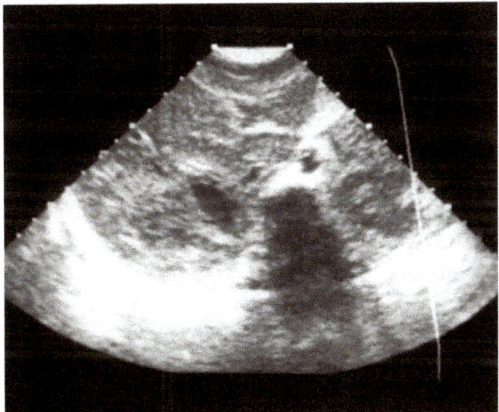

Fig. 3.9.16: An ill-defined lesion is seen in right lobe with multiple areas of hypo- and hyperechogenicity suggestive of resolving hematoma in a patient of blunt abdominal trauma.

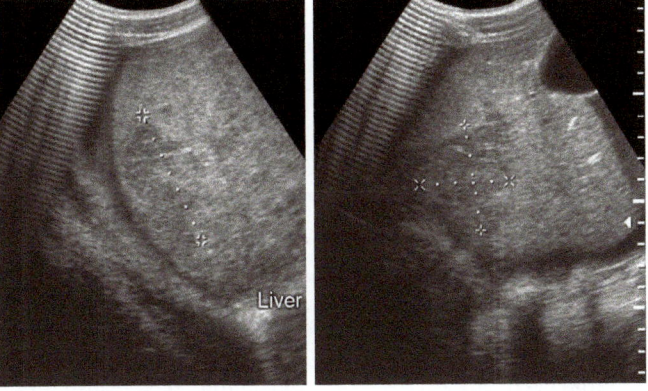

Fig. 3.9.17: US scans show hepatic laceration and contusion in a case of blunt trauma abdomen.

such as a hepatic adenoma or cavernous hemangioma.

USG—an acute hematoma tends to be highly reflective because of fibrin and erythrocytes forming multiple acoustic interfaces. Over a period of months the hematoma usually become cystic and develop internal septations.

3.10 MIXED CYSTIC AND SOLID LESIONS

- Complicated cyst—simple, hydatid (**Fig. 3.10.1**)
- Abscess
- Hepatic adenoma
- Cystadenoma and cystadenocarcinoma (**Figs. 3.10.2 to 3.10.8**)
- Hepatocellular carcinoma.

Complicated Cyst—Simple or Hydatid

Ultrasound is the best way to confirm the cystic nature of a cystic mass. Cysts complicated by infection or hemorrhage may show solid areas, septations or internal debris.

Abscess

A developing amebic or pyogenic liver abscess may show varied appearance with frankly purulent areas appearing cystic and regions of early suppuration appearing solid.

The abscess wall varies from well-defined to irregular and thick.

Hepatic Adenoma

Sonography typically demonstrates a large hyperechoic lesion with central anechoic areas corresponding to zones of internal hemorrhage, if present. But this is not specific.

Occasionally adenomas may undergo massive necrotic and hemorrhagic changes and the ultrasound appearance is that of a complex mass with large cystic areas.

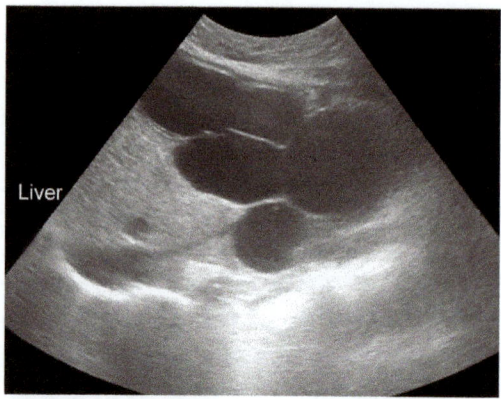

Fig. 3.10.1: Multiple simple cyst in the left lobe of liver.

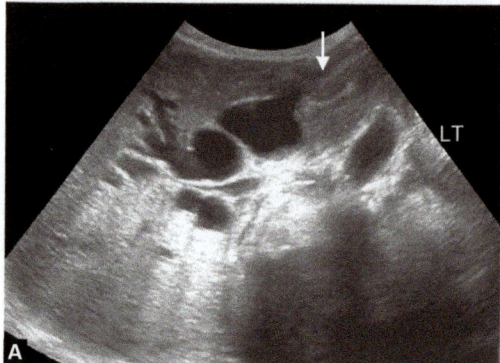

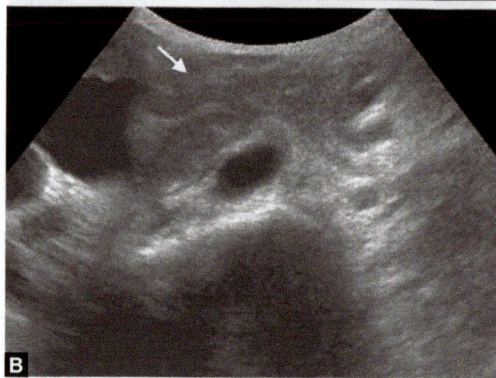

Figs. 3.10.2A and B: Cholangiocarcinoma in common bile duct (CBD)—thickened CBD wall (arrows) obliterating the lumen and causing proximal biliary dilatation.

Color Doppler may identify intratumoral veins, a finding absent in focal nodular hyperplasia may be a useful differentiating feature.

Hepatobiliary System and Abdomen

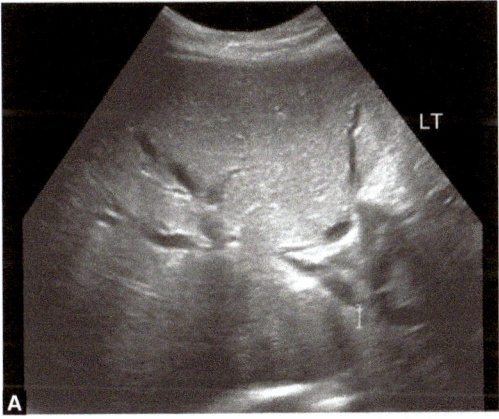
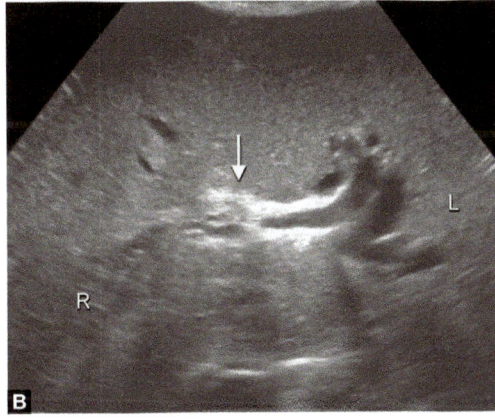

Figs. 3.10.3A and B: Hilar cholangiocarcinoma—faintly visualized hypoechoic mass (arrow) at confluence with intrahepatic biliary dilatation. (R: right lobe of liver; L: left lobe of liver)

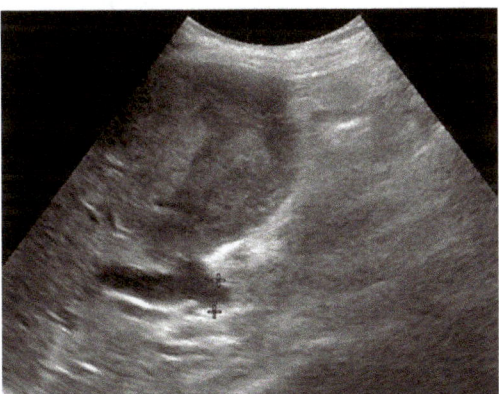
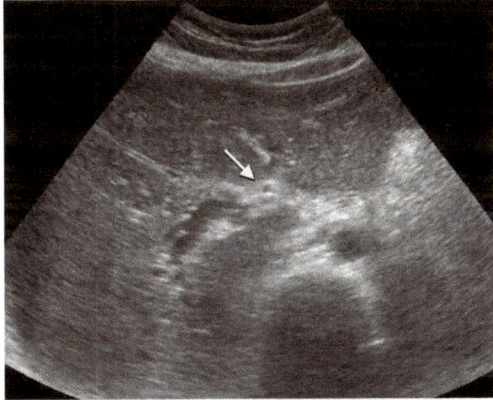

Fig. 3.10.4: Transabdominal scan showing hypoechoic GB mass which is extending into the CBD and causing narrowing of its lumen (in calipers) with dilated IHBR.

Fig. 3.10.6: Stricture in proximal CBD (arrow) with mildly dilated intrahepatic biliary radicals.

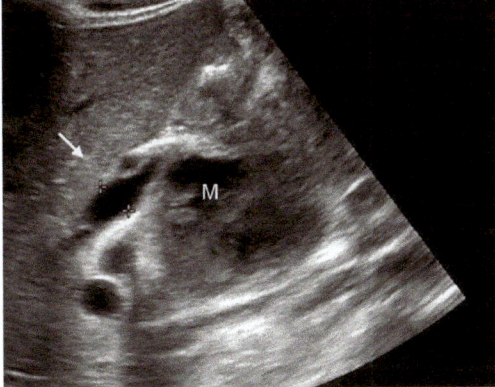
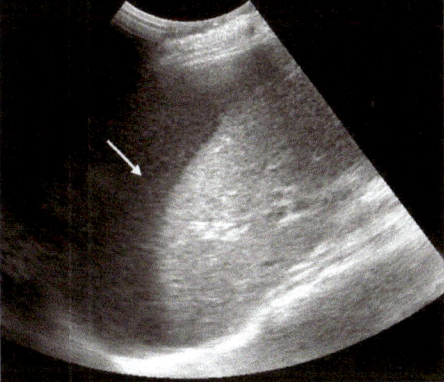

Fig. 3.10.5: Pancreatic head mass (M) causing compression of distal CBD with proximal biliary dilatation (arrow).

Fig. 3.10.7: Transabdominal scan of liver showing biloma (arrow)—a collection with low level echoes.

58 Differential Diagnosis in Ultrasound

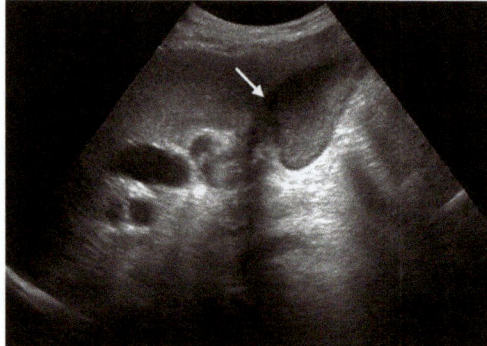

Fig. 3.10.8: Gallbladder neck mass (arrow) seen extending into the proximal CBD. CBD lumen is obliterated with proximal dilatation.

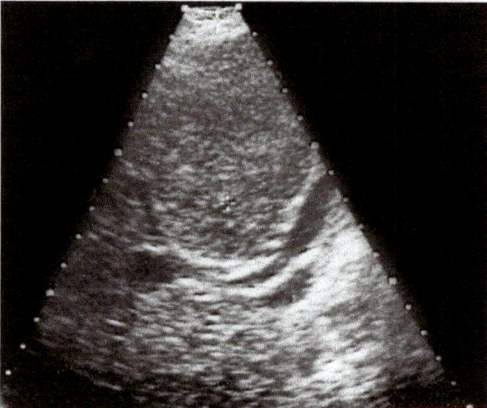

Fig. 3.10.9: Hepatocellular carcinoma: An isoechoic liver mass with ill-defined margin.

Cystadenoma and Cystadenocarcinoma

Probably congenital in origin because of presence of aberrant bile ducts.

USG—appears as multiple communicating cysts with mural nodules. Papillary projections and mural calcification may also be seen.

Combination of septation with nodularity is suggestive cystadenocarcinoma.

Hepatocellular Carcinoma (Fig. 3.10.9)

Ultrasonography can detect extremely small tumors. Small HCCs (<3 cm) often appear hypoechoic whereas tumors larger than 3 cm more often have a mosaic or mixed pattern.

Ultrasound is also capable of demonstrating the capsule in encapsulated, which appears as a thin, hypoechoic band.

3.11 PATTERNS OF HEPATIC METASTASIS

A wide range of appearances is seen in liver metastatic disease and their overlap with nonmalignant disorders inevitably results in lack of specificity.

- It is not size but the echogenicity of the lesion which determines conspicuity on sonography
- Focal lesions are the most common with most common focal pattern of echopoor masses.

The following patterns of metastatic disease has been described in **Figures 3.11.1 to 3.11.3**.

Echopoor Metastasis

These are generally hypovascular and highly cellular with internal interfaces.
- These lesions may be produced by any tumor but are typical of some of the most common malignancies like carcinoma of the breast and lung

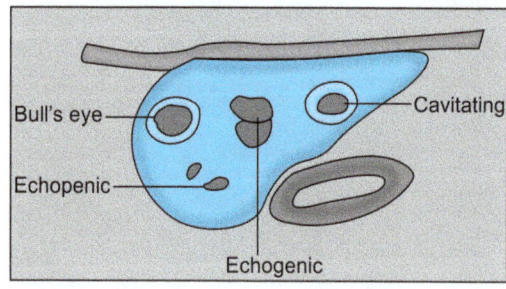

Fig. 3.11.1: Different types of metastatic lesions that may occur in the liver. Metastatic lesions shown are: 1. Bull's eye, 2. Echogenic, 3. Echopenic, 4. Cavitating cystic lesions may also be seen.

Hepatobiliary System and Abdomen

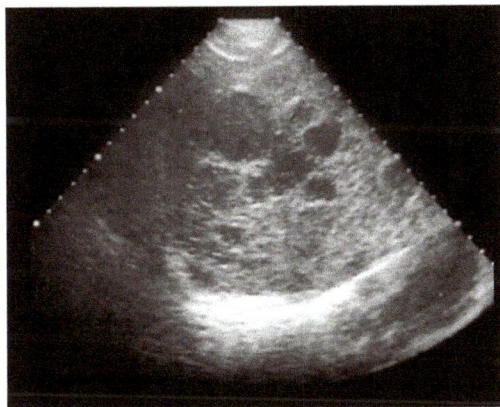

Fig. 3.11.2: Echopoor metastases are seen. Patient from a case of breast carcinoma.

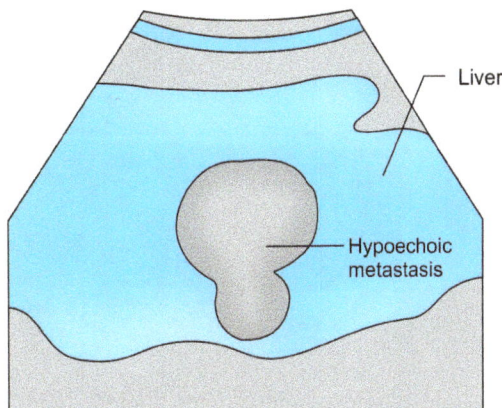

Fig. 3.11.4: Hyperechoic metastasis.

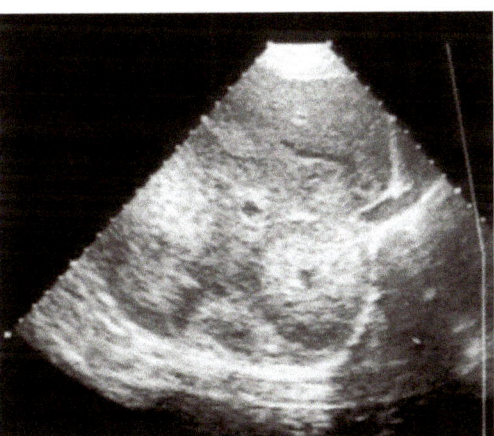

Fig. 3.11.3: Right lobe of liver shows large hyperechoic metastatic lesions. Few are showing central necrosis.

- Lymphoma, particularly when associated with AIDS, can manifest with multiple hypoechoic deposits.

Hyperechoic Metastasis (Fig. 3.11.4)

These usually arise from colon cancers and other gastrointestinal neoplasms. Vascular metastasis from islet cell tumors, carcinoid, choriocarcinoma and renal cell carcinoma tend to be echogenic as well. They are echogenic because of numerous interfaces arising from the abnormal vessels. One of the important differential diagnoses is from hemangiomas, which most commonly appear as highly reflective lesions. Although, an absolutely definite differential diagnosis is not possible, hemangiomas are typically situated in a subcapsular or perivascular position, are usually solitary, measure only a few centimeters in diameter and have uniform high amplitude echoes. There are no mass effects or evidence of invasion and they lack the echopoor halo.

"Bull's Eye" or "Target" Pattern (Fig. 3.11.5)

The anechoic, thin, poorly-defined halo that often surrounds solid liver metastasis is most often a result of peritumoral compression of normal parenchyma and less often a result of tumor infiltration into the surrounding parenchyma. Its presence usually indicates an aggressive tumor. This is frequently seen in metastasis from bronchogenic carcinoma.

Cystic Metastasis (Fig. 3.11.6)

These usually develop in patients with primary neoplasms that have a cystic component like cystadenocarcinoma of the pancreas and ovary and mucinous carcinoma of the colon.

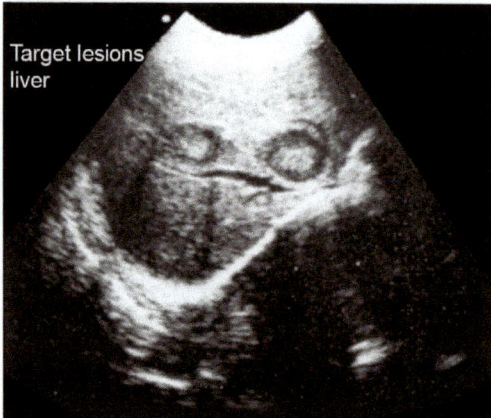

Fig. 3.11.5: "Target" or "bull's eye" seen in right lobe of liver.

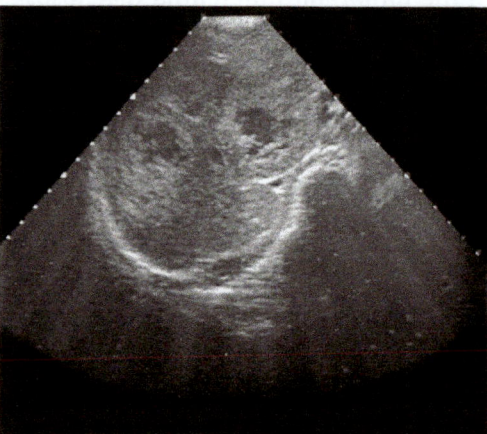

Fig. 3.11.6: Two large cystic metastatic lesions.

Usually USG reveals certain differentiating features—septa, mural nodules, debris, fluid levels and mural thickening.

Calcified Metastasis

These are relatively distinctive because of their marked echogenicity and acoustic shadowing. Mucinous adenocarcinoma of the colon is most common cause, others are osteogenic sarcoma, chondrosarcoma, teratocarcinoma and neuroblastoma.

Diffuse Infiltration

This diffuse permeative infiltration is the most difficult sonographic pattern to appreciate because the tissue texture is diffusely inhomogeneous, without the presence of well-defined mass. Diagnosis is further compromised in the presence of cirrhosis and fatty infiltration. This type of pattern is seen in carcinoma lung, breast and malignant melanoma.

3.12 NONVISUALIZATION OF GALLBLADDER ON ULTRASOUND

- Congenital absence
- Contracted
- Acute cholecystitis
- Chronic cholecystitis
- Perforation of gallbladder
- Gallbladder carcinoma
- Porcelain gallbladder.

Congenital Absence

Very rare anomaly.

Physiologically Contracted Gallbladder

Ideally scanning of gallbladder should be done after an overnight fast of 8–12 hours. Physiologically contracted gallbladder appears small and thick-walled.

Chronic Cholecystitis (Fig. 3.12.1)

Refer to symptomatic, but nonacute cholecystolithiasis.

USG shows gallbladder wall thickening that cannot be attributed to nonbiliary causes usually associated with calculus (**Figs. 3.12.2 to 3.12.5**).

Hepatobiliary System and Abdomen

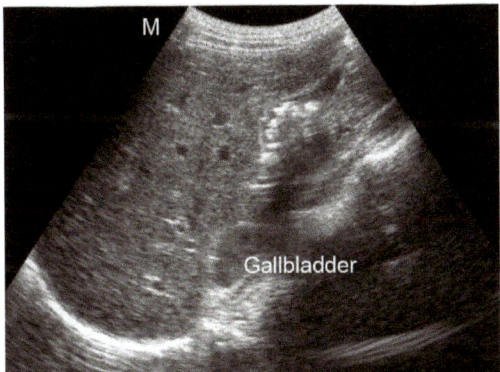

Fig. 3.12.1: US scan shows cholelithiasis with signs of chronic cholecystitis.

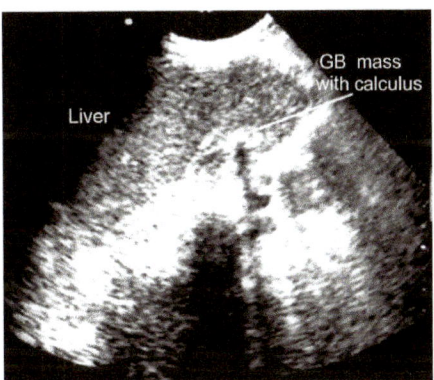

Fig. 3.12.3: The whole gallbladder (GB) is occupied by an isoechoic mass which has a calculus embedded in it. However GB wall is intact.

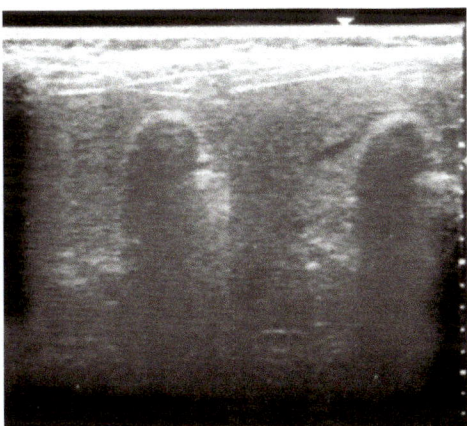

Fig. 3.12.2: Wall-echo-shadow (WES) sign—GB wall, echo from calculus with posterior acoustic shadowing are seen in the GB fossa.

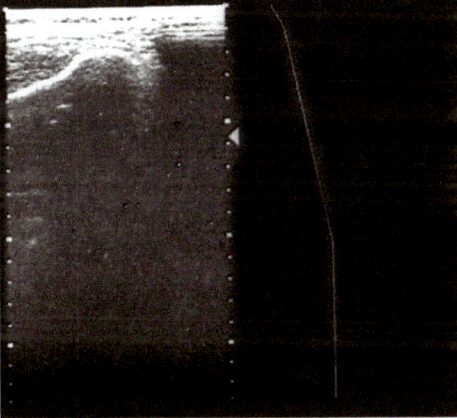

Fig. 3.12.4: Dense shadowing seen from the calcifying anterior gallbladder wall in porcelain GB.

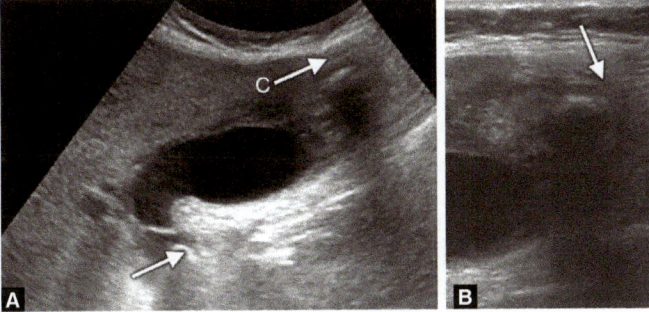

Figs. 3.12.5A and B: Gallbladder perforation—thickened GB wall with calculus in neck and a collection with calculus adjacent to the fundal region.

Gallbladder Perforation

Most perforations are subacute resulting in pericholecystic abscess.

Color Doppler may be useful and can show echogenic mass with internal vascularity.

Gallbladder Carcinoma

If a mass replaces the whole of the gallbladder (GB), it can simulate the absence of GB.

Additional features includes gallbladder wall calcification.
- Liver metastasis
- E/o direct invasion of liver or adjacent structure
- Lymphadenopathy
- Bile duct dilatation
- Cholelithiasis.

Porcelaine GB—calcification of the GB wall results in intense shadowing from the GB fossa region and causes nonvisualization of gallbladder.

3.13 DIFFUSE GALLBLADDER THICKENING

When the gallbladder thickness is more than 3 mm, wall thickening appears as a relatively hypoechoic region between two echogenic lines **(Fig. 3.13.1)**.
- Inflammation
- Hepatic dysfunction
- Congestive heart failure
- Renal diseases, AIDS sepsis
- Ascites
- Leukemic infiltration of GB
- Interleukin-2 chemotherapy
- Gallbladder wall varices.

Inflammation

- Acute cholecystitis—USG findings **(Figs. 3.13.2 and 3.13.3)**
- Gallstone—infarcted at neck
- Focally tender GB (i.e. sonographic Murphy's sign)

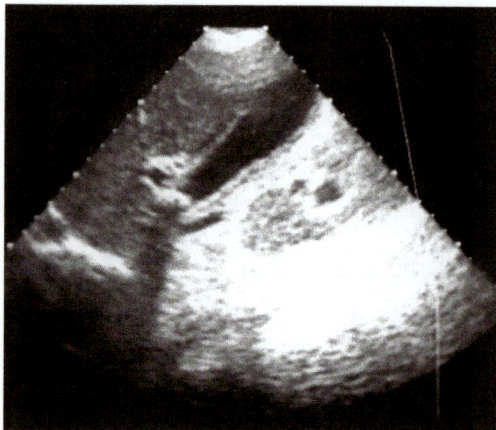

Fig. 3.13.1: Acute calculus cholecystitis—a calculus at the neck of GB is seen inside a thick-walled gallbladder.

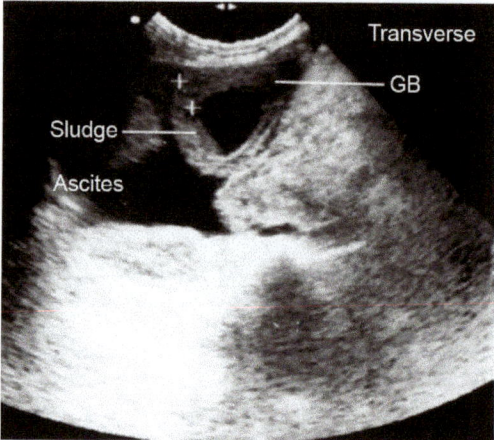

Fig. 3.13.2: Gallbladder (GB) is thickened due to ascites. Note the sludge as a debris—fluid level inside the lumen of gallbladder.

- Edema of wall gas in GB wall
- GB dilatation, rounded GB shape, pericholecystic fluid
- Sludge formation.

Hepatic Dysfunction

Associated with alcoholism, hypoalbuminemia, ascites and hepatitis.

Although hepatitis causes diffuse GB wall thickening in exceptional cases there may be

Hepatobiliary System and Abdomen

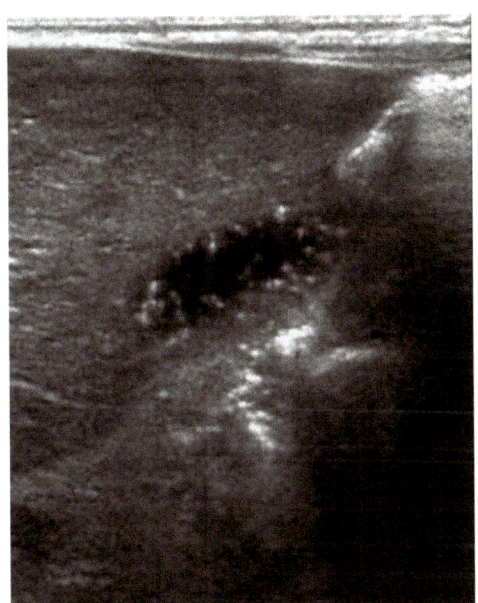

Fig. 3.13.3: Drug-induced pseudolithiasis—hyperechoic foci in gallbladder wall and lumen.

profound GB wall thickening with obliteration of GB lumen.

In some of these cases, paradoxic dilatation of GB with reduction in wall thickness may occur following administration of fat.

It has been shown that malignant ascites is usually associated with normal gallbladder wall thickness, whereas many benign causes are associated with an abnormal GB wall thickening.

Renal Diseases, Sepsis and Aids

Many of the patients have decreased intravascular osmotic pressure and elevated portal venous pressure.

Gallbladder Wall Varices

Serpentine sonolucencies transgress the gallbladder wall and extrahepatic portal vein thrombosis is present in 1/3rd of cases.

Color and duplex Doppler may show the vascularity within the GB wall.

3.14 FOCAL GALLBLADDER THICKENING

- Gallbladder carcinoma
- Metastatic nodules
- Gangrenous cholecystitis
- Polyps
- Papillary adenoma, adenomyomatosis (Figs. 3.14.1 and 3.14.2)
- Tumefactive sludge
- Villous hyperplasia, cholecystitis from TB—rare.

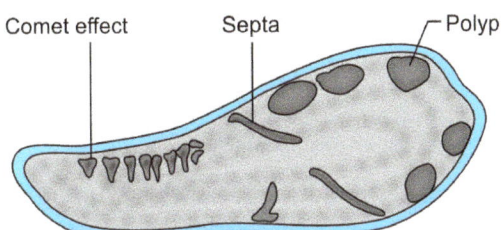

Fig. 3.14.1: Adenomyomatosis. Small stones in the gallbladder wall cause the comet effect diagnostic of adenomyomatosis. Septa may be seen. Small polyps are common.

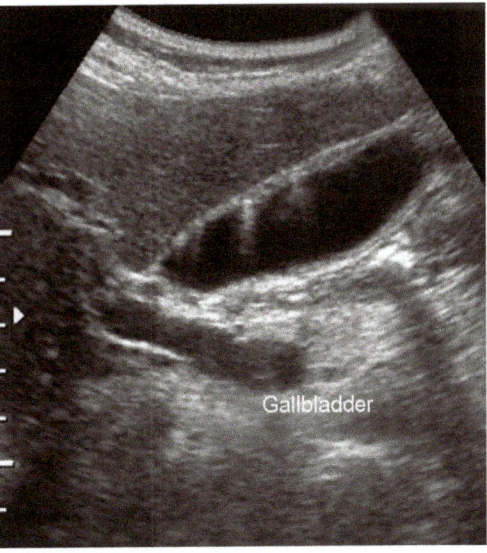

Fig. 3.14.2: US scan shows cholesterolosis with adenomyomatosis of GB.

Gallbladder Carcinoma (Figs. 3.14.3 to 3.14.7)

Gallbladder carcinoma can present as asymmetric gallbladder wall thickening.

Additional findings include:
- Gallbladder wall calcification
- Liver metastasis
- Invasion of adjacent liver or adjacent structure
- Abnormal bile duct dilatation
- Cholelithiasis
- Doppler examination—abnormally high arterial velocity originating from either the gallbladder wall or the mass in patients with primary malignancy.

Metastatic Nodules

Metastatic nodules are most often due to melanoma, GI and breast cancer. Less common malignancies include carcinoid tumor and lymphoma. Metastatic nodules often have a wide base towards the GB wall.

Complicated or Gangrenous Cholecystitis

These irregularities correspond to areas of mucosal ulceration, hemorrhage, necrosis and or microabscess formation.

Cholesterol Polyps (Fig. 3.14.8)

Seen as well-defined focal mass along the luminal wall of gallbladder, the base of these masses are relatively narrow as compared to metastatic nodules. Large polyp (>10 mm) shows aggregation of echogenic spots on endoscopic ultrasound.

Adenomyomatosis

Anechoic or echogenic foci may be seen within the thickened gallbladder wall.

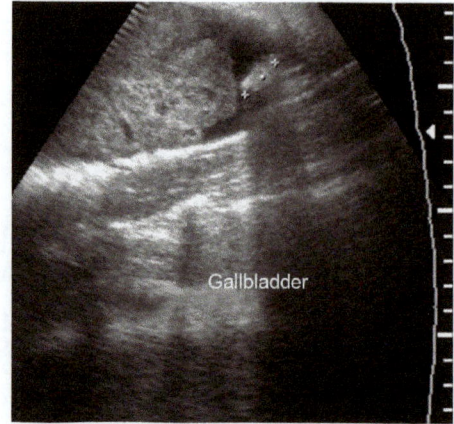

Fig. 3.14.3: US scan shows GB mass with cholelithiasis.

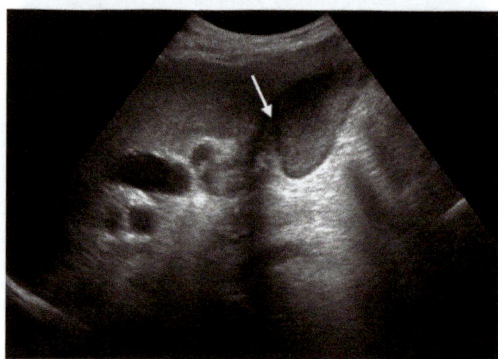

Fig. 3.14.4: GB neck mass (arrow) seen extending into the proximal CBD. CBD lumen is obliterated with proximal dilatation.

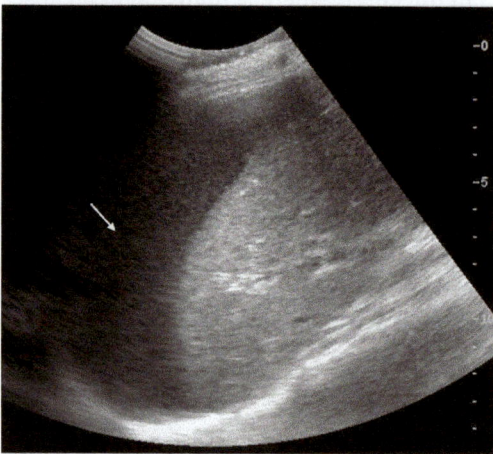

Fig. 3.14.5: Transabdominal scan of liver showing biloma (arrow)—a collection with low level echoes.

Hepatobiliary System and Abdomen

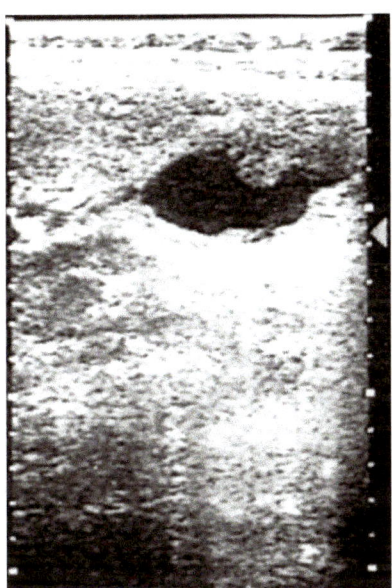

Fig. 3.14.6: Small exophytic mass seen to arise from anterior wall of gallbladder.

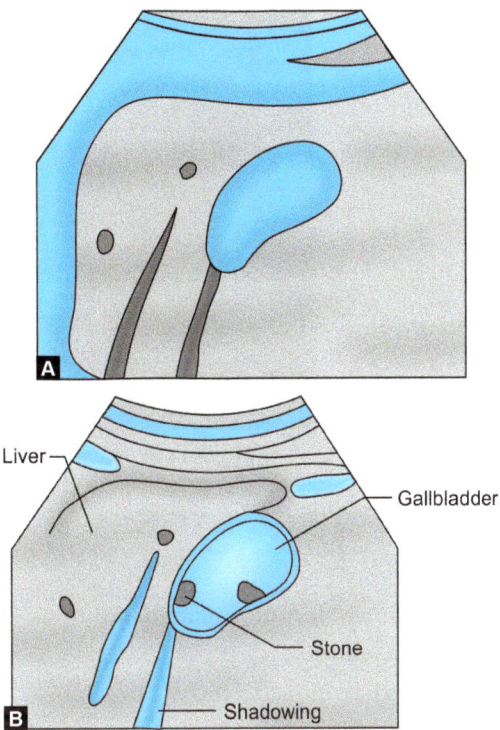

Figs. 3.14.7A and B: Gallstone with acoustic shadowing.

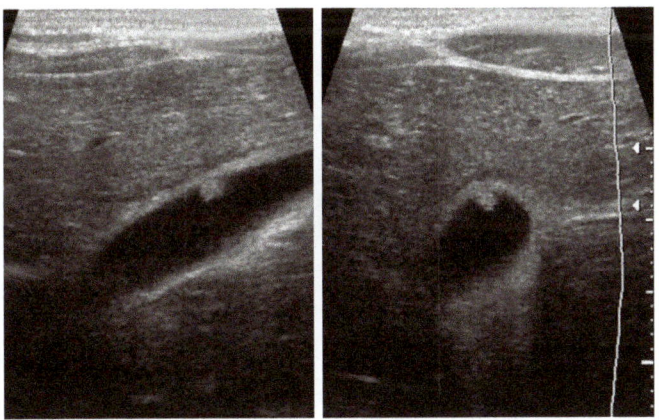

Fig. 3.14.8: US scans show evidence of GB polyp.

These irregularities correspond to areas of mucosal ulceration, hemorrhage, necrosis and or microabscess formation.

Tumefactive Sludge (Fig. 3.14.9)

Tumefactive sludge can simulate the gallbladder malignancy but repeat scan after few days can show disappearance of mass.

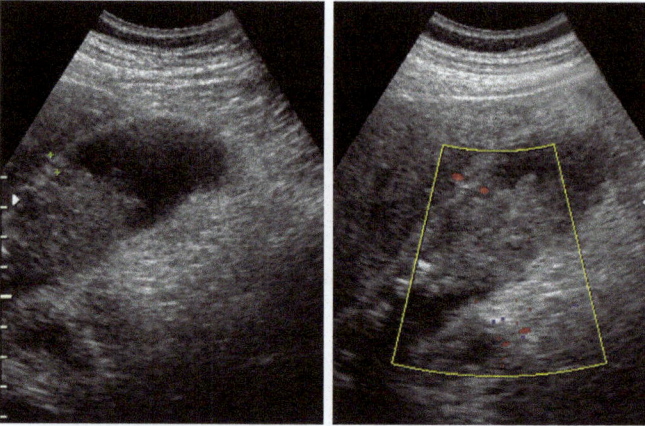

Fig. 3.14.9: US scans show tumefactive sludge in GB.

3.15 ECHOGENIC FAT IN HEPATODUODENAL LIGAMENT

Signs of pericholecystic inflammation:
- Cholecystitis
- Perforated duodenal ulcer
- Pancreatitis
- Diverticulitis.

3.16 CONGENITAL BILIARY CYST

Choledochal Cyst (Figs. 3.16.1 to 3.16.3)

Cystic dilatation of the extrahepatic biliary tree with or without dilatation of intrahepatic bile ducts, is an uncommon congenital anomaly of the biliary tree. It is 3-4 times more common in female than in male patients.

The classical clinical presentation is triad of pain, jaundice and a palpable right upper quadrant mass.

Todani et al. has described five types of choledochal cysts.
- Type 1—accounts of 80-90% of bile duct cysts. They are subdivided into three subtypes:
  - Type 1A—cystic dilatation of CBD
  - Type 1B—focal, segmental dilatation of distal CBD
  - Type 1C—fusiform dilatation of both the CHD and CBD
- Type 2 choledochal cyst—accounts for 2% of bile duct cysts and they are true diverticula arising from the CBD
- Type 3 cysts—accounts for 1-5% of bile duct cysts
  - Defined as cystic dilatation of intraduodenal portion of the CBD are defined as choledochocele
- Type 4 choledochal—accounts for 10% of bile duct cysts. Further subdivided into 2 types:
  - Type 4A—has multiple intra- and extrahepatic cysts
  - Type 4B—has multiple extrahepatic cyst only
- Type 5—comprises of remainder of bile duct cysts. This type generally involves only the intrahepatic bile ducts and may be single or multiple.

When there are multiple intrahepatic bile ducts cysts, the abnormality is known as Caroli disease.

Sonography is useful for assessing the full extent of biliary ductal dilatation and for identifying the connection of cyst with the biliary tree.

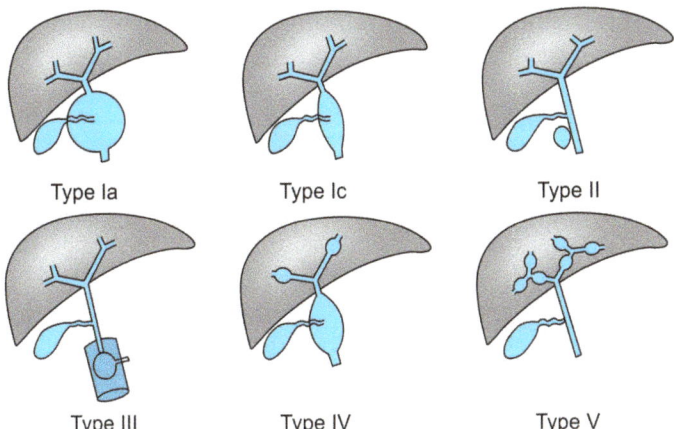

Fig. 3.16.1: Types of choledochal cyst.

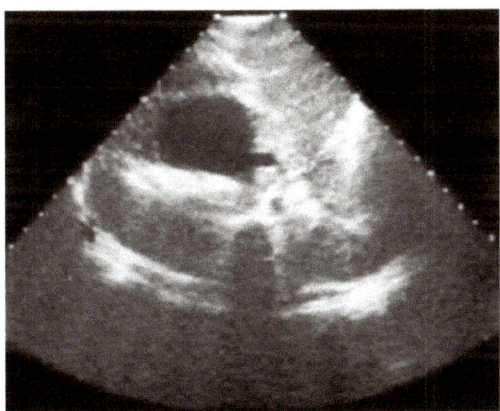

Fig. 3.16.2: A large cyst is seen in continuation with common bile duct (CBD) in this 4-year-old female.

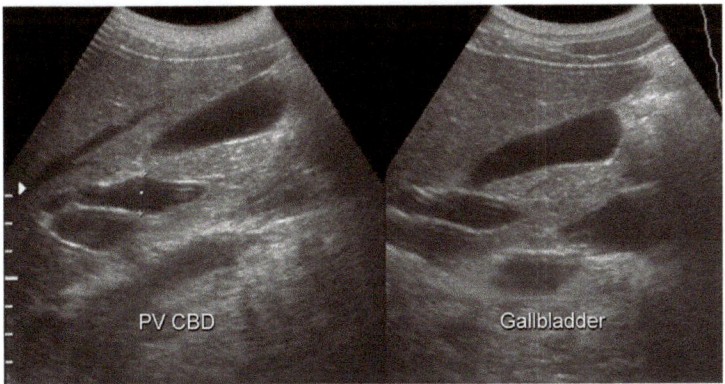

Fig. 3.16.3: US scans show Type I choledochal cyst.
(PV: portal vein; CBD: common bile duct)

The presence of stones, strictures or tumors can also be detected with sonography.

3.17 DIFFERENTIAL DIAGNOSIS OF PERICHOLECYSTIC FLUID

- *Gallbladder perforation:*
  - May be acute, subacute or chronic
  - Subacute perforation is marked by pericholecystic abscess
  - Mostly perifundic
  - Thick hypoechoic wall with cholelithiasis and septated complex fluid around is noted.
- Pancreatitis II inflammatory fluid seeps along hepatoduodenal ligament
- Peptic ulcer II duodenal ligament and major fissure up to GB fossa
- *Acalculus cholecystitis* **(Fig. 3.17.1)**:
  - Wall thickened
  - Pericholecystic fluid
  - Subserosal edema
  - Intraluminal/mural gas
  - Sloughed mucosal membranes
  - Lack of response to cholecystokinin (CCK)
  - Cystic artery length >50% length of anterior GB wall.
- Gangrenous cholecystitis
- *Pitfalls:*
  - Folded GB
  - Enteric duplication cyst.

3.18 DIFFERENTIAL DIAGNOSIS OF INTRAHEPATIC BILIARY DILATATION (FIGS. 3.18.1 TO 3.18.3)

- *Intrahepatic neoplasm:*
  - Mainly cystadenoma and cystadenocarcinoma which show like cyst with internal papillary excrescences
  - Other lesion in this category is one hilar cholangiocarcinoma also known as Klatskin tumor.
- *Sclerosing and AIDS cholangitis:*
  - Smooth/irregular wall thickening
  - Associated with ulcerative colitis
  - Narrowed and dilated segments.

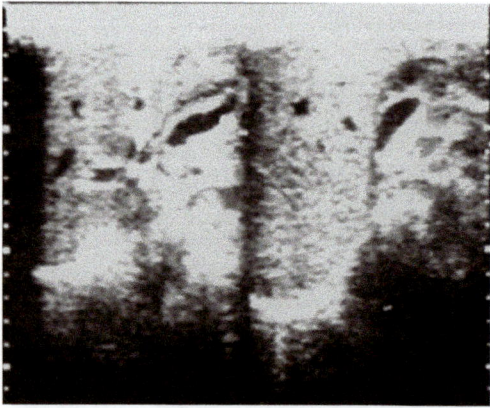

Fig. 3.17.1: Thickened gallbladder wall, pericholecystic fluid and a hypoechoic collection at the fundus is evident in this case of acute acalculus cholecystitis.

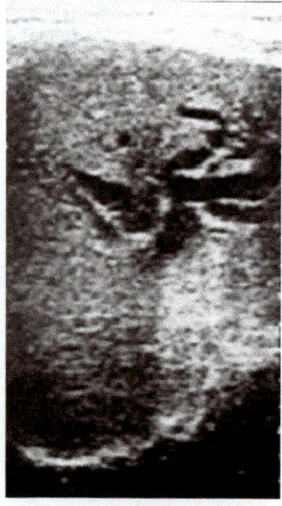

Fig. 3.18.1: Dilated intrahepatic bile ducts—stellate branching pattern seen in transverse scan.

Hepatobiliary System and Abdomen

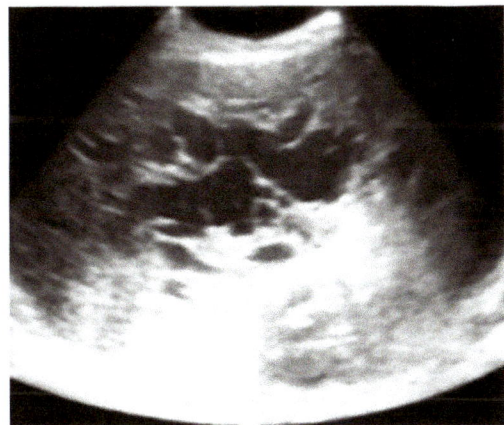

Fig. 3.18.2: Grossly dilated IHBR are seen as multiple tubular structures.

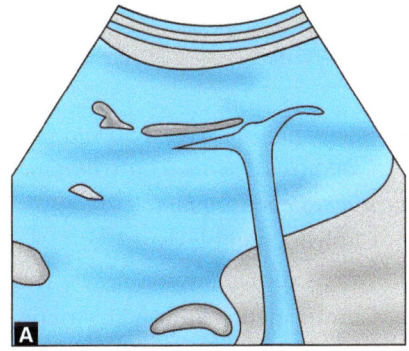

Figs. 3.18.3A and B: Gallstone with intrahepatic dilatation.

- *Intrahepatic biliary calculi:*
  - In recurrent pyogenic cholangitis
  - In oriental cholangiohepatitis
  - In intrahepatic pigment stone disease
  - In biliary obstruction syndrome of the Chinese
  - Acoustic shadows of stone may be lacking if very small.
- *Caroli's disease:*
  - Saccular communicating bile duct ectasias
  - May be associated with hepatic fibrosis
  - Associated with choledochal cysts, polycystic kidney disease.
- Bile duct hamartomas
- Peribiliary cysts
- *Pitfalls:*
  - Segmental bile duct dilatation
  - Hemobilia
  - Large vascular channels.

3.19 DIFFERENTIAL DIAGNOSIS OF EHBR DILATATION (FIGS. 3.19.1 TO 3.19.5)

- *Suprapancreatic obstruction:*
  - Primary/secondary malignancy
  - Lymph nodal enlargement
  - Parasites.
- *Posthepatic obstruction:*
  - Bile duct malignancy
  - Juxtaportal intrahepatic mass
  - Mirizzi's syndrome

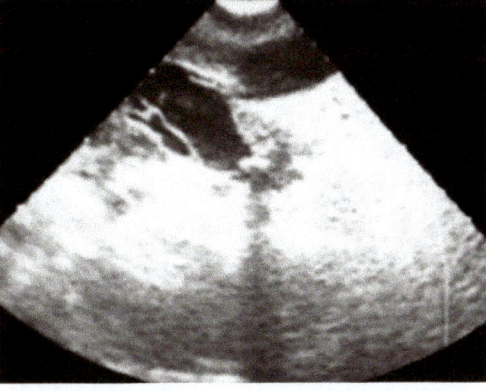

Fig. 3.19.1: CBD calculus—grossly dilated CBD (measuring 23 mm) is seen with a echogenic focus with shadowing at its distal end.

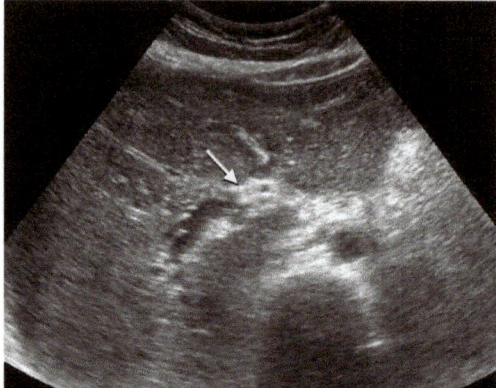

Fig. 3.19.2: Stricture in proximal CBD (white arrow) with mildly dilated intrahepatic biliary radicals.

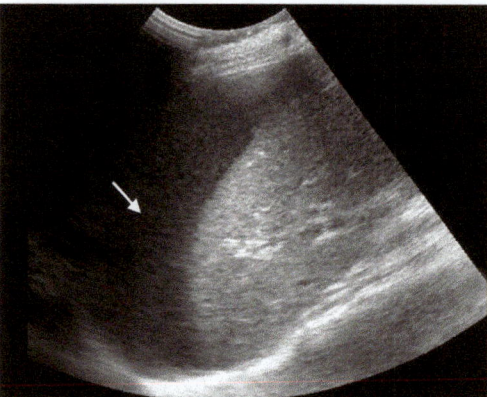

Fig. 3.19.3: Transabdominal scan of liver showing biloma (arrow)—a collection with low level echoes.

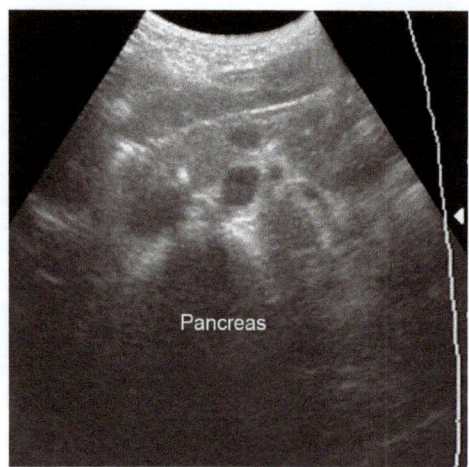

Fig. 3.19.4: US scan shows calculus at distal end of CBD.

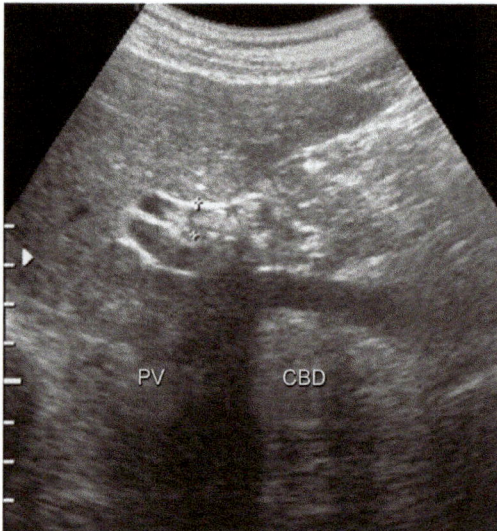

Fig. 3.19.5: US scan shows tumefactive sludge in CBD lumen. (PV: portal vein; CBD: common bile duct)

- Biliary parasites, e.g. *Fasciola hepatica, Clonorchis sinensis, Ascaris lumbricoides*.
- *Intrahepatic obstruction:*
  - Choledocholithiasis
  - Pancreatic carcinoma
  - Chronic pancreatitis with stricture.

3.20 ABDOMINAL WALL MASSES

Common

Abscesses (Fig. 3.20.1)

- Usually secondary to previous trauma, surgery
- Appear as loculated hypoechoic to anechoic collections with debris with posterior acoustic enhancement
- Occasionally, presents with thick, hypoechoic, bulky muscles in phlegmonous stage
- Septations and layering of low level echoes are characteristics.

Hematoma (Fig. 3.20.2)

- Commonly seen in rectus sheath along anterior abdominal wall

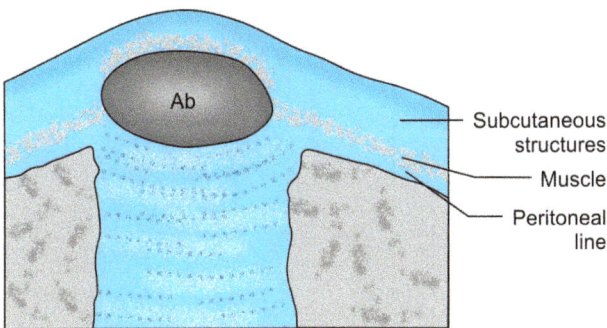

Fig. 3.20.1: Abdominal (Ab) wall abscess. The abscess has expanded and broken through the tissue planes.

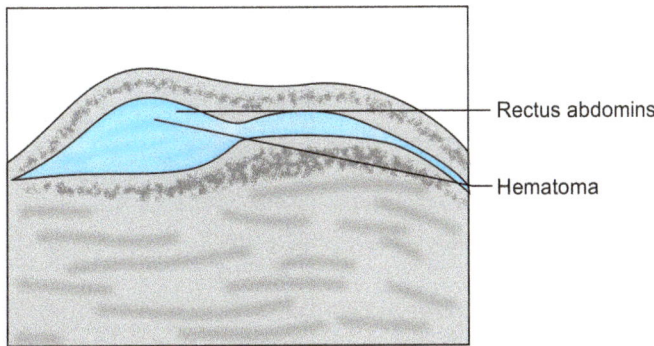

Fig. 3.20.2: Widening of the rectus abdominis muscles due to a hematoma.

- Either post-traumatic secondary to surgery, direct trauma or sudden muscular contraction as in seizures, coughing, sneezing, etc. or may be spontaneous as in patients on anticoagulant therapy
- On US, it appears as a hypoechoic or complex mass at times with layering of low level echoes due to blood cells
- Occasionally, they may appear as fluid collections due to liquefaction or clot lysis.

Hernias (Fig. 3.20.3)

- Careful scanning with a 7.5 MHz linear array transducer can demonstrate the fascial/aponeurotic hernial defect as well as the herniated contents (Omental fat or contents)
- Seen in cross-section, bowel loops appear as target lesions with strong reflective central echoes representing air in the lumen
- When obstructed, they appear as tubular fluid-filled structures with valvulae conniventes (small bowel) or Haustration, fecal matter (colon)
- Color flow imaging (CFI) may be able to give diagnosis especially the strangulation of loop
- Final diagnosis of the type of hernia depends on the site and history.

Uncommon

Seroma

- Appears as anechoic fluid collection as the site of previous surgery
- Complicated seromas may appear as abscesses.

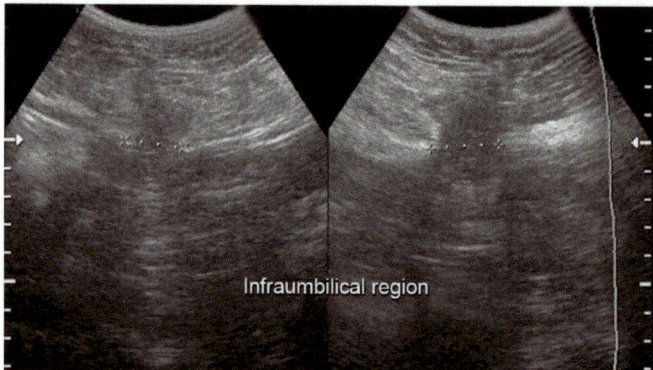

Fig. 3.20.3: US scans show evidence of hernia in anterior abdominal wall.

Urachal Cyst

- Appears as an anechoic fluid collection with posterior acoustic enhancement extending from the umbilicus to the dome of bladder. Care should be taken to differentiate from umbilical cyst **(Fig. 3.20.4)**
- May be complicated by hemorrhage or infection (urachal abscess)
- Uncommonly, tumors may arise in the urachus in children or young adults.

Endometrioma in Cesarean Scar

- On US, they appear as well-defined, unilocular or multilocular, predominantly cystic mass containing homogeneous, low level, internal echoes
- Low level echoes may be distributed homogeneously diffusely throughout the mass or may be seen in the dependent portion producing a fluid-debris level.

Foreign Bodies

- Mainly seen due to postsurgical complication
- Most common cause is sponge, which appears as echogenic mass due to the adherent blood forming multiple interfaces.

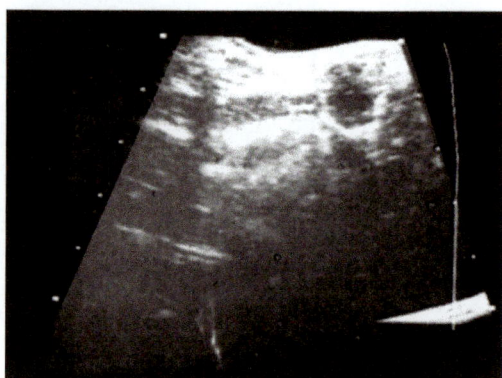

Fig. 3.20.4: Umbilical cyst—a small anechoic rounded SOL seen in the region of the umbilicus.

Parasitic Infestation

- Most common is cysticercus cyst of *Taenia solium*
- It appears as round to oval, subcentimeter anechoic collection with well-defined wall with central or eccentric speck of echogenicity **(Fig. 3.20.5)**.

Undescended Testicles

- Eighty percent are palpable and 20% are not palpable
- Of the nonpalpable testicles, 80% are in the inguinal canal and 20% are intra-abdominal
- Undescended testes is usually smaller than the normal testes

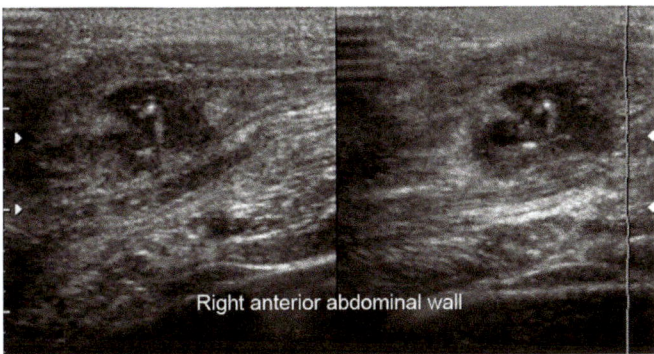

Fig. 3.20.5: High resolution ultrasound (HRUS) scans show degenerating cyst of cysticercus.

- It usually appears ovoid with its long axis parallel to the inguinal canal **(Fig. 3.20.6)**
- Visualization of an echogenic hilum differentiates lymph node from testicle.

Vascular Masses

- *Varices:*
  - Recanalized umbilical vein—it appears, irregular, tortuous and can be traced inferiorly. Color flow imaging can demonstrate the blood flow pattern.
  - Varicoceles and saphenous varices are compressible and have typical venous Doppler characteristics.
- *Subcutaneous arterial bypass grafts:*
  - High resolution sonography is ideal in imaging subcutaneous axillofemoral and femorofemoral arterial bypass grafts
  - Postgraft complications especially seromas can be easily detected
  - Thrombosis and pattern of blood flow can be demonstrated
  - Other complication as graft aneurysms can be detected.
- *Pseudoaneurysms and AV fistulas:*
  - Commonly seen as complication of catheterization
  - Pseudoaneurysms is a pulsatile hematoma secondary to bleeding in soft tissues, with fibrous encapsulation and a persistent communication between the vessel and fluid space
  - Most are seen within 2 cm of the arterial injury
  - Real time criteria of pseudoaneurysm includes echogenic swirls within a cystic cavity, expansile pulsatility, hypoechoic mass and a visible tract
  - When present, echogenic swirls are diagnostic of pseudoaneurysm.

Doppler characteristics include arterial flow within a mass separate from the artery and to and fro flow between the artery and the mass.

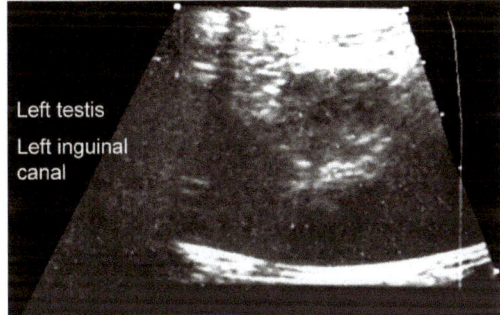

Fig. 3.20.6: Left ectopic testis lying in the inguinal canal.

Lymph Nodes

- They appear on US as hypoechoic masses with central echogenicities

- With extensive lipomatosis, they may become indistinguishable from surrounding subcutaneous tissue
- Lymphomatous nodes are extremely hypoechoic and may even be anechoic, especially in non-Hodgkin's lymphoma (NHL) with a central artery of 1-3 mm diameter
- Central artery is not seen in carcinomatous nodes as it is infiltrated.

Tumors

- *Desmoid:*
    - It arises from fascia or aponeurosis of muscle
    - Most common location is anterior abdominal wall
    - Usually seen in patients with previous surgery and often at the site of scar
    - Also occur in patients with familial polyposis and is associated with pregnancy.
      Females outnumbers males in the ratio of 3 : 1
    - Appears as hypoechoic masses with foci of distal acoustic shadowing due to fibrous collagenous tissue and not due to calcification.
- Lipomas—appear as well encapsulated, highly echogenic septae in a predominantly hypoechoic mass **(Fig. 3.20.7)**
- Rarely—neuromas, neurofibromas may be seen
- *Metastasis—most commonly metastatic melanoma:*
    - Other tumors that can produce metastatic subcutaneous nodules include lymphoma, Ca lung, breast, ovary, colon, etc.
    - Local metastases from malignancies of pleura, peritoneum, diaphragm or intra-abdominal organs such as the colon

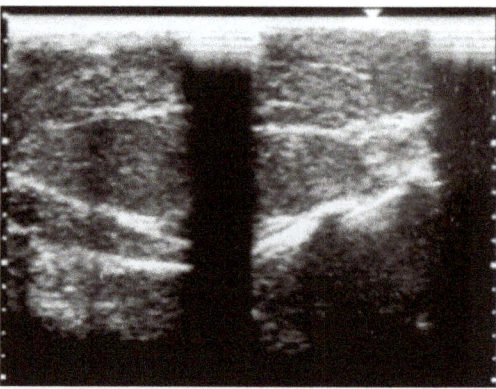

Fig. 3.20.7: Axillary scan showing predominantly hypoechoic solid mass with echogenic septae in it. Fine-needle aspiration cytology (FNAC) revealed adipocytes—lipoma.

- Most melanomas appear hypoechoic masses with enhancement through transmission.

Artefactual Masses

- Ghost artifact or split image artifact
- It arises due to the presence of extraperitoneal fat deep to linea alba and rectus abdominis muscle
- Scanning in sagittal and oblique plane will settle the issue.

3.21 ACUTE ABDOMEN

The abdomen is divided into 9 quadrants by 2 horizontal lines and 2 vertical lines **(Fig. 3.21.1)**.

- Upper horizontal line is at the level of transpyloric plane
- Lower horizontal line is at the level of transtubercular plane
- Vertical line is drawn on either side of midline through the midpoint between anterior superior iliac spine and symphysis pubis.

The division of quadrants is as given in **Figure 3.21.1**.

Hepatobiliary System and Abdomen

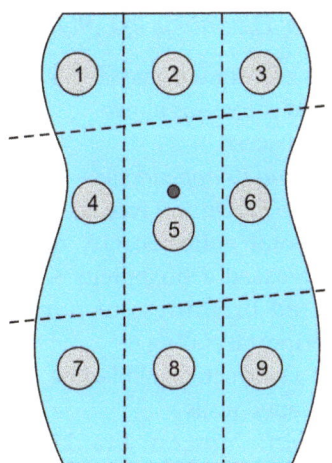

Fig. 3.21.1: Division of quadrants: (1) Right hypochondrium; (2) Epigastrium; (3) Left hypochondrium; (4) Right lumbar; (5) Umbilical; (6) Left lumbar; (7) Right iliac; (8) Hypogastrium; (9) Left iliac.

Differential Diagnosis in Cases of Right Hypochondrial Involvement

Structures and conditions related are:
- Liver—hepatitis, abscess, hemorrhage into cyst or tumor, etc. **(Fig. 3.21.2)**
- Gallbladder—cholecystitis, empyema, cholangitis
- Subphrenic space—abscess
- Pylorus and duodenum—perforated ulcer-loculated fluid collection or free peritoneal fluid may be seen
- Hepatic flexure of colon—acute colitis, diverticulitis, intussusception
- Right kidneys—calculi, abscess **(Fig. 3.21.3)**
- Right suprarenal—hemorrhage.

Differential Diagnosis for Epigastrium

Structures and conditions related are:
- Liver and subphrenic space—as above
- Stomach and duodenum—as above
- Transverse colon—intussusception, diverticulitis and abscess
- Omentum—infarction
- Pancreas—pancreatitis
- Aorta—dissecting aneurysm
- Retroperitoneum—hemorrhage.

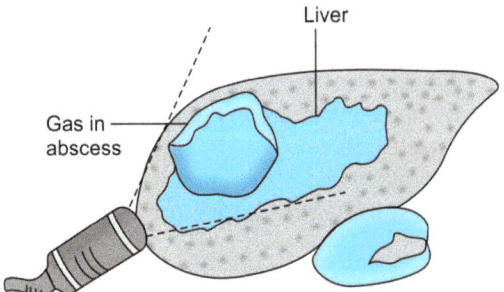

Fig. 3.21.2: Abscess in the liver with gas rising to the anterior margin, scan from a posterolateral approach with the patient in a supine position so the beam passes behind the gas.

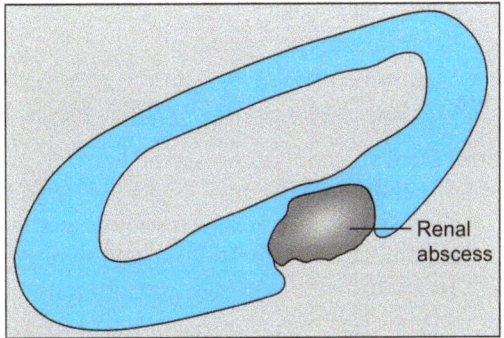

Fig. 3.21.3: Abscesses in the kidney tend to have some internal echoes and irregular walls.

Differential Diagnosis for Left Hypochondrium

Structures and conditions related are:
- Spleen—abscess, hemorrhage (spontaneous)
- Liver and subphrenic space—as above
- Splenic flexure of colon—as above
- Tail of pancreas—as above
- Stomach—as above
- Left kidney—as above
- Left adrenal—as above.

Differential Diagnosis for Lumbar Quadrants (Right and Left)

Structures and conditions related are:
- Ascending or descending colon—abscess, diverticulitis

- Right and left kidney—perinephric abscess, calculi
- Adjacent structures—liver, GB and appendicular conditions on right side and spleen on left side.

Differential Diagnosis for Umbilical Region

Structures and quadrant related are:
- Stomach and duodenum—as above
- Transverse colon—as above
- Omentum—as above
- Small intestine and mesentery—intussusception, closed loop obstruction infarction
- Pancreas—as above
- Aorta—as above
- Retroperitoneum—as above.

Differential Diagnosis in Right Iliac Region

Structures and conditions related are:
- Appendix and cecum—appendicitis and abscess; typhlitis and perityphlitis, cecal/appendicular perforation, cecal volvulus
- Terminal ileum—enteritis and perforation, intussusception
- Iliopsoas—abscess
- Kidney—undescended or descended—as above
- Uterus and appendages—endometritis, salpingitis, ovarian torsion, pyosalpinx, ectopic pregnancy, abscess of broad ligament, cyst hemorrhage
- Urinary bladder—cystitis and urinary retention
  Thickened nodular walls with debris in lumen
- Pelvic abscess.

Differential Diagnosis in Hypogastrium

Structures and conditions related are:
- Urinary bladder—as above
- Small intestine—as above
- Sigmoid colon—sigmoiditis, diverticulitis, volvulus, abscess
- Uterus and appendages—as above
- Pelvic abscess.

Differential Diagnosis in Left Iliac Region

Structures and conditions related are:
- Sigmoid colon—as above
- Pelvic abscess
- *Uterus and its appendages—as above:*
  - *Acute hepatitis*: Liver is enlarged with normal echogenicity or diffusely decreased echogenicity with accentuated brightness of portal triads, periportal cuffing
    - Contracted gallbladder with thickened walls
  - *Hepatic abscess*: Frankly purulent abscesses appear cystic with fluid ranging from echo-free to highly echogenic
    - Early abscesses appear solid, hypoechoic regions of altered echogenicity with posterior acoustic enhancement
    - Wall may be well-defined or irregular and thick
    - Fluid—fluid interfaces, internal septicus and debris may be observed
  - *Hemorrhagic SOLs*: Appear as complex, heteroechoic SOL'S, at times with organized clot or fluid-debris levels
  - *Acute cholecystitis:* Primary signs include gallstones, focally tender GB (sonographic Murphy's sign) and impacted gallstone
    - Secondary signs include—GB dilatation, sludge and diffuse wall thickening
  - *Colitis:* Thickened, hypoechoic bowel walls
    - Hyperemia as seen with CFI
    - Creeping fat seen as hyperechoic mass effect
    - Mesenteric adenopathy
    - Free fluid may be present
  - *Diverticulitis:* Segmental concentric thickening of gut wall with reduced echogenicity of walls reflecting muscular hypertrophy

- Inflamed diverticulum is seen as echogenic foci within or beyond gut wall with acoustic shadowing or ring down artifact
- Hyperechoic mass effect reflecting inflammation of pericolonic fat
- Abscess formation seen as loculated fluid collection
- Intramural sinus tracts seen as linear hyperechoic lesion within gut wall
- Thickening of mesentery
- Hypo to hyperechoic linear tracts from gut to bladder, vagina or adjacent loops signifies fistulous tracts
- *Intussusception*: Appearance of multiple concentric rings, related to the invaginating layers of telescoped bowel, seen in transverse section is pathognomonic
- 'Hay-fork' appearance on longitudinal scans
- Renal abscess—appear as a round thick-walled hypoechoic complex mass often with some through transmission
  - Internal debris may be seen
  - Gas with dirty shadowing may be seen
  - Septations may be present
  - May spontaneously decompress into the collecting system or perinephric space
- Adrenal hemorrhage—acute hemorrhage appear as a bright echogenic mass in the adrenal bed, which becomes smaller and anechoic with time (**Figs. 3.21.4A to C**)
- With resolution, focal areas of calcification may develop.

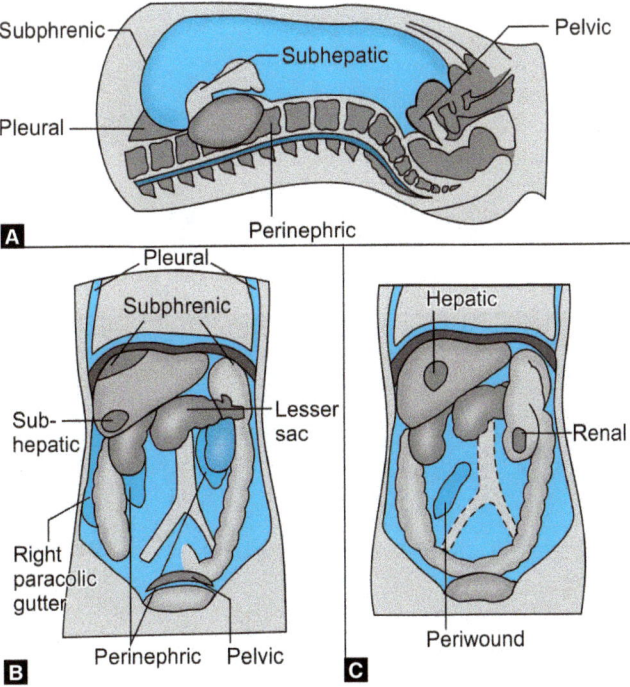

Figs. 3.21.4A to C: (A and B) A number of spaces exist in the abdomen where fluid collect. Common sites for fluid collection are the pelvic, subhepatic, paracolic gutter, and lesser sac areas. Fluid may collect around the kidneys or the pleural space; (C) Sites where abscesses may form are the spaces already mentioned, as well as within the liver, of kidney and around incisions.

Subphrenic Abscess (Fig. 3.21.5)

Loculated fluid collection containing gas bubbles.

Septations or debris may be present.

Omental Infarction

On US, appears as a plaque or cake-like area of increased echogenicity suggesting inflamed or infiltrated fat.

Usually seen in right flank superficially with adherence of peritoneum **(Fig. 3.21.6).**

Pancreatitis (Fig. 3.21.7)

Focal disease is seen as isoechoic or hypoechoic enlargement of pancreas.

- In diffuse disease, the pancreas become increasingly hypoechogenic relative to normal liver and increases in size
- Focal hemorrhage appears as an echogenic mass
- Retroperitoneal hemorrhage—US appearance is variable, solid or cystic
  - Cystic lesions may be sonolucent or echogenic with debris producing a layering effect. With time become more echogenic and show progressive with time
- Aortic dissection—classical appearance of a thin membrane fluttering in the lumen at different phases of cardiac cycle **(Figs. 3.21.8A and B)**

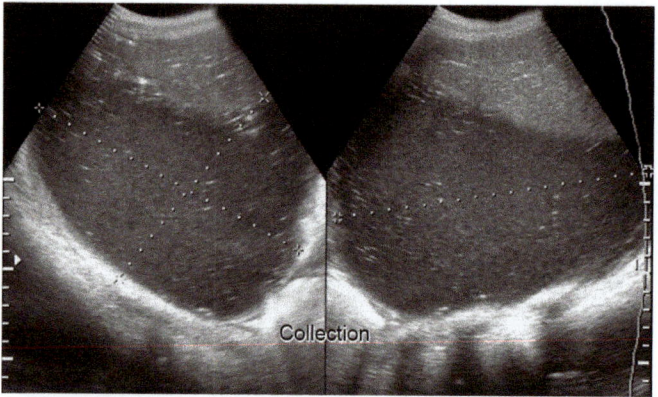

Fig. 3.21.5: US scans show subphrenic abscess.

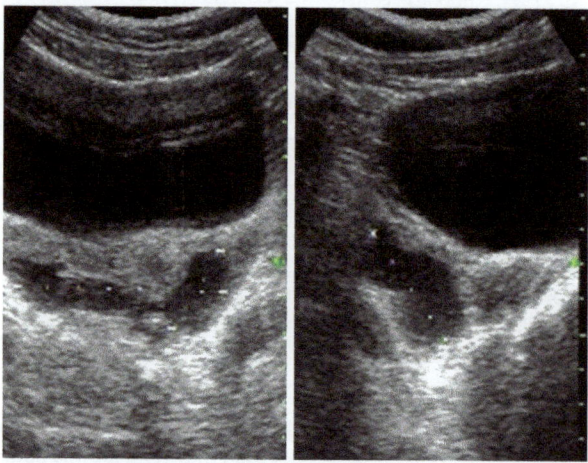

Fig. 3.21.6: US scans show collection in pelvis in a case of pelvic inflammatory disease (PID).

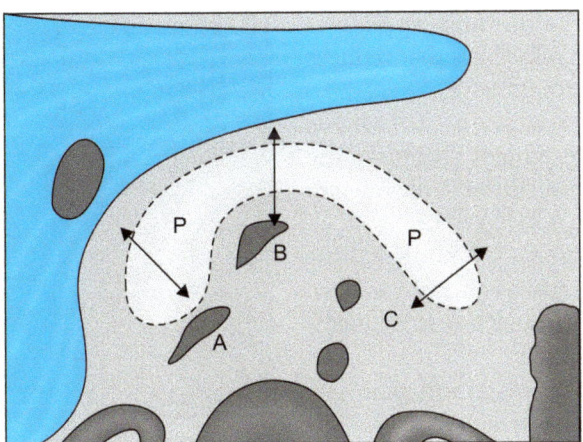

Fig. 3.21.7: In pancreatitis, the pancreas swells and becomes more sonolucent than usual. The dotted lines show the normal size of the pancreas; the arrows (A, B, C) show the increase that occurs with pancreatitis. The pancreas is normally considered to have an upper size limit of 1.5 cm at the level of the body and of 3 cm at the head and tail.

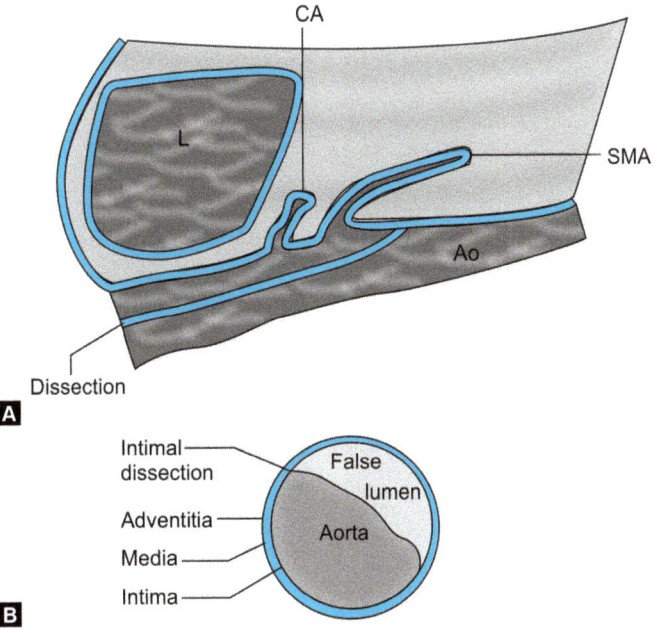

Figs. 3.21.8A and B: Longitudinal and transverse sonographic views of a dissecting aneurysm. Note the line from the intima that represents one border of the dissection. (CA: celiac artery; SMA: superior mesenteric artery; Ao: aorta; L: liver)

- CFI shows blood flow in both channels but with different rates
- Spleen abscess—appearance varies from simple cystic lesion to complex or hypoechoic lesions; diagnosis made in conjunction with clinical findings
- Frequently, gas is seen within an abscess cavity

- Splenic hemorrhage—may appear as echogenic or complex mass that reduces in echogenicity with time
- Closed-loop obstruction—US shows dilated involved segment and often the normal caliber bowel distal to the point of obstruction **(Figs. 3.21.9A to C)**
- Acute appendicitis—US show blind-ended, aperistaltic tube with gut signature measuring greater than 6 mm in diameter **(Fig. 3.21.10)**
    - Inflamed perienteric fat with pericecal collection and appendicolith.

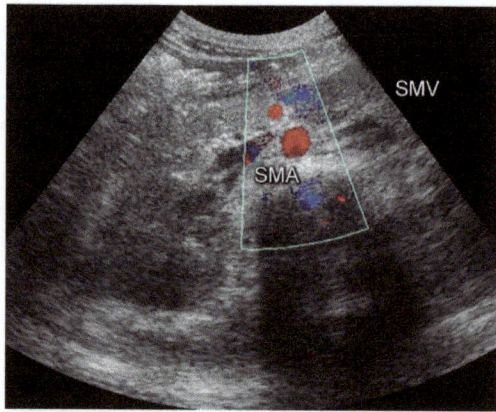

Fig. 3.21.9C: Reversal of SMA and SMV relationship. (SMV: superior mesenteric vein; SMA: superior mesenteric artery)

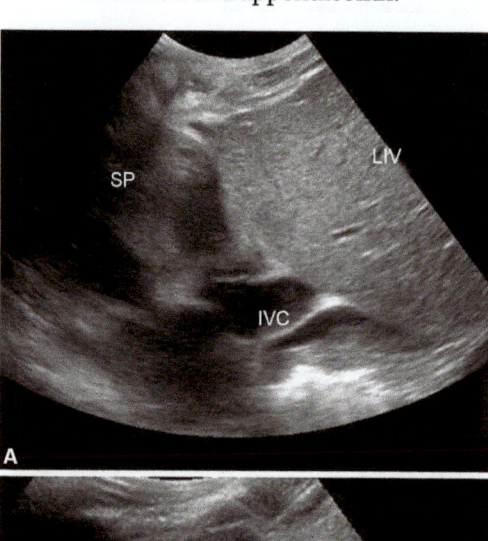

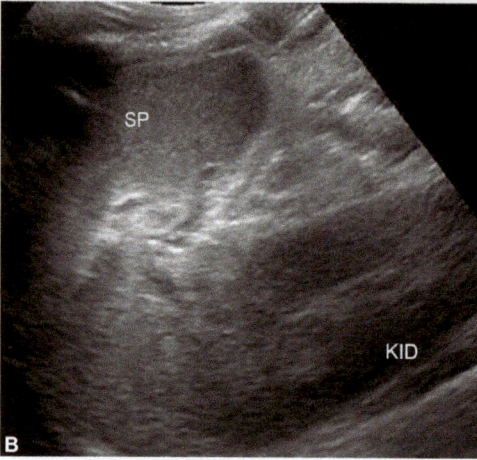

Figs. 3.21.9A and B: Situs inversus—liver located in left upper quadrant (LUQ) and spleen in the right upper quadrant (RUQ). (LIV: liver; IVC: inferior vena cava; SP: spleen; KID: kidney)

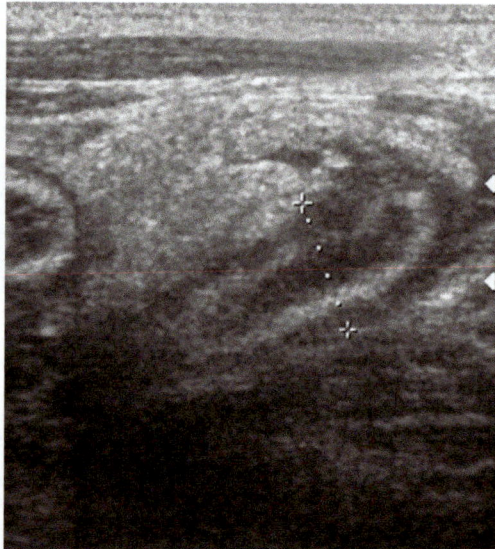

Fig. 3.21.10: High resolution ultrasound scan shows acute appendicitis.

Pelvic Inflammatory Disease

- *Endometritis:* Endometrium appears thickened and irregular
    - Fluid/gas may or may not be present
- Pus in cul-de-sac—appears as particulate fluid

Hepatobiliary System and Abdomen

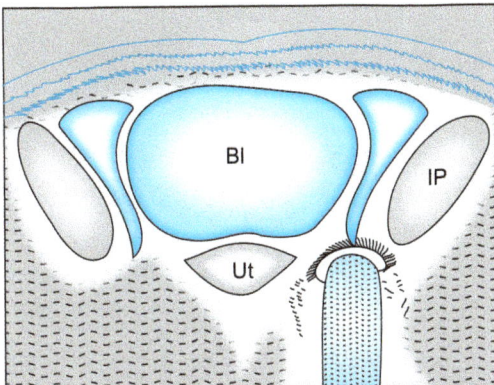

Fig. 3.21.11: A transverse view of the female pelvis with a left-sided tubo-ovarian abscess. The abscess contains air, which rises to the top and casts a strong acoustic shadow. (Bl: bladder; Ut: uterus; IP: iliopsoas)

- Periovarian inflammation—enlarged ovaries with multiple cysts and indistinct margin
- Pyosalpinx or hydrosalpinx—fluid-filled tubes with or without internal debris
- Tubo-ovarian complex—fusion of the inflamed tube and ovary
- Tubo-ovarian abscess—complex multiloculated mass with variable septations, irregular margins and scattered internal echoes **(Fig. 3.21.11)**.

3.22 ABDOMINAL LYMPHADENOPATHY

Benign	Malignant
Oval, beam-shaped	Round
Roundness index >2 (longitudinal/transverse ratio)	<2
Echogenic hilum/present	Absent or narrow
No eccentric cortical thickening	Eccentric cortical thickening presence
Normal arrangement of intranodal vessels on Doppler	On Doppler—avascular intranodal regions with displacement or distortion of intranodal vessels

Criteria for Assessing Nodal Disease (Figs. 3.22.1 to 3.22.5)

Abdominal	<1.0 cm—normal
	>1.0 cm, single—suspicious
	>1.5 cm, single—abnormal
	>1.0 cm, multiple—abnormal
Retrocrural	>0.6 cm—abnormal
Pelvic	>1.5 cm—abnormal.

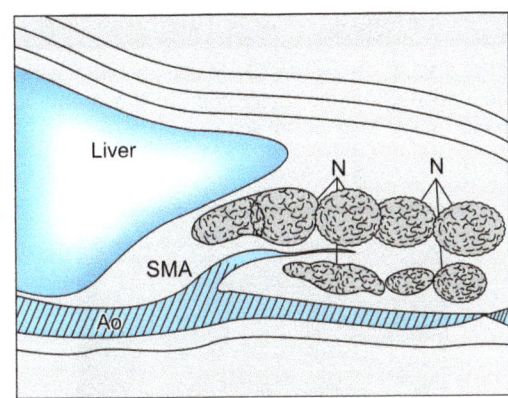

Fig. 3.22.1: The sandwich sign. Nodes (N) lie anterior and posterior to the superior mesenteric artery (SMA) and the mesenteric sheath in the mesentery.

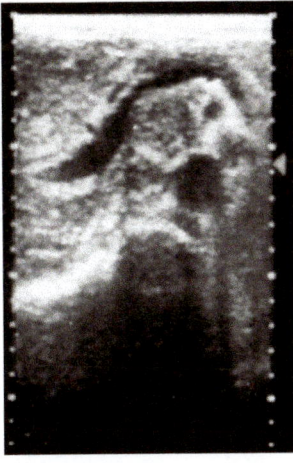

Fig. 3.22.2: A single rounded echogenic lumen seen anterior to the aorta. SMA is seen on the left side. PV is anterior to the LN. It was a metastatic LN from adenocarcinoma colon.

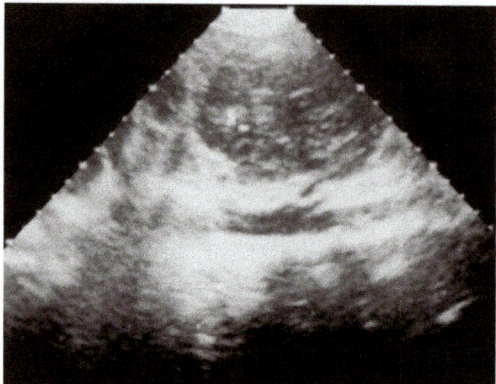

Fig. 3.22.3: Preaortic LN mass—a large well-defined hypoechoic mass seen in the preaortic region in this longitudinal scan.

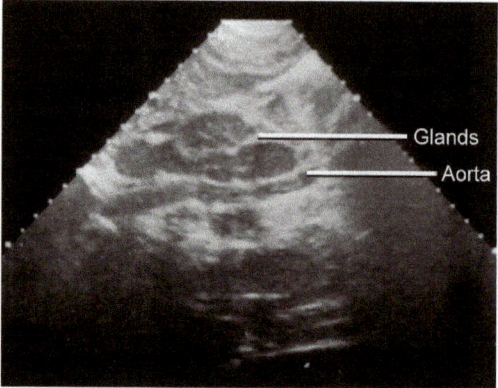

Fig. 3.22.5: Discrete hypoechoic nodular lesions seen in preaortic region suggestive of lymph nodes. Fine-needle aspiration cytology (FNAC) revealed lymphoma.

Lymphomatous Lymph Nodes

- Extremely hypoechoic or may be anechoic, with absence of posterior acoustic enhancement (helps to differentiate from cyst)
- A 1-3 mm central artery may be seen within enlarged lymphomatous nodes, which is:
  - Not seen in carcinomatous nodes
- Lymphomatous nodes may fuse to form a hypoechoic mantle of tissue, that surrounds the aorta and there may be loss of aortic outline (Silhouette sign) and may elevate it from the spine (floating aorta sign).

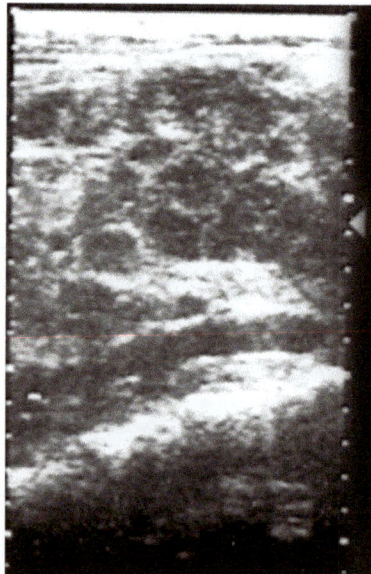

Fig. 3.22.4: Multiple hypoechoic nodular lesions with evidence of matting and necrosis suggestive of tubercular lymphadenopathy in para-aortic region.

CHAPTER 4

Spleen

4.1 NONVISUALIZATION OF SPLEEN ON ULTRASOUND

- Asplenia syndrome
- Polysplenia syndrome
- Wandering spleen
- Traumatic fragmentation of spleen.

Asplenia Syndrome

- It is a part of the spectrum of anomalies known as visceral heterotaxy.
- Patients with asplenia may have bilateral rightsidedness. They may have two morphologically right lungs, midline location of liver, reversed position of abdominal aorta and IVC, anomalous pulmonary venous return, and horseshoe kidney.
- In this condition, absence of spleen *per se* causes impairment of the immune response, and such patients can present with serious infections such as bacterial meningitis.

Polysplenia

- It is also a part of visceral heterotaxy.
- Patients with polysplenia have bilateral leftsidedness or a dominance of leftsided over right-sided body structures, they may have two morphologically left lungs, left-sided azygos continuation of interrupted IVC, biliary atresia, absence of gallbladder, GIT malrotation.

- Nuclear studies are the most sensitive methods for localizing the splenic tissue in this condition.

Wandering Spleen

- The spleen may have a long mobile mesentery, if the dorsal mesentery may fail to fuse with the posterior peritoneum.
- The wandering spleen can be found in unusual location and may be mistaken for a mass.

Traumatic Fragmentation of Spleen

Traumatic fragmentation of spleen may associate with perisplenic hematoma and hemoperitoneum.

4.2 CYSTIC LESION OF SPLEEN

Like elsewhere splenic cyst appears as well-defined, echofree lesions with smooth sharp borders and posterior acoustic enhancement.

- *Congenital:* Epidermoid cyst.
- *Vascular:*
  - Splenic laceration or fracture (**Figs. 4.2.1A and B**)
  - Hematoma
  - Cystic degeneration of infarct.
- Post-traumatic cyst.

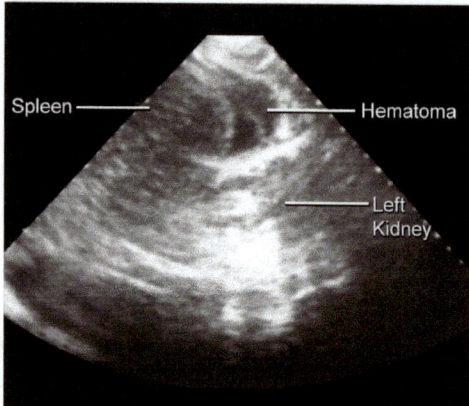

Fig. 4.2.1A: Splenic trauma—splenic laceration with hematoma.

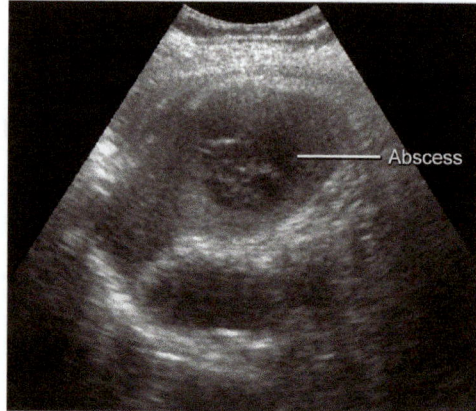

Fig. 4.2.3: US scan shows an abscess in splenic parenchyma.

- *Infection or inflammation:*
  - Pyogenic abscess (**Figs. 4.2.2 and 4.2.3**)
  - Microabscess
  - Granulomatous infection
  - *Pneumocystis carinii* infection
  - Parasitic cyst
  - Pancreatic pseudocyst.
- *Cystic neoplasm:*
  - Necrotic metastasis.

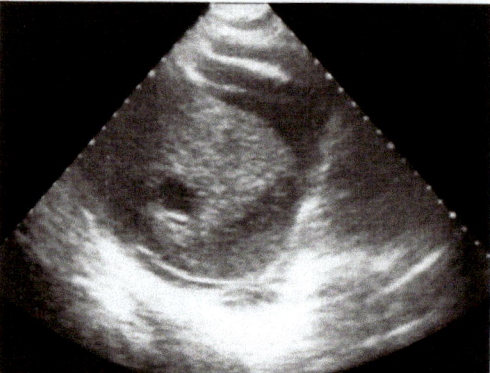

Fig. 4.2.1B: An anechoic collection around the spleen—perisplenic hematoma. There is also a parenchymal laceration with hematoma of the spleen.

Epidermoid Cyst

- It is also known as primary congenital cysts.
- It can be differentiated from post-traumatic cysts by the presence within them of an epithelial or endothelial lining.

Vascular

- *Splenic laceration or fracture:*
  - History of blunt abdominal trauma
  - Intraparenchymal hematoma—initially inhomogeneous, later on become anechoic in appearance.

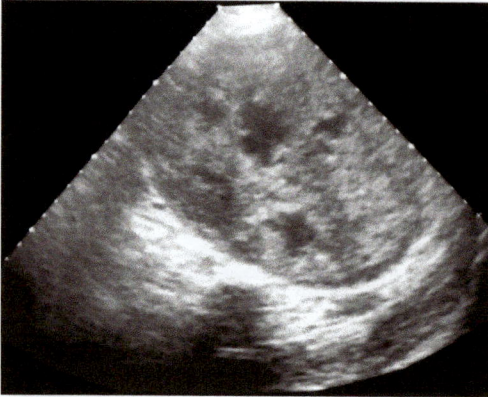

Fig. 4.2.2: A case of splenic abscess—a large space-occupying lesion (SOL) of heterogeneous echotexture with anechoic areas and slight posterior acoustic enhancement.

- *Cystic degeneration of infarct (embolic or thrombosis):*
  If a typical peripheral, then wedge-shaped echofree lesion is seen, splenic infarct is the most likely possibility.

Post-traumatic

Post-traumatic are in fact pseudocysts as they are devoid of a cellular lining. They contain low level echoes due to cholesterol crystals or debris. The wall may show calcification.

Infection or Inflammation

Pyogenic abscess.

Causes

Hematogenous spread (75%), infarction (10%), trauma (15%) abscess may have an appearance similar to that of a simple cyst, but the diagnosis can be made in conjunction with the clinical findings.

Frequently, there may be gas within an abscess cavity which will cause acoustic shadow or ring down artifacts.
- *Microabscess:*
  - Organism (especially *Candida, Aspergillus, Cryptococcus*, etc.)
  - About 26% of splenic abscess.

Splenomegaly

Multiple hypoattenuating lesion of 5 to 10 mm often associated with hepatic and renal involvement.
- *Granulomatous infection:*
  - *Mycobacterium tuberculosis*—miliary tuberculosis.
  - Mild splenomegaly uncommon:
    - *Mycobacterium avium intracellulare*
    - Marked splenomegaly seen in 20% **(Fig. 4.2.4)**.
- *Pneumocystis carinii* infection—splenomegaly with multiple hypoattenuating lesion
- *Parasitic cyst (Echinococcus)* **(Figs. 4.2.5 to 4.2.7)**—Spleen is one of the least common

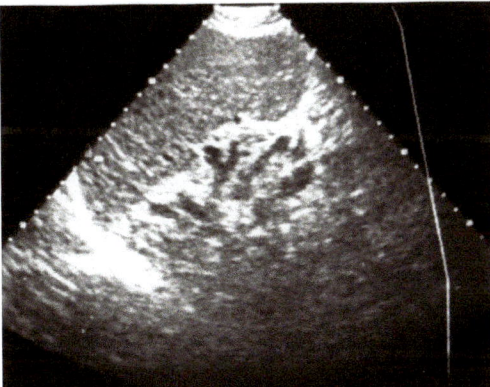
Fig. 4.2.4: A splenomegaly with cavernous transformation of splenic vein.

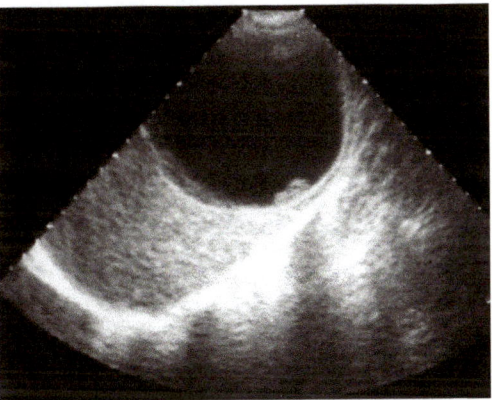
Fig. 4.2.5: Splenic hydatid—large cyst with a daughter cyst and hydatid sand.

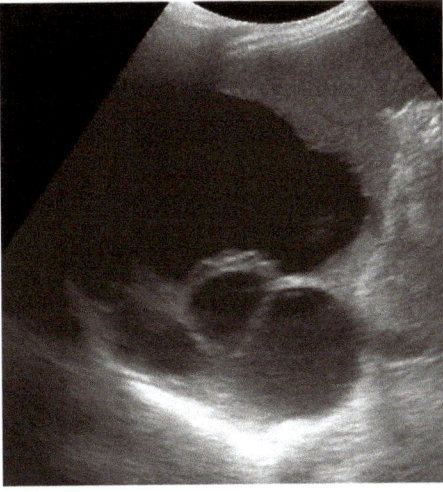
Fig. 4.2.6: Multiple hydatid cysts in spleen.

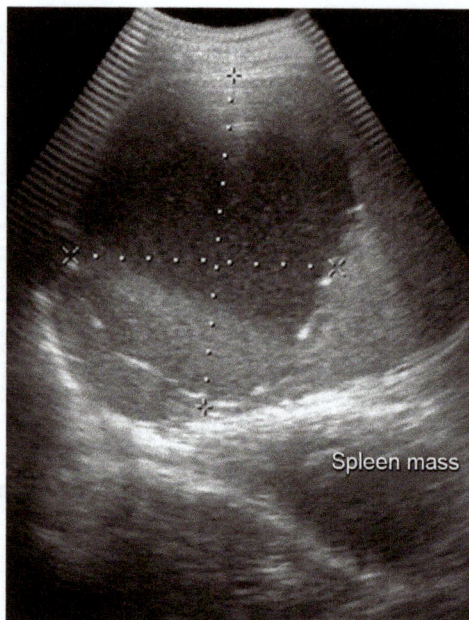

Fig. 4.2.7: US scan shows hydatid cyst with fluid-debris level in spleen.

sites for the development of the hydatid cyst. Calcification may be seen within the wall of the cyst.
- *Pancreatic pseudocyst*—extending into the spleen can be diagnosed with the associated features of pancreatitis.

Cystic Neoplasm

Necrotic metastasis of malignant melanoma, ovarian, pancreatic, endometrial, colonic, mammary carcinoma, chondrosarcoma and lymphoma.

4.3 SOLID SPLENIC LESION

Benign Lesion

- Hamartoma (splenoma)
- Hemangioma
- Sarcoidosis
- Gaucher's diseases
- Candidiasis
- Miliary tuberculosis
- Inflammatory pseudotumors
- Lymphangioma.

Malignant Lesion

- Lymphoma
- Metastasis
- Angiosarcoma
- Malignant fibrous histiocytoma, leiomyosarcoma, fibrosarcoma.

Benign Lesions

Splenic Infarction (Figs. 4.3.1A and B)

They are usually embolic (in IV drug abuses or atrial fibrillation) or occur spontaneously in splenomegaly due to vascular compromise. It is a feature of sickle cell disease. A well-defined wedge-shaped area with apex towards hilum. It is an echopoor in acute stage, later becoming heterogeneous in appearance.

Hamartoma (Splenoma)

Solid/cystic splenic mass of low attenuation.

Hemangioma

- It is most common primary splenic tumor.
- Age—20 to 50 years.
- It may be associated with Klippel-Trenaunay-Weber syndrome—multiple hemangiomas.

Sonography

- It may have well-defined echogenic appearance similar to liver hemangioma.
- Lesions of mixed echogenicity with cystic spaces of variable sizes have also been demonstrated.
- Foci of speckled snowflake like calcification can also be seen.

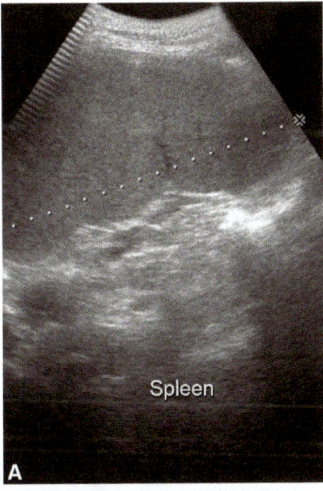
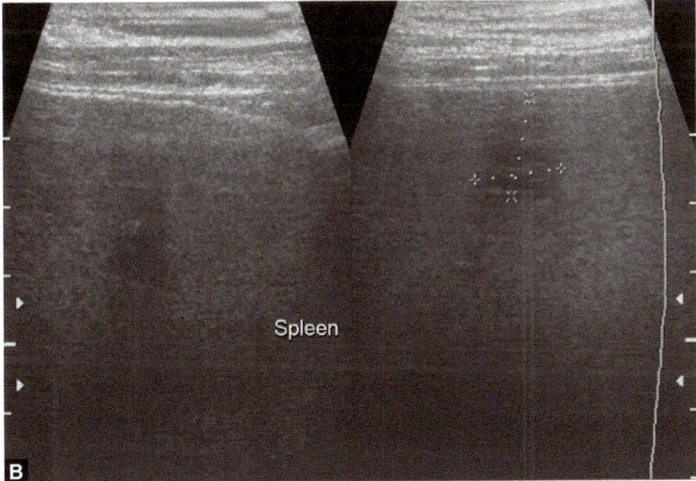

Figs. 4.3.1A and B: US scans show splenomegaly with splenic infarcts.

Sarcoidosis

Granulomatous lesions (focal hyperechoic lesion) common in tuberculosis and histoplasmosis but rare in sarcoidosis.

Gaucher's Disease

Sonographic findings:
- Splenomegaly—almost always seen.
- One-third patients have multiple splenic nodules—usually well-defined hypoechoic lesion, but may also be irregular, hyperechoic, or of mixed echogenicity.

Candidiasis

- Typical wheel within wheel appearance is seen.
- The outer wheel is thought to represent a ring of fibrosis surrounding the inner echogenic wheel of inflammatory cells and a central hypoechoic necrotic area.

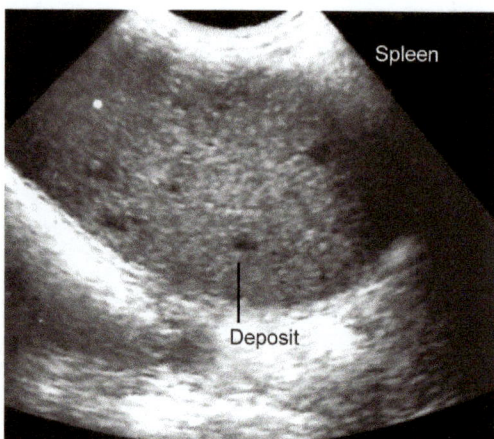

Fig. 4.3.2: Multiple hypoechoic lesions are seen in an enlarged spleen in this case of disseminated tuberculosis.

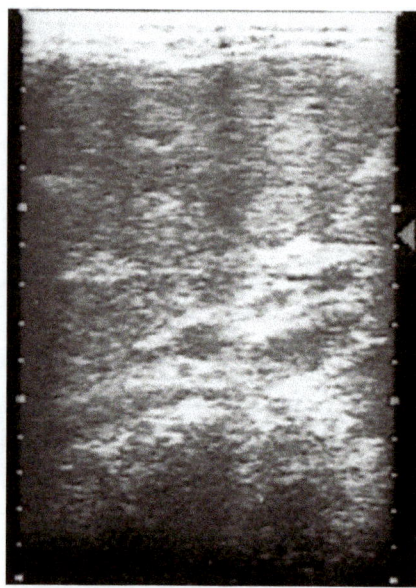

Fig. 4.3.4: Metastases. Multiple echogenic areas seen in the spleen—case of adenocarcinoma colon.

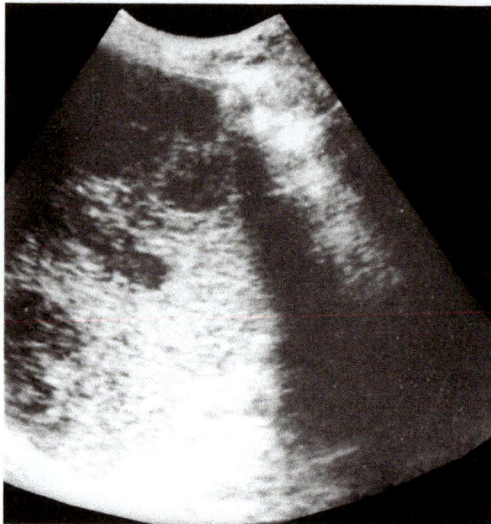

Fig. 4.3.3: Multiple echopoor SOLs seen in spleen. Similar lesions were seen in the liver and there was generalized lymphadenopathy.

Miliary Tuberculosis (Fig. 4.3.2)

- Innumerable tiny echogenic foci can be seen diffusely throughout the spleen in active TB, echopoor or cystic lesion representing TB abscess may be seen.

- Lymphangioma may have an appearance similar to the hemangioma.

Malignant Lesion

Lymphoma (Fig. 4.3.3)

- Can be—Hodgkin's lymphoma
- Non-Hodgkin's lymphoma
- *Primary splenic lymphoma:*
    - Homogeneous splenomegaly (differential diagnosis from diffuse infiltration of spleen)
    - Miliary nodules
    - Large 2–10 cm nodules in 10–25% cases
    - Nodes in splenic hilum (50%) in NHL.

Metastasis (Fig. 4.3.4)

Metastasis seen in melanoma (6–34%), breast carcinoma (12–21%), bronchogenic carcinoma

(9–18%), colon carcinoma (4%), renal carcinoma (3%), ovary (8%), prostate (6%) carcinoma.

Angiosarcoma
- *Incidence:* rare.
- *Age:* 50 to 60 years.
- Multiple nodules of varying sizes usually enlarging the spleen.
- Metastasizes to liver in approx 70%.
- Spontaneous rupture seen in 30% of cases.

4.4 HYPERECHOIC SPLENIC LESION

- Granulomas **(Figs. 4.4.1 and 4.4.2)**
- Lymphoma and leukemia
- Myelofibrosis
- Gamna-Gandy nodules
- Granulomas—miliary tuberculosis, histoplasmosis.

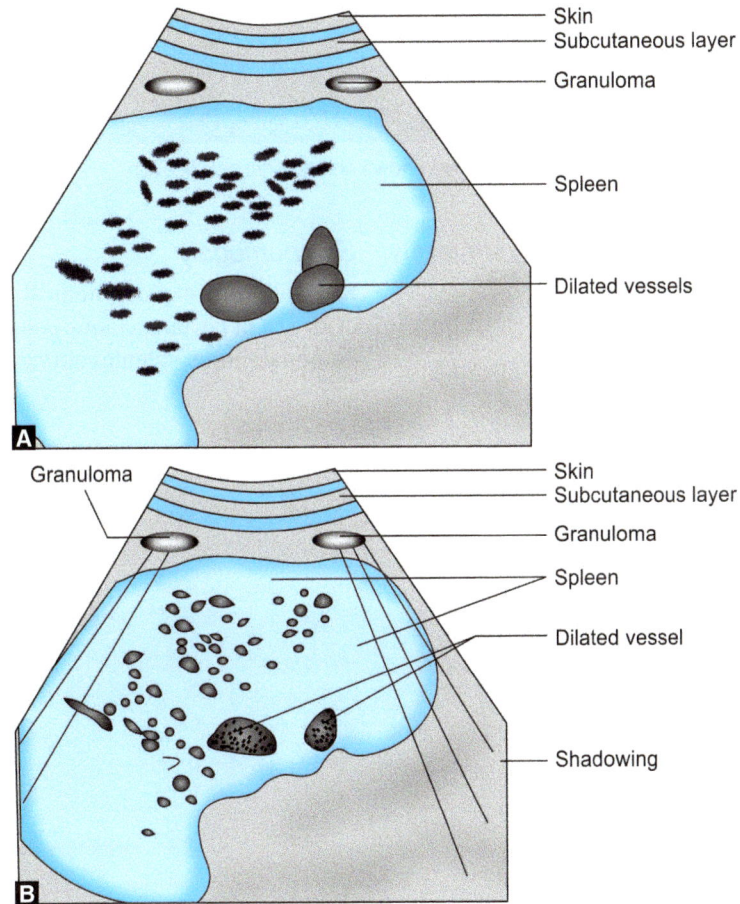

Figs. 4.4.1A and B: Multiple echogenic areas—"star-sky spleen."

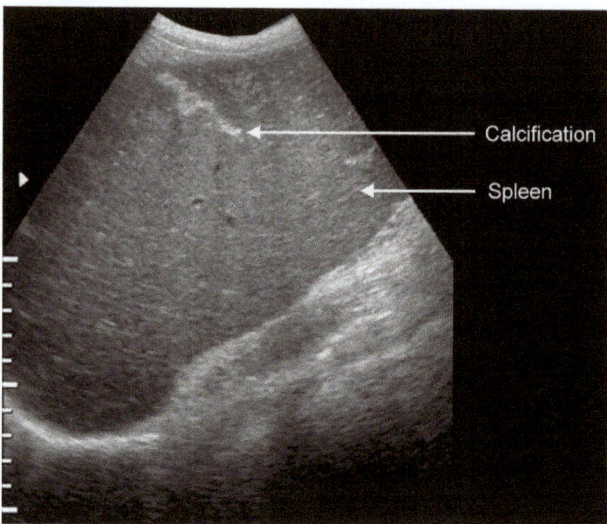

Fig. 4.4.2: US scan shows soft splenic calcification.

- Myelofibrosis—massive splenomegaly seen in myelofibrosis.
- Gamna-Gandy nodules—seen in portal hypertension.

Splenomegaly

Recanalization of paraumbilical vein, and other evidence of portal systemic collaterals such as linorenal shunts, splenic vein varices, or ascites.

CHAPTER 5

Pancreas

5.1 DIFFERENTIAL DIAGNOSIS OF CYSTIC PANCREATIC MASSES

Cystic tumors of pancreas arise from ductal epithelium mainly. The benign/inflammatory lesions may represent extra/intrapancreatic collection of pancreatic juice or even areas of necrosis caused by extravasation of such juices.

Classification

- Benign microcystic serous cystadenoma also known as glycogen rich cystic tumor.
- Malignant/premalignant macrocystic mucinous cystadenoma/carcinoma.

The differentiation between microcystic and macrocystic tumors is very important.

Microcystic	Macrocystic
Female equal male	Female more than male
Old	Young
Head	Body and tail
Numerous cysts >6	Few <6
Small cysts <2 cm	Large >2 cm
Benign	Malignant/premalignant
Central sunburst calcification in the fibrotic scar	Peripheral calcification
No internal nodule	Papillary projection in cavity may be present
Serous glycogen rich content	Mucin rich content present

Contd...

Contd...

Microcystic	Macrocystic
May even appear heterogeneous solid or spongy mass on USG	Has many USG appearances: a. Cyst with debris b. Cyst with solid c. Clear cyst d. Totally solid
Nonobstructive	Obstructive

- *Intraductal papillary tumors:*
    - Large, well-defined
    - Intraductal in origin
    - Young age; black; females
    - May have solid component
    - Calcification may be present
    - Low-grade malignancy
    - May send cystic secondaries
- *Cystic change in any other lesion:*
    - Cystic teratomas
    - Islet cell tumor (described in solid tumors)
    - Lymphoma (described in solid tumors)
    - Adenocarcinoma (described in solid tumors)
    - Sarcomas
- *Simple cysts and congenital cysts in conditions such as von Hippel-Lindau disease:*
    - Develop from embryonal ductal remnants
    - Usually uncomplicated in nature
    - May/may not have an echogenic lining of ductal epithelium
- *Retention cyst:* Any condition causing obstruction of large or small ducts leads to

formation of small cysts of multiple sizes due to pooling of fluid in ducts.
- *Pseudocyst:*
  - Most common cystic lesion of pancreas
    1. Encapsulated peri-pancreatic or remote fluid collection which develop after 4 weeks of onset of pancreatitis
    2. Appears as a cystic collection associated with changes of pancreatitis in any part of abdomen or intra-abdominal **(Figs. 5.1.1 and 5.1.2)**.

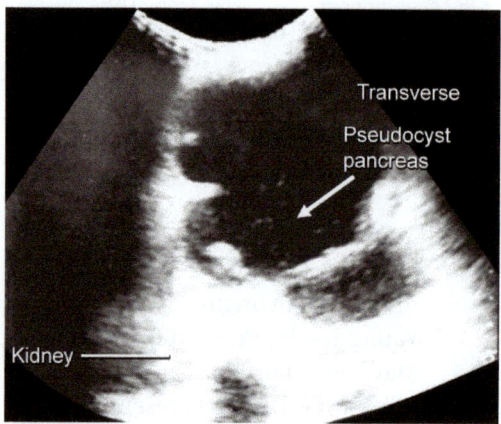

Fig. 5.1.1: Pseudocyst pancreas—a large multi-loculated collection seen in lesser sac with evidence of debris in it.

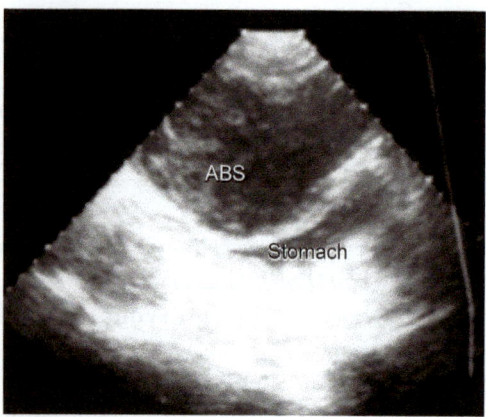

Fig. 5.1.2: Transverse scan of epigastrium show a large, well-defined rounded space-occupying lesion (SOL) with internal contents and posterior enhancement in the lesser sac. (ABS: abscess)

- Internal debris, gas or thickened wall may be seen due to secondary infection or intervention.
- *Mucinous ductal ectasia:*
  - Old; men, heavy smokers
  - Mainly head of pancreas
  - Viscid secretions fill up the ducts leading to their dilatation, pancreatitis such as symptoms and pathology
  - Patients of cystic fibrosis have similar features on ultrasound.
- *Lymphangioma:*
  - Multicystic lesion
  - Diagnosis always pathological.
- *Hemangioma:*
  - Complex cystic lesion with or without Doppler signal, with normal surrounding parenchyma.
- *Cavernous transformation of portal vein:*
  - Characterized by multiple, tortuous serpentine, cystic lesions in portal, periportal and head of pancreas areas **(Fig. 5.1.3)**.
  - Diagnosis helped by color Doppler examination showing multidirectional flow.
- *Vascular aneurysms and pseudoaneurysm:*
  - Celiac artery

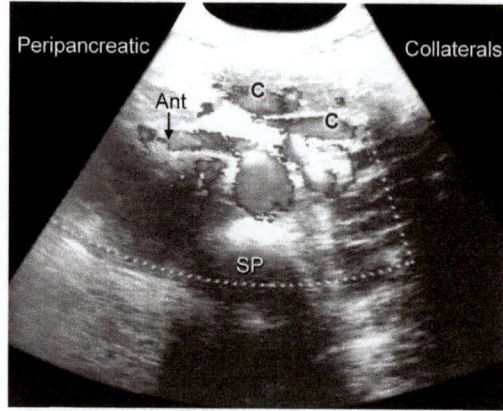

Fig. 5.1.3: Peripancreatic collaterals. (C: collaterals; SP: spinous process)

- Hepatic artery
- Superior mesenteric artery
- Splenic artery.

All are seen as cystic structures in relation to various parts of pancreas. Internal flow and pulsatality may be noted on gray scale while color Doppler examination is diagnostic.

5.2 DIFFERENTIAL DIAGNOSIS OF SOLID/COMPLEX LESION

Classification

Primary

- *Nonendocrine:*
  - Adenosquamous carcinoma
  - Adenocarcinoma **(Figs. 5.2.1 to 5.2.5)**
  - Adenoma
  - Acinar cell tumor
  - Epithelial tumor
  - Connective tissue tumor
  - Pancreaticoblastoma
  - Inflammatory pancreatic masses
- *Endocrine:*
  - Gastrinoma
  - Glucogenoma
  - Insulinoma
  - VIPoma
  - Somatostatinoma.

Secondary

- *Metastasis:*
  - Rare, usually direct invasion by stomach
  - Other sites are breast, melanoma, ovary, lung
  - Multiple, small, hypoechoic lesion.
- *Lymphoma:*
  - NHL histiocytic
  - May appear as a single nodule, multiple nodular lesions, infiltrative heterogeneous lesion increasing the pancreatic bulk.

Adenocarcinoma

- Male; old
- Head most commonly involved, tail least common
- About 20% multifocal
- Appears as a hypoechoic, heterogeneous mass lesion on USG having ill-defined/irregular margins
- Calcification is absent
- Necrosis and formation of retention cysts is rare. There is smooth dilatation of main pancreatic duct and its side branches
- Loss of peripancreatic planes and planes with mesenteric vessels
- Dilated PS P DV—venous involvement
- Gastrocolic vein >5 mm—splenic vein involvement.

Pancreaticoblastoma

- Solid pediatric neoplasm
- Nesidioblastosis is a tumor-like condition of pediatric pancreas characterized by diffuse proliferation and persistence of primitive ductal epithelium. It is associated with hypoglycemia and Beckwith-Wiedemann syndrome.

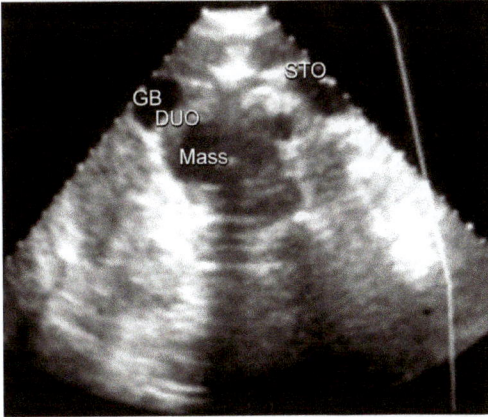

Fig. 5.2.1: A well-defined rounded hypoechoic space-occupying lesion (SOL) seen in the region of head of pancreas. Fine-needle aspiration cytology revealed it to be a well-differentiated adenocarcinoma. (GB: gallbladder; STO: stomach; DUO: duodenum)

94 Differential Diagnosis in Ultrasound

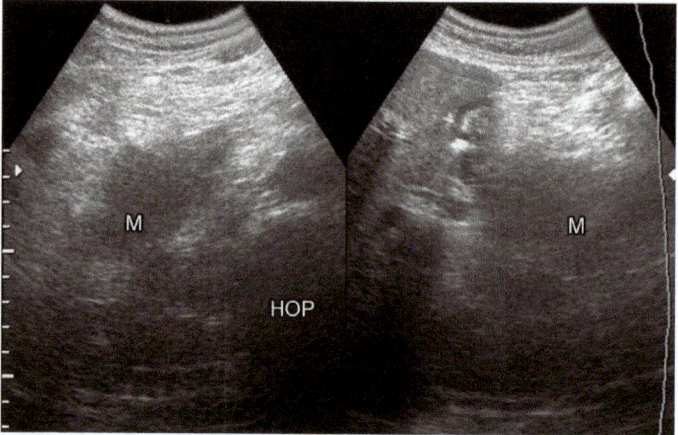

Fig. 5.2.2: US scans show focal pancreatitis of head presenting as focal mass. (HOP: head of pancreas; M: mass)

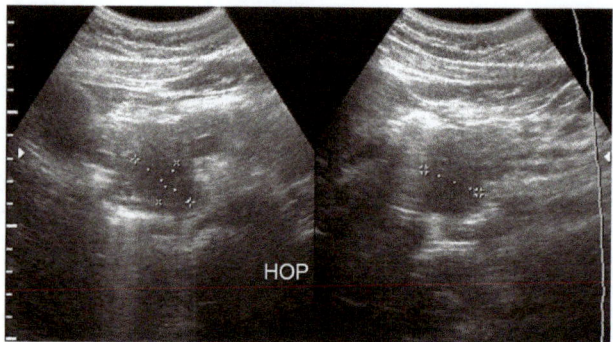

Fig. 5.2.3: US scans show phlegmon in head of pancreas. (HOP: head of pancreas)

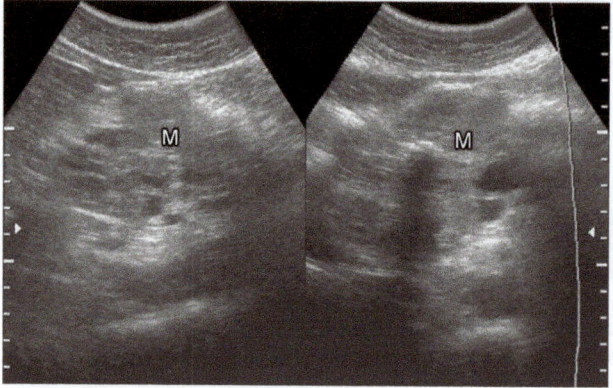

Fig. 5.2.4: US scans show microcystic adenoma in head of pancreas. (M: mass)

Inflammatory Pancreatic Mass

- Infiltrative mass like **(Fig. 5.2.6)**
- Fat planes with vessels present
- Extensive perilesional fat stranding
- Moderate irregular dilatation of pancreatic duct
- Smooth, gradual dilatation of common bile duct
- Side branches are normal.

Insulinoma

- Head more common site
- Size <2 cm
- Single > multiple
- About 10% malignant
- About 10% metastasize
- Calcification rare
- Hypervascular on Doppler.

Gastrinoma

- Body and tail more common
- Large size
- Multiple > solitary
- About 60% malignant

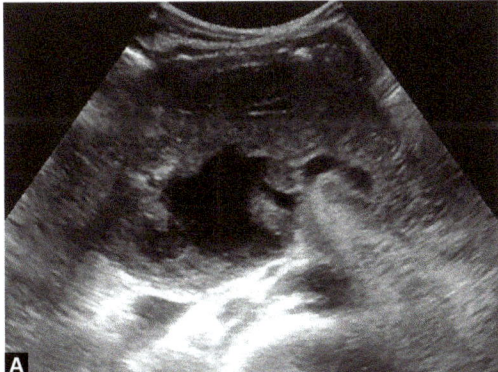
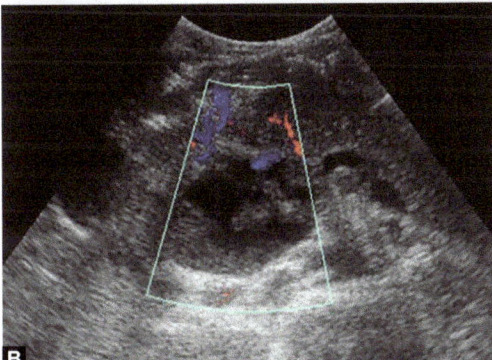

Figs. 5.2.5A and B: US scans showing heteroechoic necrotic mass in head of pancreas showing no vascularity in a case of carcinoma head of pancreas.

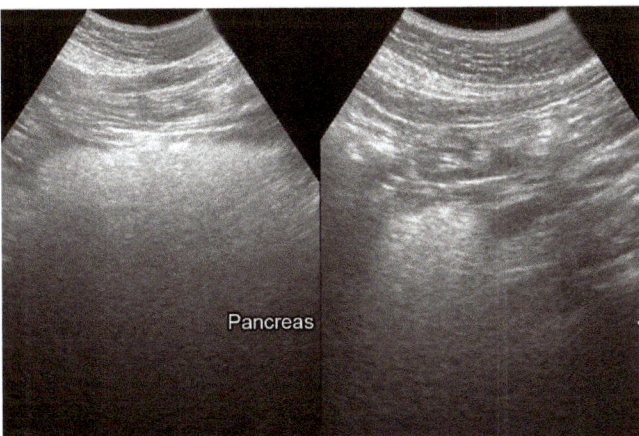

Fig. 5.2.6: US scans show diffuse fatty infiltration of pancreas.

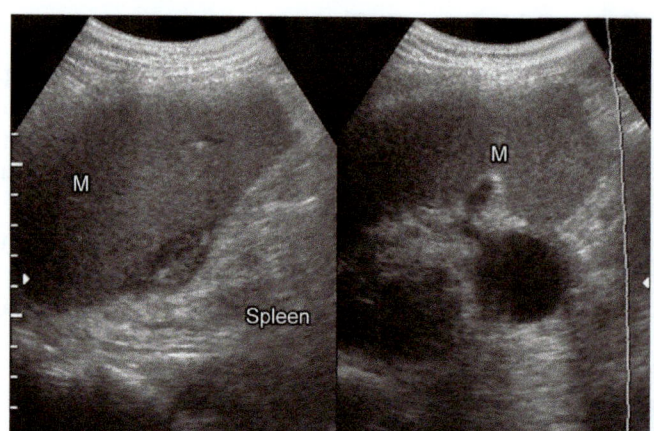

Fig. 5.2.7: US scans show cystic mass in tail of pancreas at the splenic hilum in a case of chronic inflammatory mass. (M: mass)

- Sends many secondaries
- Calcification most common
- Hypovascular.

VIPoma

- Iso/hyperechoic on USG with a peripheral hypoechoic halo
- Cystic change **(Fig. 5.2.7)** and calcification common
- Contour deformed
- Intraoperative USG is the gold standard
- Never do a biopsy as hormones may suddenly increase.

Somatostatinoma

- Heteroechoeic on USG
- Frequently seen in pancreas or periampullary region
- Present with hepatic metastases.

Nonfunctioning Islet Cell Tumors

- Benign remain obscure
- Malignant ones are large
- Calcification are more common
- Mainly in head
- More common
- Present as a mass of variable echogenicity on USG.

CHAPTER 6

Gastrointestinal Tract

6.1 ULTRASOUND DIFFERENTIAL DIAGNOSIS OF GASTROINTESTINAL TRACT

Esophagus (Endoscopic Ultrasound)

On ultrasound, gastrointestinal tract (GIT) has got different features as illustrated in **Figures 6.1.1A to C**.

Esophageal Tumors

Endoscopic ultrasound is a highly accurate modality for imaging the different layers of esophageal wall and localization of the lesions.

Epithelial Tumors

- *Esophageal carcinoma*: Seen on U/S as (a) poorly reflective tissue, (b) are homogeneous when small and more disorganized, (c) when large, there is loss of appearance of gut wall with spread into different layers
  - EUS is fairly accurate in assessment of extent/depth of spread of tumor as well as longitudinal spread
  - Specificity of diagnosing regional nodal metastases and for diagnosing recurrence at anastomotic site
- *Papillomas*: Small squamous tumors, usually single. On US appears as a mass projecting into the lumen with rounded surface
- *Adenomas*: Can be pedunculated; have predilection for lower esophagus. Appears sonologically as sessile or pedunculated hypoechoic masses.

Intramural Lesions

Endoscopic ultrasound has a potentially greater role in these lesions as overlying mucosa is normal.
- Leiomyomas are the most common intramural lesions. On US it is seen as a poorly,

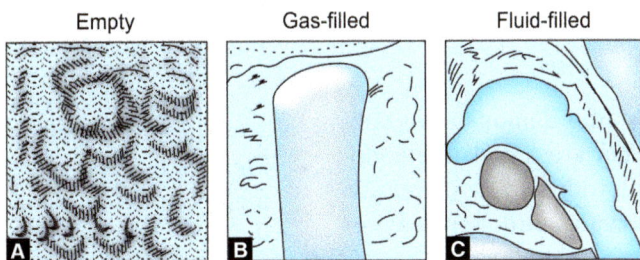

Figs. 6.1.1A to C: Gut can have a number of different manifestations. (A) when empty, there is an echo-free wall around and echogenic center; (B) When gas-filled, there is acoustic shadowing; (C) When fluid-filled, one may be able to make out the haustral markings of the colon or valvulae conniventes of the small bowel in the wall of the fluid-filled bowel.

echogenic mass continuous with the layer of muscularis propria. It may bulge the lumen when large
  - Not seen below 20 yr, may be single or multiple and can calcify
- Fibromas, hemangiomas, lymphangiomas are other benign intramural lesions. Hemangiomas and lymphangiomas show tortuous cystic spaces with color flow in hemangiomas
- Cystic lesions—congenital foregut duplication cysts—often localized, but may extend all along the esophagus
  - Mucus retention cysts—generally smaller. Both of these appear as cystic, echo-free well-defined lesions beneath the mucosal layer. Duplication cysts often contain debris.

Inflammatory Conditions/ Infections

Nonspecific wall thickening with preserved structure of layers.

Differentiation of Primary and Secondary Achalasia (Pseudoachalasia)

Endoscopic ultrasound aids differentiation of secondary achalasia due to malignancy by showing submucosal infiltration of gastroesophageal junction and cardia with evidence of growth.

Submucosal Varices

Endoscopic ultrasound demonstrates submucosal varices that are not visible endoscopically in patients with portal hypertension and identifies azygos and hemiazygos connections.

On US, varices are seen as dilated tortuous venous channels with color flow in submucosal region (**Fig. 6.1.2**).

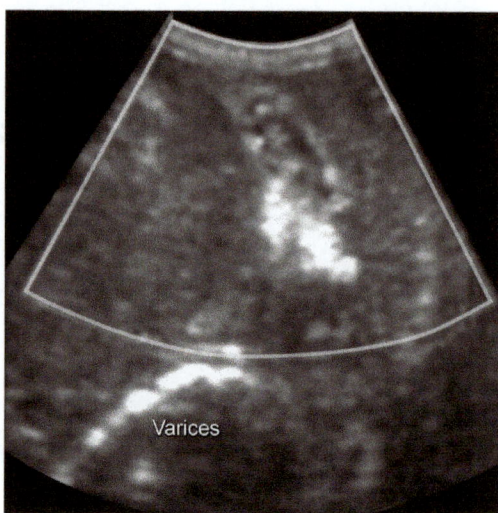

Fig. 6.1.2: Tortuous varices at gastroesophageal junction.

6.2 STOMACH

Thickening of Gastric Wall

Normal stomach wall measures 3–5 mm in thickness when distended.

Thickening >1 cm is usually due to malignancy.
- *Gastric carcinoma* (**Figs. 6.2.1 and 6.2.2**): Initially seen as localized thickening of the inner wall with hypoechoic soft tissue lesion

  With progression, there is loss of layered structure with infiltration of muscularis propria, eventually producing circumferential thickening
- *Gastric lymphoma* (**Fig. 6.2.3**):
  - Hypoechoic wall thickening >4 cm or large hypoechoic ulcerated masses
  - Transpyloric spread
  - Extensive lymphadenopathy
- *Metastases:* Usually from breast and melanoma appear as hypoechoic well-defined masses with ulceration which appears as bright foci with ring down artifacts. Associated ascites, gut serosal nodules, omental and peritoneal nodules may be positive

Gastrointestinal Tract

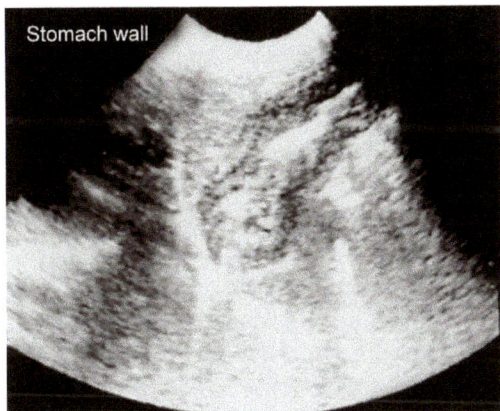

Fig. 6.2.1: Coronal scan showing thickened stomach wall in the region of the fundus in a case of carcinoma stomach.

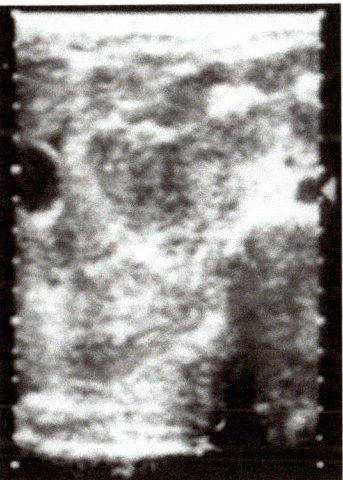

Fig. 6.2.3: A small hypoechoic lesion is seen (shown by cursor) suggestive of lymph node.

On US, there is nonspecific thickening of the gastric wall.

6.3 GASTRIC DILATATION

Mechanical Obstruction

- Malignancy growth involving pylorus and antropyloric regions may cause gastric outlet obstruction
  - Duodenal, pancreatic malignancy may cause duodenal obstruction and gastric dilatation, history is shorter, history of weight loss, hematomas
  - US may show polypoidal tumors growing into the lumen **(Fig. 6.3.1)**
  - There may be annular carcinomas with concentric thickening of the stomach
  - Extrinsic malignancies/masses may be seen involving the stomach
- Fibrosis secondary to ulceration, long history of dyspepsia, US—ulcers may be seen as echogenic foci with ring down artefacts due to entrapped air
- Volvulus—acutely painful condition with vomiting. Meal study is diagnostic. It may occur as an isolated lesion or combined with obstruction due to adhesive bands

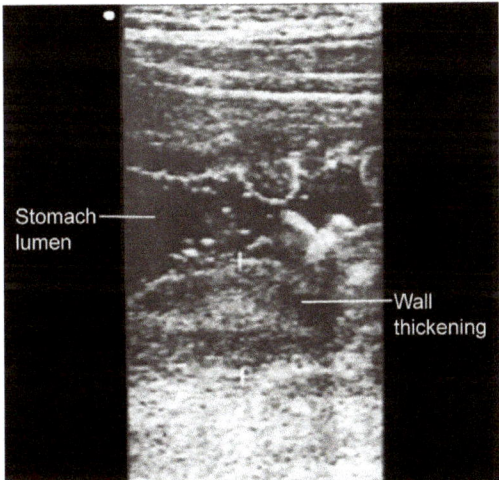

Fig. 6.2.2: Anterior and posterior wall of stomach irregularly thickened in a case of linitis plastica.

- Ménétrier's disease—disease of adult males. There is glandular hyperplasia with marked mucosal and submucosal thickening
  - EUS aids in diagnosis by showing sparing of muscularis propria and serosal layers
- Granulomatous gastritis, e.g. tuberculosis, syphilis, Crohn's disease, sarcoidosis and fungal infections.

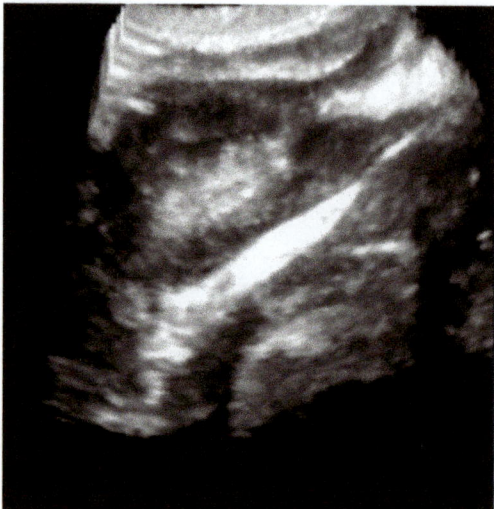

Fig. 6.3.1: 3D US scan shows adenocarcinoma of pyloric antrum.

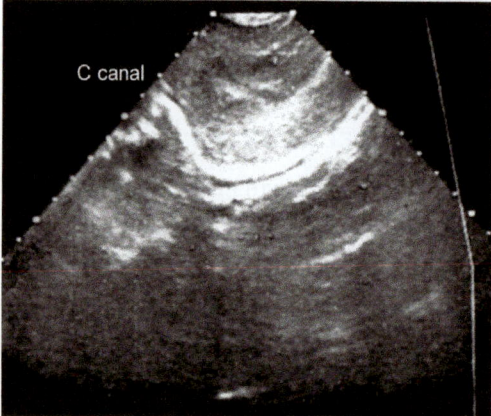

Fig. 6.3.2: Infantile hypertrophic pyloric stenosis. The total length of the C-shaped canal is 24 mm. The diameter of the antrum is 15 mm. The muscle thickness is 10 mm.

- It is often associated with congenital anomalies of the mesentery and malrotation
- US may show a dilated stomach with breaking at the point of twist. Stomach appears as a spherical viscus displaced up and to the left. Distal small bowel is collapsed. There may be free fluid associated with it

- *Hypertrophic pyloric stenosis:*
  - Adult—infantile. Hypertrophic pyloric stenosis (**Figs. 6.3.2 and 6.3.3**). Males 2-6 weeks. Hypoechoic thickening of the muscle of pylorus >3 mm, elongated pyloric canal >1.5 cm
  - Stasis of food contents in stomach for longer direction. Hyperperistalsis of stomach
    Adult—stomach wall is thickened >1 cm with, hypoechoic wall (**Figs. 6.3.4A and B**)
  - Extensive food residue in stomach hyperperistaltic stomach
  - Proximal small bowel obstruction
  - Shows dilated duodenum/jejunum.

Paralytic Ileus

- Postoperative
- Drugs—anticholinergics
- Metabolic—uremia, hypokalemia.
  There is aperistalsis of almost all bowel loops, including colon with dilated bowel.

Gas in Stomach Wall

Seen as linear echogenic foci with dirty shadowing in gastric wall.
- *Interstitial gastric emphysema:*
  - Peptic ulcer seen as defect in mucosal layer (by EUS) or as highly reflective focus in wall
  - Postgastroscopy
  - Necrotizing enterocolitis—On US, dilated loops of bowel, ascites, gas in portal veins may be present
  - Raised intragastric pressure due to gastric obstruction and distension
- *Emphysematous gastritis:*
  - Due to gas-forming organisms in stomach wall
    There is severe pain, hematemesis
  - Diabetes
  - Alcohol abuse

Gastrointestinal Tract

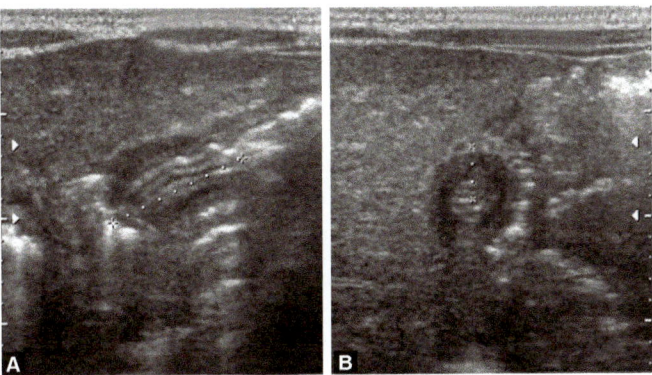

Figs. 6.3.3A and B: US scans show hypertrophic pyloric stenosis in an infant.

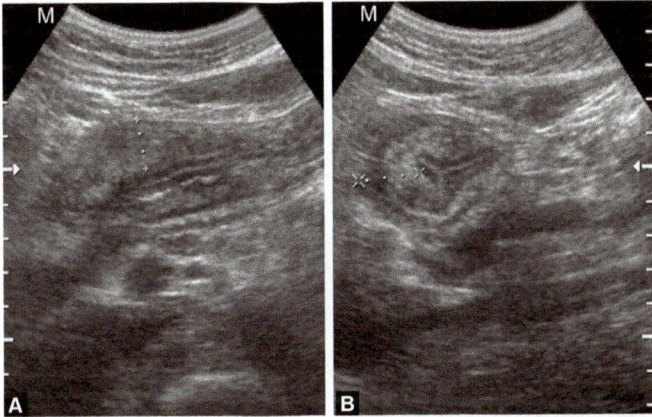

Figs. 6.3.4A and B: US scans show hypertrophic gastric wall in an adult (M: mass)

- Corrosive ingestion.

Ultrasound shows air in stomach wall as echogenic foci.

Bezoars

Masses of foreign material in the stomach as after ingestion of undigestible organic substances or hairs (Trichobezoar). US shows intraluminal density with intense distal acoustic shadowing.

6.4 DUODENUM

Dilatation of duodenum (double bubble sign) in pediatric ultrasound due to dilated stomach and duodenum.

Mechanical Obstruction

- Bands—most frequent cause of neonatal duodenal obstruction. Band of Ladd may cause compression of duodenum
  - US—there is linear abrupt cut-off of the dilated stomach and duodenum at the site of compression by band with distal normal or collapsed bowel. Associated with malrotation and midgut volvulus
- Atresia, webs, stenosis, often associated with Down's syndrome, US may be able to show the cause in atresia, the distal bowel will be completely collapsed
  - In duodenal stenosis, small amount of fluid will pass into the distal bowel which may thus be visualized

- Annular pancreas—enlarged pancreatic head on USG with double bubble sign
  - Clinically child presents as persistent vomiting, abdominal pain, jaundice (50%)
- Superior mesenteric artery syndrome: Narrowing of angle between SMA and aorta to 10-22ºC (Normal—45-65º, and abrupt change in caliber distal to compression
- Distal small bowel obstruction due to thickening of duodenal wall **(Fig. 6.4.1)**/volvulus
- Paralytic ileus particularly due to pancreatitis associated with dilated small and large bowel
- Malrotation with volvulus—malrotation implies incomplete rotation of bowel. This gives rise to symptoms of associated band of Ladd and shortening of mesenteric attachments. On US, duodenojejunal junction is displaced medially and downward and cecum medially and upward
  - Superior mesenteric vein lies medial towards left of the SMA
  - There is dilatation of gut.

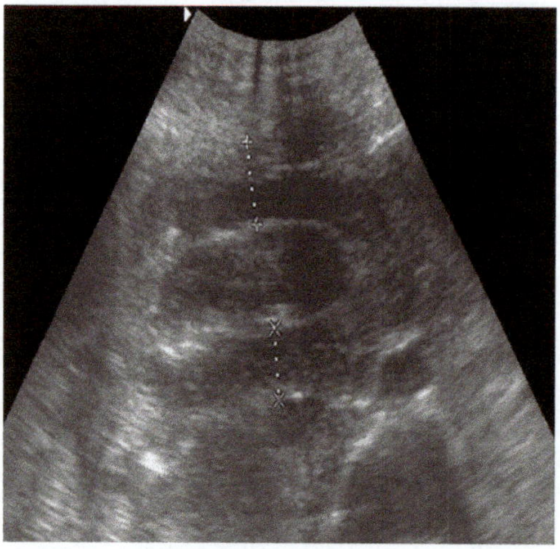

6.5 SMALL BOWEL AND COLON

Dilated Small Bowel (Figs. 6.5.1 and 6.5.2)

- Mechanical obstruction—dilated large bowel US can tell the approximate level of obstruction because there is dilatation proximal to the obstruction. There is accumulation of large quantities of fluid and/or gas with hyperperistalsis

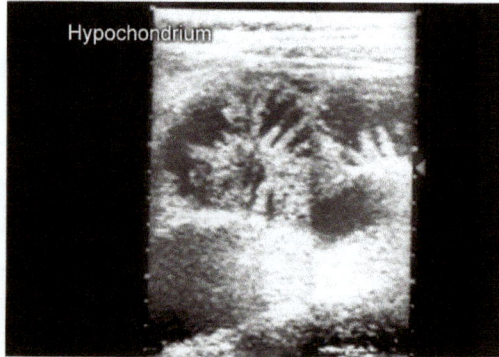

Fig. 6.5.1: Dilated fluid-filled jejunal loops: Valvulae conniventes are well seen.

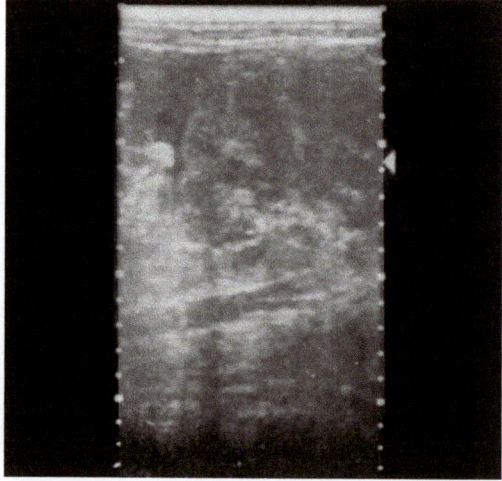

Fig. 6.5.2: Matted bowel loop: Clumped small bowel loops are seen in right iliac fossa (RIF) with surrounding free fluid in a case of abdominal tuberculosis.

Fig. 6.4.1: Extensive thickening of the duodenal wall (in calipers) by lymphomatous infiltration in lymphoma. Thickening was in continuation to stomach wall thickening.

- Paralytic ileus—dilated fluid-filled hypo or aperistaltic bowel loops involving almost whole of the bowel (small and large)
- Iatrogenic—post-vagotomy and gastrectomy due to rapid emptying of stomach contents
- Ischemia—thickened bowel loops with free fluid, lack of color flow on Doppler imaging
- Extensive small bowel resection—compensatory dilatation and thickening of folds.

Thickening of Terminal Ileum and/or Cecum

Inflammatory/Infective

- Tuberculosis—most common cause in Indian population. Continuity of involvement, with cecum and ascending colon can occur **(Fig. 6.5.3)**
  - Cecum is predominantly involved, associated mesenteric thickening, lymph nodes, ascites, omental cake formation
- Amebic typhlitis—thickening of terminal ileum and/or cecum with ameboma formation with lump in right iliac fossa. Presence of cysts of *E. histolytica* in stool **(Fig. 6.5.4)**
- Actinomycosis—very rare, predominantly cecum

- Crohn's disease
- Ulcerative colitis due to backwash ileitis.

Neoplastic

- Lymphoma—hypoechoic wall thickening, lymph nodes ±
- Carcinoid—most ileal carcinoids originate in distal ileum, are malignant if >2 cm cecum may be involved
- Metastasis—malignant melanoma and lung and breast tumors are the most common sites
- Ischemic—acute severe pain in abdomen, nonstratified thickened bowel wall absent, barely visible color flow.

Pseudokidney Sign (Target Sign)

Normal bowel wall thickness in nondistended state is 5 mm and 3 mm in distended state. When bowel is thickened **(Fig. 6.5.4)**, there is formation of pseudokidney sign **(Figs. 6.5.5 and 6.5.6)** due to central highly reflective contents and hypoechoic surrounding wall.

Causes

- Tumors
  - Adenocarcinoma—most common GI malignancy, colon is a very common site **(Figs. 6.5.7 and 6.5.8)**.

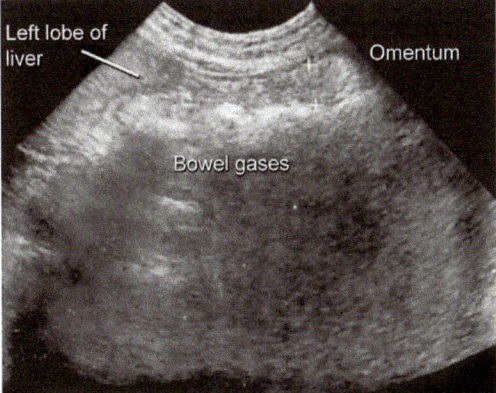

Fig. 6.5.3: Thickened omentum (1.6 cm) in a case of abdominal Koch's.

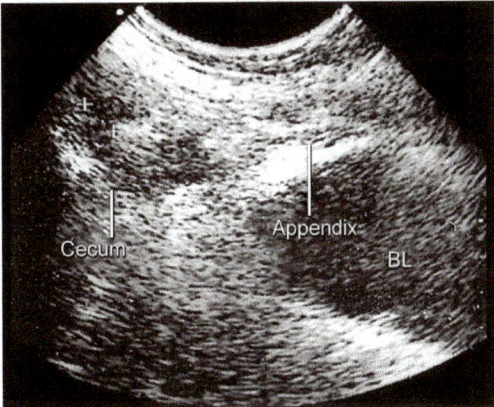

Fig. 6.5.4: Inflammatory thickening of cecum and appendix is seen in a case of typhilitis. (BL: bladder)

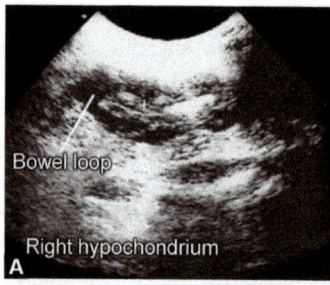
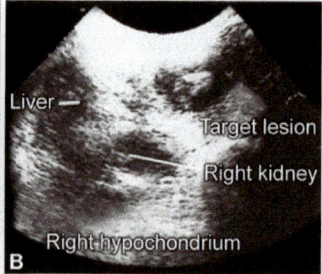

Figs. 6.5.5A and B: Target lesion: Longitudinal and transverse scan showing bowel thickening.

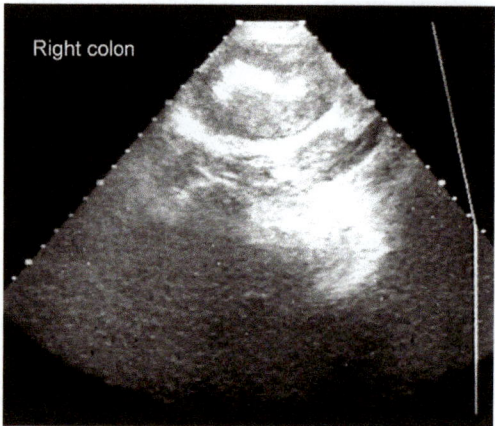

Fig. 6.5.6: Pseudokidney sign seen in a case of bowel thickening.

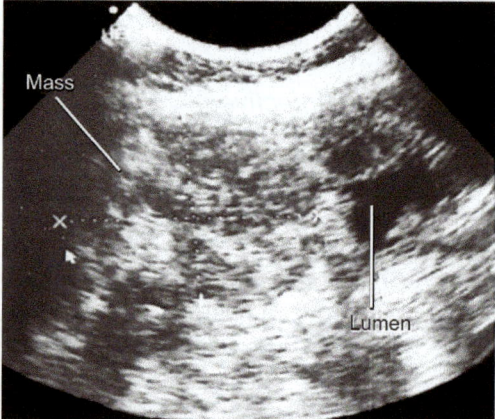

Fig. 6.5.7: Carcinoma colon—a large soft tissue mass, predominantly hypoechoic is seen arising from the hepatic flexure.

It can be exophytic, annular or intraluminal. There may be symmetric or asymmetric wall thickening which is usually hypoechoic lymph nodes, metastasis may be present.
- Lymphoma—hypoechoic wall thickening lymphadenopathy
- Leiomyosarcoma—mainly exophytic, outwards ulceration and cavitation is common, calcification may occur and is heterogeneous in echotexture
- Carcinoid
- Metastasis—known primary is present, other metastatic lesions
• Inflammatory
  - Tuberculosis—lymph nodes, mesenteric thickening ascites, etc. (**Figs. 6.5.9 to 6.5.14**)

- Crohn's disease—ultrasonographic features are:
  - Gut wall thickening—mostly concentric and quite marked. Involved gut appears rigid and fixed with no peristalsis
  - Strictures—appear as linear echogenic central area within a thickened bowel loop
  - Creeping fat—edema and fibrosis of adjacent mesentery forms a mass which creeps over the border of abdominal gut. On US, it appears as a hyperechoic mass effect or halo around the mesenteric border of gut. It causes separation of loops
  - Hyperemia—increased flow on Doppler

Gastrointestinal Tract

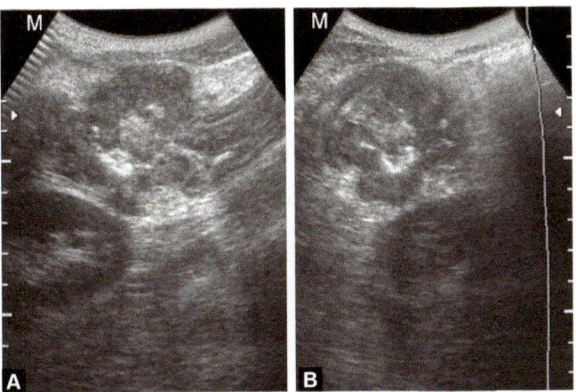

Figs. 6.5.8A and B: US scans show mass in ascending colon. (M: mass)

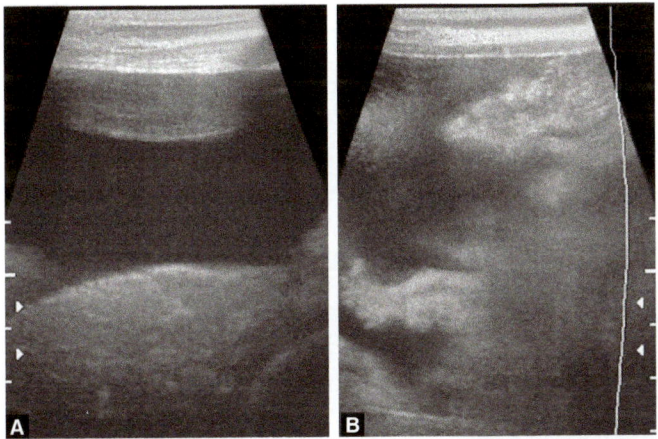

Figs. 6.5.9A and B: US scans show omental and peritoneal thickening with ascites in tubercular abdomen.

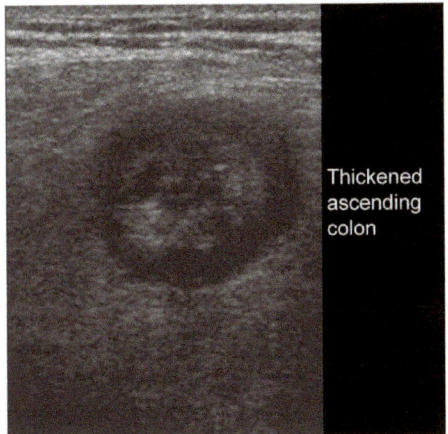

Fig. 6.5.10: Abdominal tuberculosis—circumferential thickening of the ascending colon with pericolic fat proliferation.

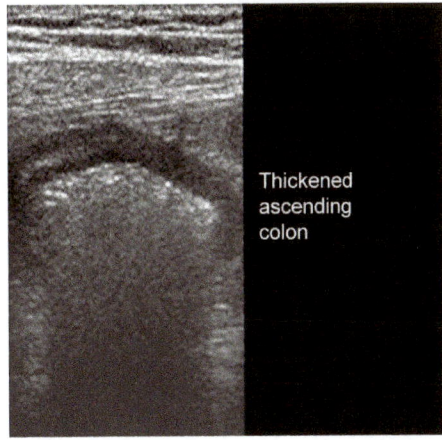

Fig. 6.5.11: Thickening of the ascending colon.

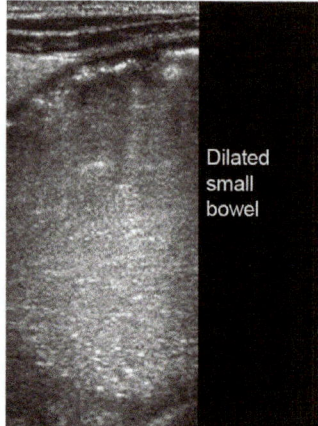

Fig. 6.5.12: Dilated small bowel loop with internal echogenic contents proximal to a stricture (not shown) in a case of abdominal tuberculosis.

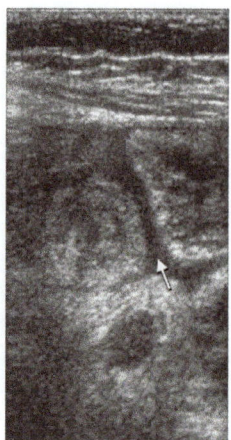

Fig. 6.5.14: Interbowel loop fluid (arrow). Also seen is a mesenteric lymph node—abdominal TB.

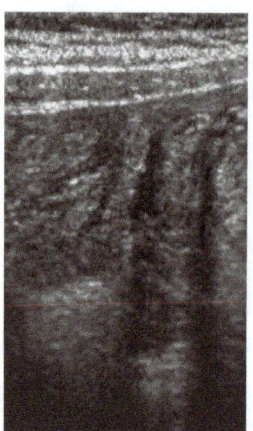

Fig. 6.5.13: Tubercular peritonitis—matted bowel loops giving 'sliced bread' appearance.

- Inflammatory conglomerate masses formed by clumps of matted bowel, mesentery, fat and lymph node
- Complex or fluid-filled phlegmons or abscess may be present
- Fissures in gut wall may be seen as linear echogenic areas penetrating into the wall
- Diverticular disease—segmental, concentric bowel wall thickening, echogenic foci within bowel wall due to air, localized collections, thickening of mesentery **(Fig. 6.5.15)**
- Chronic granulomatous diseases, e.g. syphilis, sarcoidosis, etc.
- Pseudomembranous colitis—thickening of colon wall with exaggerated haustra. Watery diarrhea is the most common symptom with fever and abdominal pain
- Appendicitis—dilated (>6 mm) tubular, noncompressible, aperistaltic blind-ended structure in right iliac fossa with localized fluid collection, probe tenderness, fever, vomiting, etc.

- Miscellaneous
  - Intussusception **(Figs. 6.5.16 and 6.5.17)**: Sonographic appearance of multiple concentric rings with features of intestinal obstruction
    - Invagination of a bowel segment into the next distal segment
    On US:
    - Multiple concentric rings due to layers of invagination bowel with attenuate echogenic and hypoechoic layers may be seen

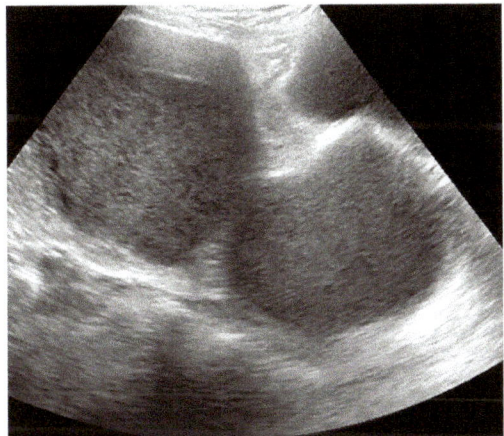

Fig. 6.5.15: Two duplication cyst in the peritoneal cavity.

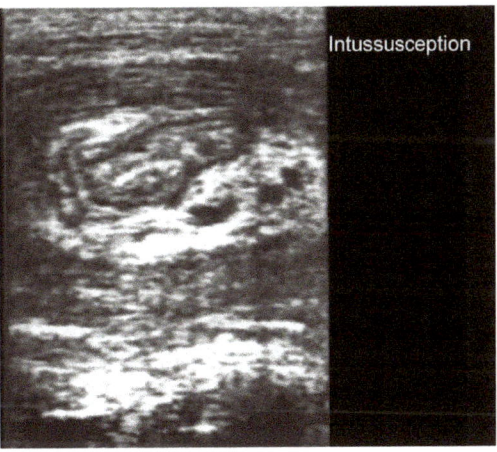

Fig. 6.5.16: Intussusception is seen as target sign—hypoechoic solid mass with a central echogenic component.

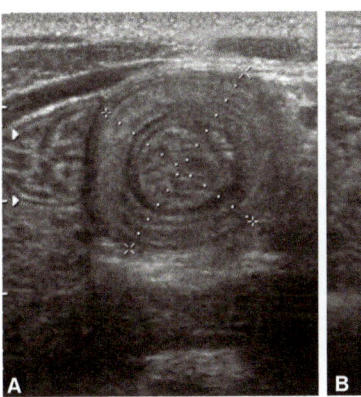 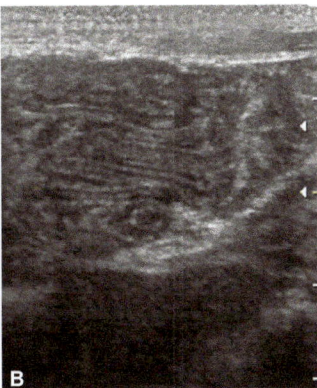

Figs. 6.5.17A and B: US scans show evidence of intussusception.

- Target sign with center echogenic and thick hypoechoic wall
- Longitudinal scan may show fork appearance

  The mesentery with the mesenteric vessels seen invaginate into the mass is a specific sign.
- Ischemia—due to thickening of bowel wall
- Amyloidosis—pathological evidence with immunohistochemical
- Radiation enteritis—history of radiation therapy

- Mimicks
  - Normal kidney in ectopic position—renal sinus is echogenic with surrounding kidney tissue
  - Multiple loops of fluid-filled bowel
  - Ovarian dermoid due to echogenic fat and surrounding fluid which is hypoechoic
  - Normal colon—surrounding wall with echogenic lumen
  - Gas in head of pancreas
  - Mesenteric lymph nodes—due to echogenic fatty intum
  - Gallstones in thick-walled gallbladder
  - Hemorrhage in bowel wall.

6.6 DIFFERENTIAL DIAGNOSIS OF ACUTE APPENDICITIS (APPENDICEAL LESIONS)

Acute Appendicitis (Figs. 6.6.1 to 6.6.3)

The underlying factor is obstruction of appendiceal lumen causing retention of secretions, increasing intraluminal pressure—compromising venous return—hypoxia and ischemia—gangrene and perforation.

US
- Blind-ended, aperistaltic tube arising from the tip of cecum with gut signature and diameter >6 mm
- Supportive evidence of inflamed perienteric fat, pericardial collection appendicolith.

Appendiceal Perforation (Figs. 6.6.2 to 6.6.9)

- Loculated pericecal fluid
- Phlegmon
- Abscess
- Prominent pericecal fat
- Circumferential loss of submucosal layer of appendix.

Appendicular Lump (Fig. 6.6.10)

Inflamed appendix (Fig. 6.6.11) is encased by inflamed bowel loops, mesentery, omentum, fluid and lymph nodes.

US
- An ill-defined mass heterogeneous in appearance with adherent hypoperistaltic thickened bowel
- Mesentery and omentum appear echogenic due to fat

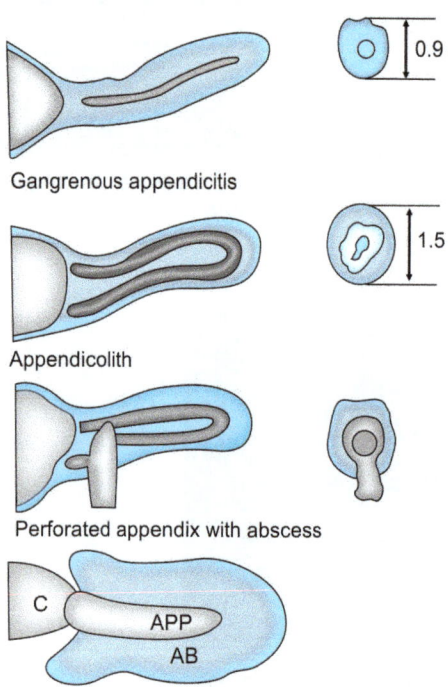

Fig. 6.6.1: Diagram showing the patterns adopted by the appendix during the various phases of development of appendicitis. (C: cecum; APP: appendix; AB: abscess)

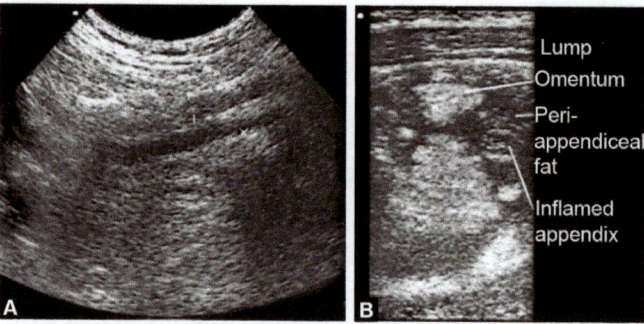

Figs. 6.6.2A and B: Longitudinal and transverse scans of right iliac fossa (RIF) show inflamed appendix, however, no periappendicular collection is seen.

Gastrointestinal Tract

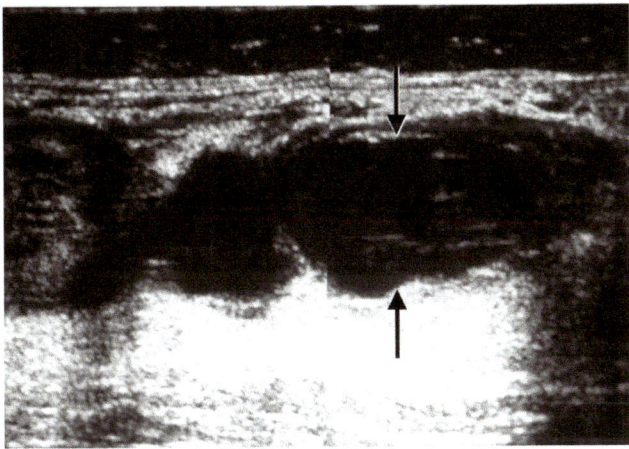

Fig. 6.6.3: Mucocele of the appendix (arrows).

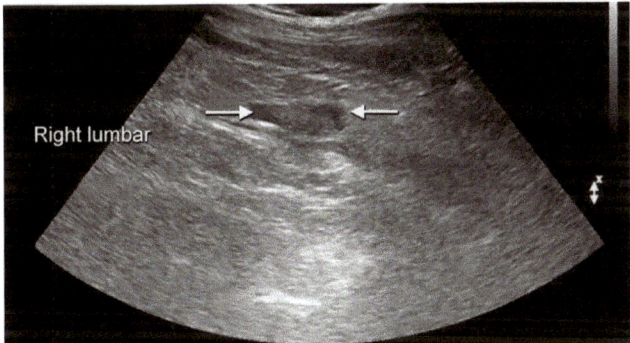

Fig. 6.6.4: Minimal loculated fluid collection in the right lumbar region in a case of suspected appendicular perforation.

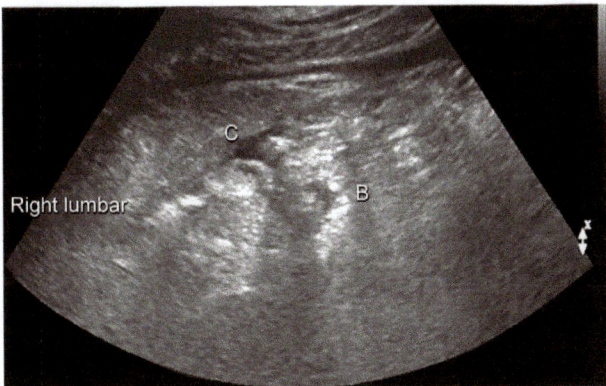

Fig. 6.6.5: Minimal loculated fluid collection in the right lumbar region with surrounding inflammation of mesentery in a case of suspected appendicular perforation. (C: cecum; B: bladder)

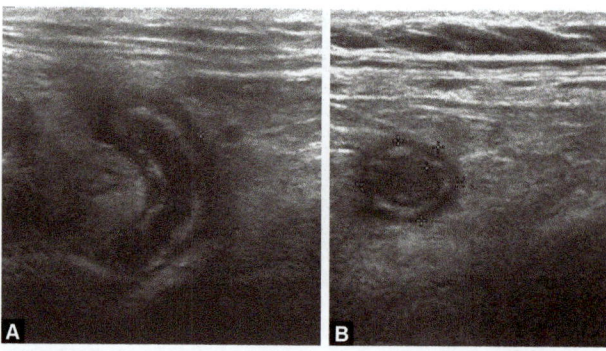

Figs. 6.6.6A and B: Thickened appendix with surrounding increased echogenic fat in a case of acute appendicitis.

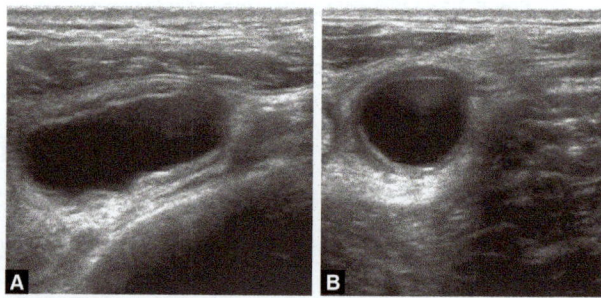

Figs. 6.6.7A and B: LS and TS of a case of mucocele of appendix—note the dilated anechoic lumen.

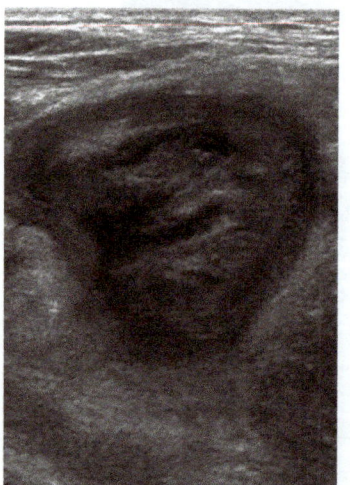

Fig. 6.6.8: Circumferential thickened cecal wall in case of appendicitis.

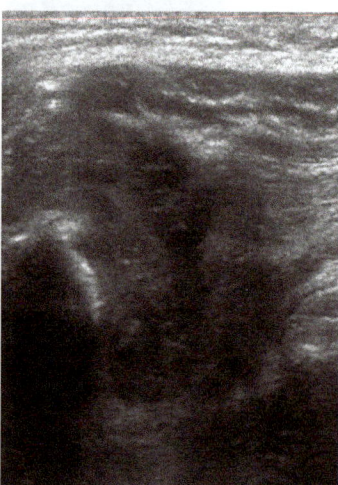

Fig. 6.6.9: Abscess in the right iliac fossa following perforation of inflamed appendix.

Gastrointestinal Tract

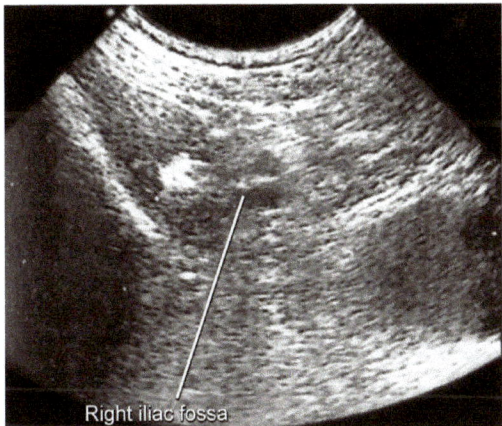

Fig. 6.6.10: Appendicular lump: Seen as an ill-defined complex SOL in the right iliac fossa. Inflamed appendix, periappendiceal fat and omentum are seen in the lump, adherent bowel loops are also seen.

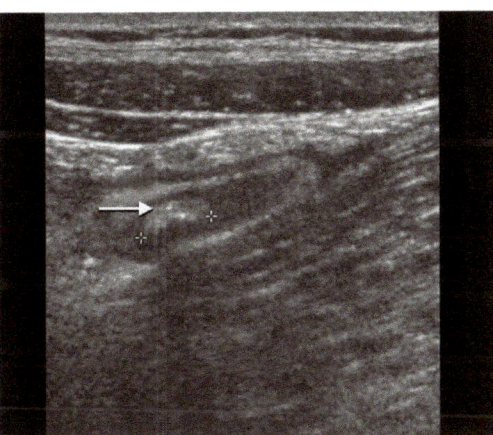

Fig. 6.6.11: A case of appendicitis—appendicolith (arrow) is also seen in the lumen.

- Loculated fluid collections and LN may be seen.

US Differential Diagnosis

Thickened terminal ileum shows peristalsis and is not blind-ended. It is compressible.

6.7 ROLE OF RECTAL ENDOSONOGRAPHY

- Staging of detected rectal carcinomas
  Rectal carcinoma arises from mucosal surface of the gut
  - Tumors appear as relatively hypoechoic masses that may distort the rectal lumen
  - Loss of continuity of different layers of rectal wall
  - Surface ulceration may be seen as echogenic foci with ring down artefact
  - LN appears as round or oval hypoechoic masses in perirectal fat
- Differentiates extrinsic, intramural and mucosal lesions
- Anal evaluation: To show integrity of sphincters with documentation of the degree and size of muscle defects.

CHAPTER 7

Retroperitoneum

RETROPERITONEAL PATHOLOGIES

- Most common manifestation of a retroperitoneal pathology is "Presence of a Mass"
- Sonographic signs apart from above that localize the mass and differentiate mass from pseudomass are:
  - Displacement of normal structures
  - Direct invasion of adjacent organ
  - Asymmetry of normal paired structures
  - Silhouetting of normal structures
  - Loss of retroperitoneal details.

7.1 DIFFERENTIAL DIAGNOSIS OF SOLID MASSES

Signs for Organ of Origin of Solid Masses in Retroperitoneum

Phantom sign: Mass completely surround and envelops the organ. The organ is typically not seen sonographically.

Embedded organ sign: The organ is embedded in the mass.

Beak sign or claw sign: The mass is arising from the organ man makes acute angle with the organ suggesting origin from the organ.

Prominent feeding artery sign: Hypervascular masses are often supplied by prominent feeding arteries which are usually identified on CT/MRI, but may be sometimes seen on ultrasound.

Lymphadenopathy

- Inferior to CT for this purpose as it is poorly reproducible and the image is degraded by gas
- *Size <1 cm = Normal:*
  - >1 cm, single = Suspicious abdominal nodes
  - >1 cm, multiple = Abnormal
  - >1.5 cm, single = Abnormal
  - >.6 cm = Abnormal-retrocrural
  - >1.5 cm = Pelvic
- *Signs of malignancy:*
  - Longitudinal to transverse ratio <2, i.e. round/oval
  - Eccentric cortical thickening Narrow/absent echogenic hilum
  - Displaced/distorted intranodal vessels
  - Intranodal avascular areas
- *Causes:*
  - Malignant deposits—testes, Gastrointestinal (GI), lung, pelvic tumors
  - Lymphoma **(Figs. 7.1.1A and B)**
    - Multiple hypoechoic masses **(Fig. 7.1.2)**
    - May fuse to form a mantle
    - May invade the retroperitoneum
- Infections.

Primary Retroperitoneal Tumors

- Adult mainly
- Mostly malignant
- Mostly mesenchymal
- More in men

Retroperitoneum

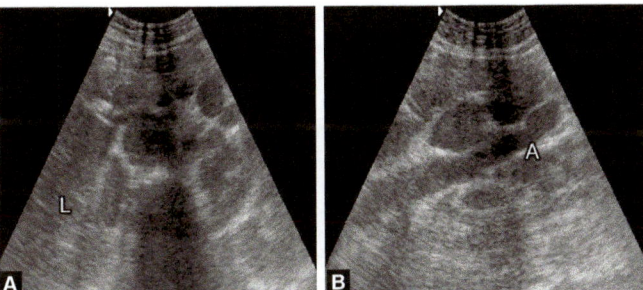

Figs. 7.1.1A and B: (A) TS and (B) LS—retroperitoneal lymphadenopathy in a case of lymphoma. (A: aorta; L: liver)

- *Main lesions are:*
  - Lipoma sarcoma—has echogenic fat
  - Leiomyosarcoma—hypoechoic
  - Malignant fibrous histiocytoma
  - *Teratoma:*
    - Fat fluid levels
    - Calcification
  - Germ cell tumors.

Secondary Deposits

- Intranodal **(Figs. 7.1.3 and 7.1.4)**
- Extranodal
- Direct invasion.

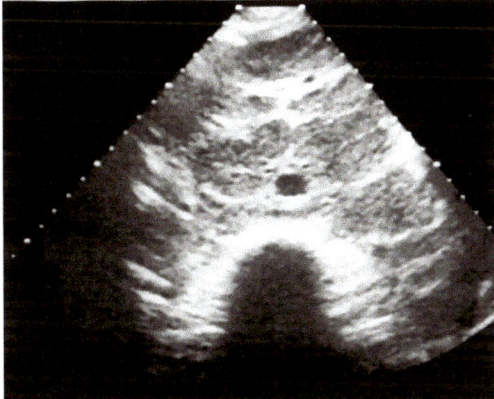

Fig. 7.1.2: Conglomerate lymph nodes mass seen in the preaortic region.

Retroperitoneal Fibrosis

- Also known as Ormond's disease
- *Causes:*
  - Idiopathic (68%)
  - Malignancies (8%) (stomach, lung, breast, colon, prostate, kidney), Methisergide (12%)
  - Crohn's disease
  - Riedel's struma
  - Sclerosing cholangitis
  - Radiotherapy
  - Aneurysm leak/surgery
  - Infection
  - Urine leak
  - Hypoechoic, smooth marginated homogeneous fibrous clumps are noted
  - Ureters medially deviated due to psoas abscess **(Figs. 7.1.5 to 7.1.8)**.

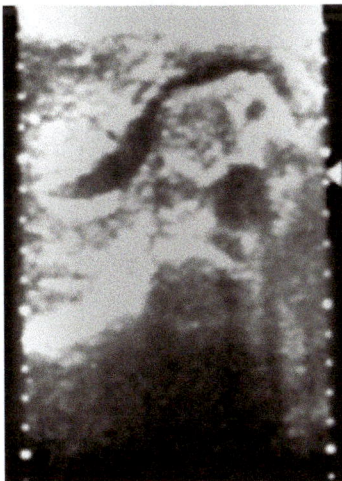

Fig. 7.1.3: A single rounded echogenic lumen seen anterior to the aorta. SMA is seen on the left side. PV is anterior to the LN. It was a metastatic LN from adenocarcinoma colon. (SMA: superior mesenteric artery; PV: portal vein; LN: lymph nodes)

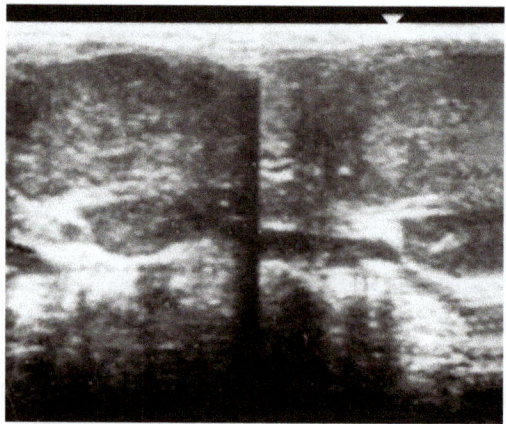

Fig. 7.1.4: A large ill-defined solid hypoechoic lesion seen anterior to the compressed aorta turned out to be a retroperitoneal sarcoma.

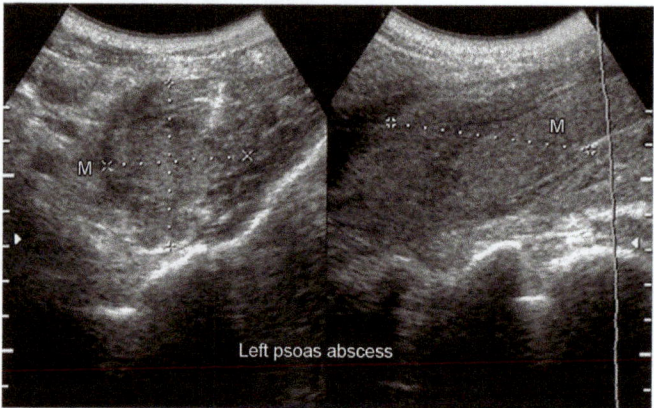

Fig. 7.1.5: US scans show psoas abscess in iliac fossa. (M: mass)

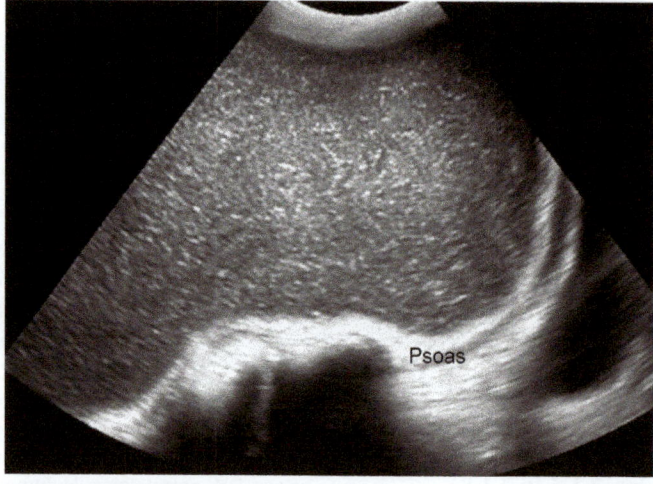

Fig. 7.1.6: A large psoas abscess filling the retroperitoneum and displacing the bowel loops.

Retroperitoneum

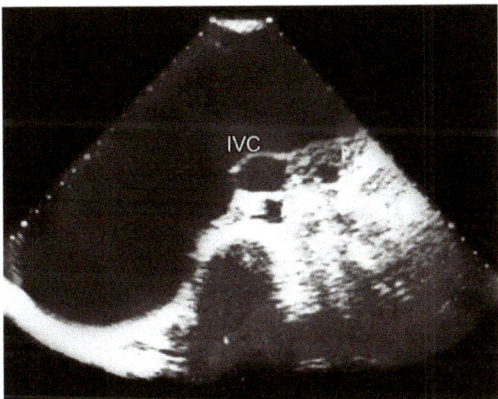

Fig. 7.1.7: A huge completely anechoic retroperitoneal cyst is seen in this transverse scan. (IVC: inferior vena cava).

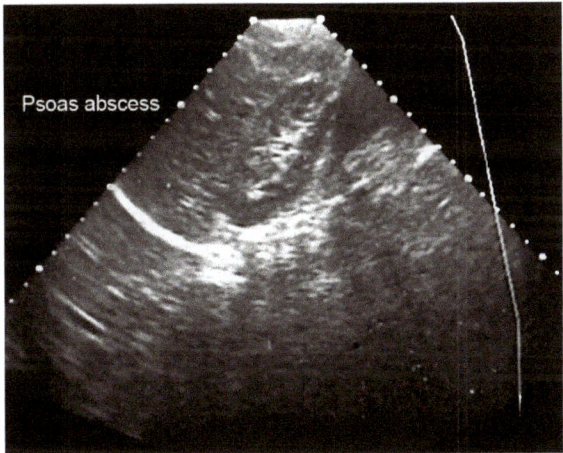

Fig. 7.1.8A: Psoas abscess—there is a hypoechoic collection in right psoas muscle.

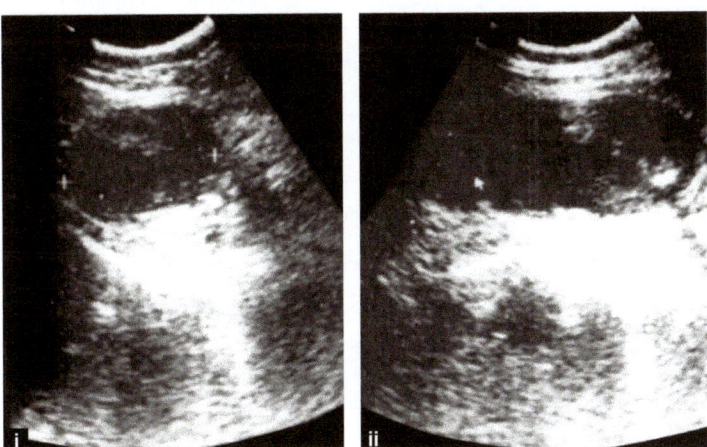

Fig. 7.1.8B: Psoas abscess—(i) transverse, (ii) longitudinal scan showing a collection in psoas muscle with evidence of internal echoes, thick posterior wall and calcification.

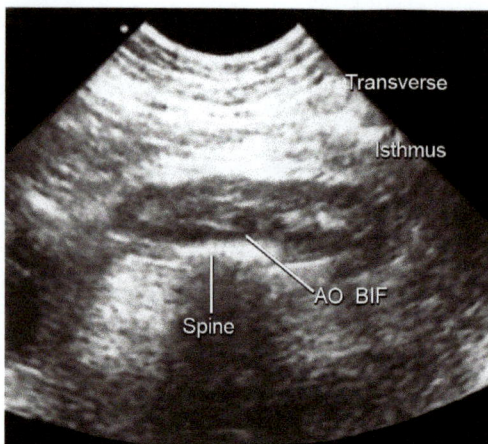

Fig. 7.2.1: Horseshoe kidney: Transverse scan shows the isthmus connecting the lower poles of the right and left kidneys anterior to the aorta. (AO BIF: aortic bifurcation)

7.2 DIFFERENTIAL DIAGNOSIS OF PSEUDOMASSES

- *Horseshoe kidney* **(Fig. 7.2.1):**
  - Intravenous pyelogram (IVP) diagnostic
  - Mild to moderate hydronephrosis
- *Ptotic kidney:*
  - Also called as floating or wandering kidney
  - Descent of kidney more than 5 cm or two vertebral levels when a person moves from supine to upright position
  - IVP diagnostic
- Low-lying pancreas
- Varix
- Extramedullary hematopoiesis
- Hematoma
- Duplication cyst of gut.

7.3 DIFFERENTIAL DIAGNOSIS OF CYSTIC LESIONS AND FLUID COLLECTION

- Primary retroperitoneal cysts
- *Lymphangioma:*
  - Congenital
  - Cyst with multiple thick septa or unilocular
- *Lymphoceles:*
  - Like simple cysts
  - Lateral to bladder within 3 cm of abdominal wall
  - Mostly postsurgical
- *Urinoma:*
  - Hypoechoic loculated collection
  - Perilesional fibrosis
  - Following obstruction, trauma, surgery
- Varix
- *Pancreatic pseudocyst:*
  - In any space but mostly anterior pararenal space
  - Definite evidence of pancreatitis present
- *Hematoma/hemorrhage:*
  - Due to trauma intervention, aneurysm, bleeding diathesis, tumor bleed
  - Heterogeneous fluid collection
  - Changing appearance with time
- *Infections:*
  - Psoas abscess in Pott's spine
  - Spread of infection from adjacent organ
  - Predisposed by diabetes, AIDS, trauma, surgery, alcohol.

CHAPTER 8

Renal

CAUSES OF LOCALIZED BULGE IN RENAL OUTLINE

- Dromedary hump
- Prominent septum of Bertin
- Hilar lip—hyperplasia of parenchyma adjacent to the renal hilum
- Pseudotumor in reflux nephropathy
- Renal cyst
- Renal tumor.

8.1 DIFFERENTIAL DIAGNOSIS OF RENAL PSEUDOTUMOR

- *Hypertrophied column of Bertin (HCB) (Fig. 8.1.1):*
  - A normal variant that occurs due to unresorption of polar parenchyma from one or both of the two subkidneys that fuse to form the normal kidney
  - Indentation of renal sinus laterally
  - Bordered by junctional parenchymal defects
  - Location at junction of upper and middle thirds
  - Continuous with renal cortex
  - Contains renal pyramids
  - Less than 3 cm in size
- *Renal duplication artifacts:*
  - Due to refraction of sound beam between the lower portion of spleen or liver and adjacent fat
  - Left; obese
  - Change transducer position; scan in deep inspiration
- *Fetal lobulations:*
  - Usually persist in all pediatric kidneys but may also be seen in 51% of adult kidneys
  - No associated cortical loss is noted
- *Compensatory hypertrophy:*
  - Diffuse—in cases of contralateral nephrectomy, renal agenesis, renal hypoplasia, dysplasias, atrophy
    - Generalized renal involvement
  - *Focal/nodular:*
    - When residual island of normal tissue hypertrophy in an otherwise diseased kidney, e.g. reflux nephropathy
    - Nodular areas of hypertrophy resembling mass lesions are seen

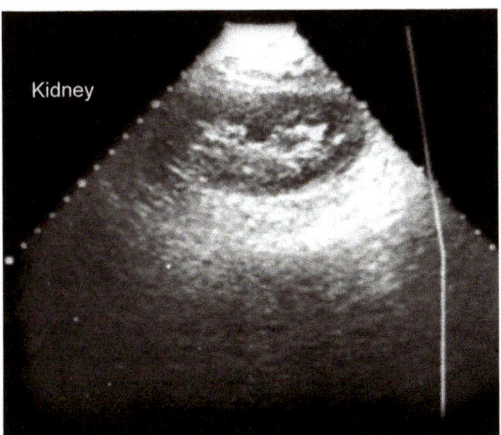

Fig. 8.1.1: Pseudotumor—the pelvicalyceal (PC) system is indented by a mass isoechoic to the cortex—hypertrophied column of Bertin.

- *Renal malakoplakia:*
  - Cortical and medullary granulomatous masses of the Hansemann's giant cells containing Michaelis-Gutmann inclusion bodies are seen
  - *E. coli, Klebsiella*
  - Multifocal masses, enlarging the kidney, bilateral in 50%
  - Masses are hypoechoic and distort the central renal sinus
- *Xanthogranulomatous pyelonephritis:*
  - A chronic suppurative renal infection leading to destruction of renal parenchyma and replacement of it with lipid laden macrophages
  - Unilateral, diffuse/segmental/focal
  - 70% have a staghorn calculus
  - Proteus, *E. coli*
  - Focal/segmental varieties are difficult to differentiate from renal abscess or tumor
- *Vascular malformations and aneurysm:* Color Doppler is the helping investigation
- *Parasitic infection:* Hydatid, filaria, schistosoma
- *Fungal infection: Candida* forming fungal balls.

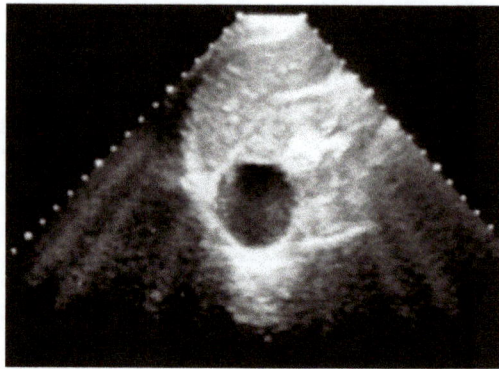

Fig. 8.2.1: Simple cortical cyst—a well-defined anechoic space-occupying lession (SOL) with posterior acoustic enhancement seen in upper pole of right kidney.

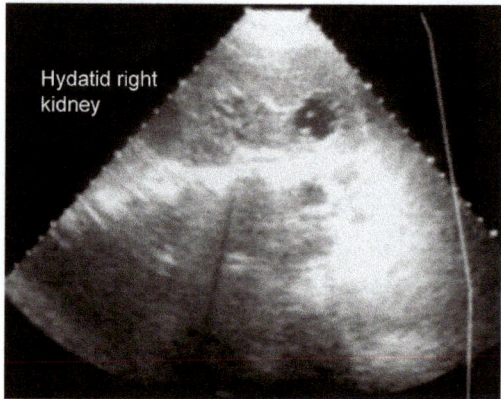

Fig. 8.2.2: Right kidney shows the presence of hydatid cyst with 3 daughter cysts inside it.

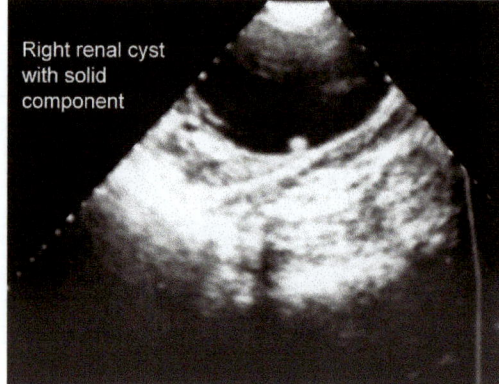

Fig. 8.2.3: A large anechoic cyst is seen occupying the lower and middle pole of right kidney with a mural nodule inside it—renal cell carcinoma.

8.2 DIFFERENTIAL DIAGNOSIS OF CYSTIC RENAL DISEASE

A kidney having 3–5 cysts of any kind is known as "kidney with cystic disease **(Figs. 8.2.1 to 8.2.3)**."

Classification (by Elkin)

Renal Cystic Dysplasia

- Multicystic dysplastic kidney (Potter-2)
- Focal and segmental cystic dysplasia
- Multiple cysts associated with lower urinary tract obstruction
- Hereditary and familial cystic dysplasia.

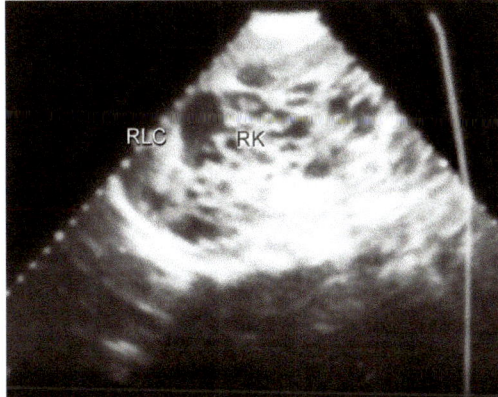

Fig. 8.2.4: Adult polycystic kidney disease—a classical case of APKD showing innumerable cyst with complete architectural distortion of the right kidney. The kidney is also enlarged. (RLC: right lower calyx; RK: right kidney; APKD: adult polycystic kidney disease)

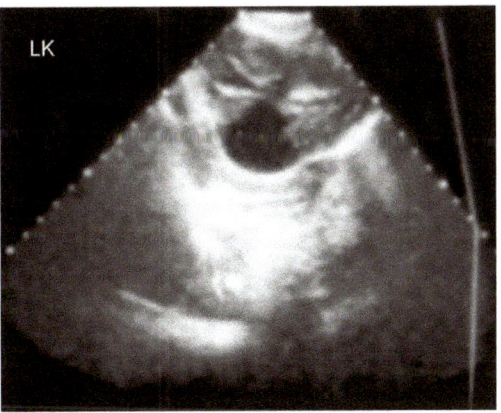

Fig. 8.2.5: Urinoma—a small anechoic collection is seen to communicate with pelvicalyceal system of right kidney. (LK: left kidney)

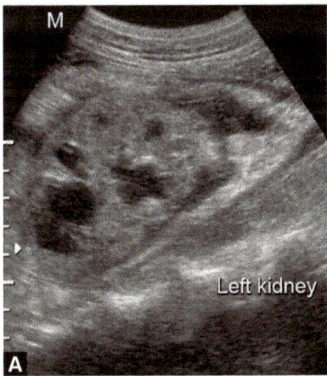 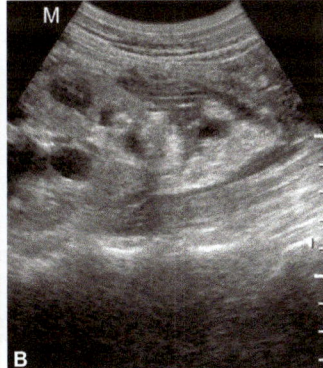

Figs. 8.2.6A and B: US scans show dilated PC system with rupture of lower pole calyx and formation of perinephric urinoma. (M: mass)

Polycystic Kidney Disease (Fig. 8.2.4)

- Polycystic kidney disease (PKD) of young (Potter-1)
- PKD of adult (Potter-3).

Cortical Cysts

- Simple-serious (typical), atypical, complicated (**Figs. 8.2.5 and 8.2.6**)
- Multilocular
- Trisomy associated
- Tuberous sclerosis, von Hippel-Lindau disease.

Medullary Cysts

- Medullary sponge kidney
- Cysts associated with uremia/dialysis
- Pyelogenic cysts
- Papillary necrosis.

Miscellaneous

- Inflammatory (TB, hydatid)
- Neoplastic (Renal cell carcinoma, Wilms' tumor, multilocular cystic nephroma)
- Trauma (resolved hematoma).

Extrarenal Cysts

- Peripelvic
- Parapelvic
- Perinephric.

Multicystic Dysplastic Kidney

- Most common cystic disease in infant and fetus
- Associated with oligohydramnios
- About 20% bilateral
- Lobulated kidney having multiple small to large cysts separated by strands of abnormal parenchymal.

Infantile Autosomal Recessive Polycystic Kidney Disease

- Bilateral, symmetrical
- Tiny radial cysts due to dilated collecting tubules
- Large and echogenic kidneys with a hypoechoic rim
- In mild disease only the medulla is affected.

Adult Autosomal Dominant Polycystic Kidney Disease

- Occurs due to a defect in formation of basement membrane collagen
- Multiple, bilaterally, asymmetrical cysts of different sizes are seen
- Kidney size is increased
- Both cortex and medulla are affected
- Normal renal parenchyma is seen.

Ravines Modification of Bear's Criteria for Diagnosis of ADPCKD

Age	Family history	Number of cyst	Kidney affected
<30 years	+	>2	U/L or B/L
31–59 years	+	>2 + 2	B/L
>60 years	+	>4 + 4	B/L

Medullary Sponge Kidney

- Occur due to ectasia and elongation of medullary tubules
- Dystrophic calcification in walls
- Rarely cysts are seen separately only echogenic kidney are seen.

Uremia Associated Cystic Disease

- Occurs due to ischemia associated with dialysis
- Cyst may occur both in cortex and medulla and increase in size with time
- Association of adenoma and renal cell carcinoma are well-known.

8.3 DIFFERENTIAL DIAGNOSIS OF COMPLEX/SOLID RENAL MASSES

Benign

- Oncocytoma and adenoma
- Angiomyolipoma
- Reninoma
- Mesoblasticnephroma
- Multilocular cystic nephroma (Fig. 8.3.1)
- Hemangioma, aneurysm, arteriovenous malformation (AVM), hematoma.

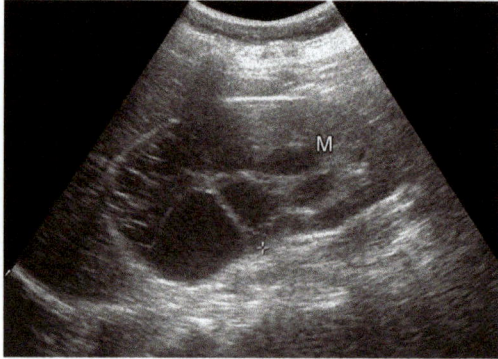

Fig. 8.3.1: US scans show multilocular nephroma of kidney. (M: mass)

Malignant

- Wilms' tumor
- Renal cell carcinoma
- Squamous cell carcinoma
- Soft tissue sarcomas
- Lymphoma
- Leukemia
- Metastasis
- Transitional cell carcinoma (**Figs. 8.3.2 and 8.3.3**).

Oncocytoma/Adenoma

- Oncocytoma is an eosinophilic adenoma, both are usually benign tumors arising from proximal convoluted tubules
- Sharply-defined masses of variable echogenicity and peripheral spoke wheel pattern of blood vessels.

Mesoblastic Nephroma

- The most common solid tumor in first month of life hence known as congenital Wilms' tumor
- Appearance is similar to Wilms' and differentiation on ultrasonography (USG) is not possible
- Calcification is rare.

Multilocular Cystic Nephroma

- Known as cystic Wilms' tumor and benign cystic nephroma
- May have calcification in wall and indent the pelvicalyceal system causing obstruction.

Angiomyolipoma

- Females, solitary
- About 20% associated with tuberous sclerosis
- Locally invasive
- Fat is a very specific feature.

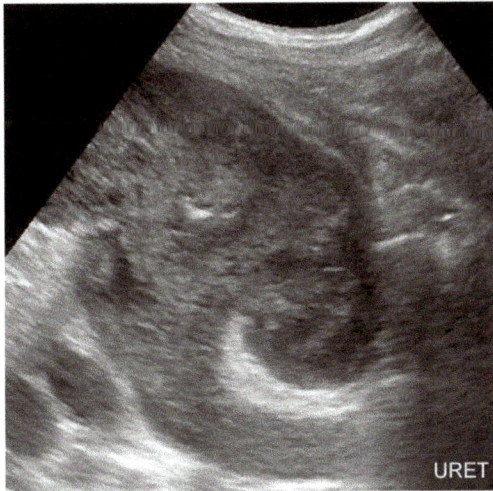

Fig. 8.3.2: Transitional cell carcinoma—mass involving middle and lower pole calyx and extending into upper ureter. (URET: ureter)

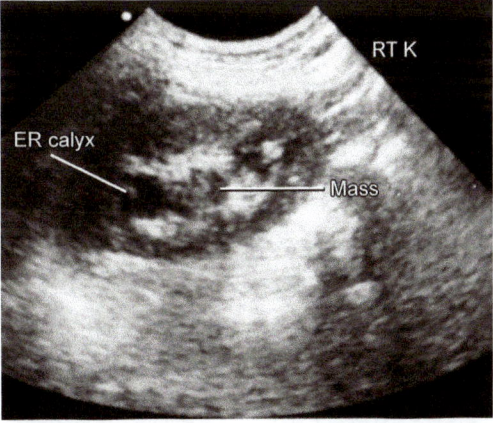

Fig. 8.3.3: Transitional cell carcinoma—a hypoechoic mass is seen splitting the central sinus echocomplex and causing focal caliectasis of the upper pole of right kidney. (ER: lower; RT K: right kidney)

Transitional Cell Carcinoma

- Punctate coarse calcification
- Hypovascular
- Intrapelvic/intracalyceal mass invading the parenchyma
- May form a terminal dilated calyx known as *oncocalyx*.

Wilms' Tumor

- Most common intrarenal malignancy of childhood
- About 5–10% are bilateral, 5–10% have calcification
- Echogenic mass, well-defined with a halo of compressed tissue around it
- Sonolucent lakes of large size are common.

Renal Cell Carcinoma (Figs. 8.3.4 to 8.3.7)

- Most common (86%) of all renal tumors
- Arising from tubular epithelium
- Peak age = 50–70 years
- Males three times more
- Basically an echogenic lesion with hypoechoic rim

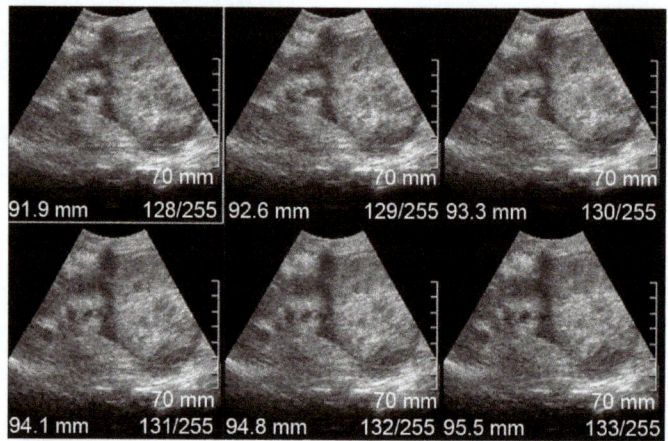

Fig. 8.3.4: 3D US scans show presence of renal cell carcinoma at lower pole of kidney.

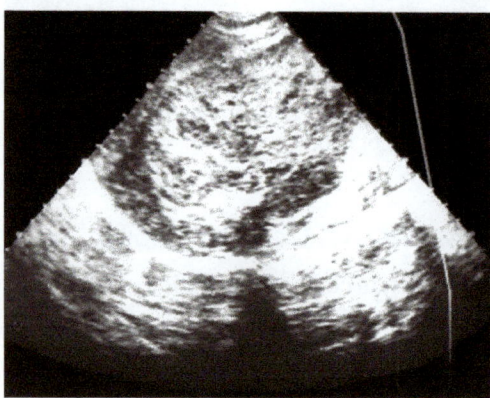

Fig. 8.3.5: A heterogeneous echotexture SOL is seen in the region of upper middle pole of right kidney.

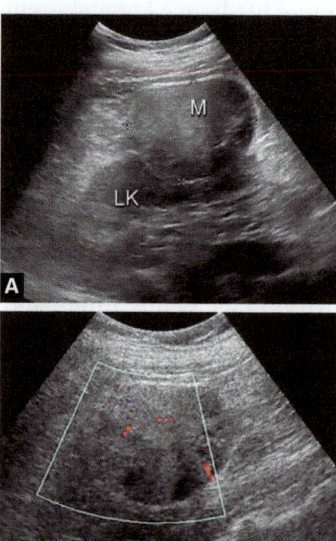

Figs. 8.3.6A and B: Renal cell carcinoma mass bulging out from the lower pole of kidney with internal vascularity on Doppler. (M: mass; LK: left kidney)

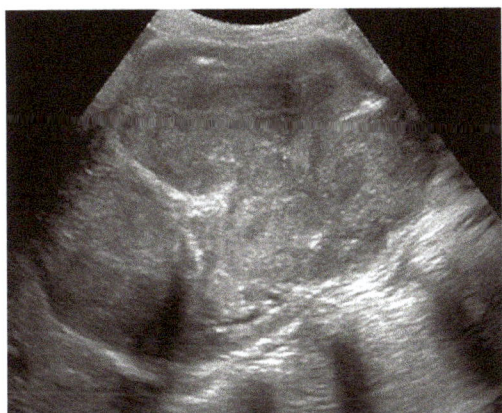

Fig. 8.3.7: Renal cell carcinoma—large iso- to hyperechoic mass from lower pole of kidney.

- Areas of necrosis may be seen
- *About 3–7% lesions are near totally cystic:* All the malignant lesions have a nonspecific appearance of a hypoechoic space occupying lesion.

8.4 DIFFERENTIAL DIAGNOSIS OF HYPOECHOIC RENAL SINUS

- All causes of pelvicaliectasis
- Transitional cell carcinoma
- Pyonephrosis **(Fig. 8.4.1)**
- Prominent vessels in sinus
- Parapelvicperipelvic cyst
- *Blood clot at pelvis:* Description of these conditions are given in respective sections.

8.5 DIFFERENTIAL DIAGNOSIS OF HYPERECHOIC RENAL NODULES

- *Complicated cystic lesion:* When there is hemorrhage within a cyst
- Inflammatory masses in kidney formed in cases of tuberculosis, malakoplakia, xanthogranulomatous pyelonephritis, fungal infection, schistosomiasis
- AIDS-related conditions like calculus **(Fig. 8.5.1)** nephro-calcinosis **(Fig. 8.5.2)**, acute tubular necrosis, interstitial nephritis, *Candida*, CMV, *Cryptococcus*, *Pneumocystis*, MAIC, lymphoma, Kaposi's sarcoma
- Gas loculi seen in cases of emphysematous pyelonephritis
- Calcified tumoral components in Wilms' tumor, RCC, TCC, etc.
- Calcified vascular lesions like AVM, aneurysm
- Fat containing tumors like Wilms' tumor, oncocytoma and angiomyolipoma

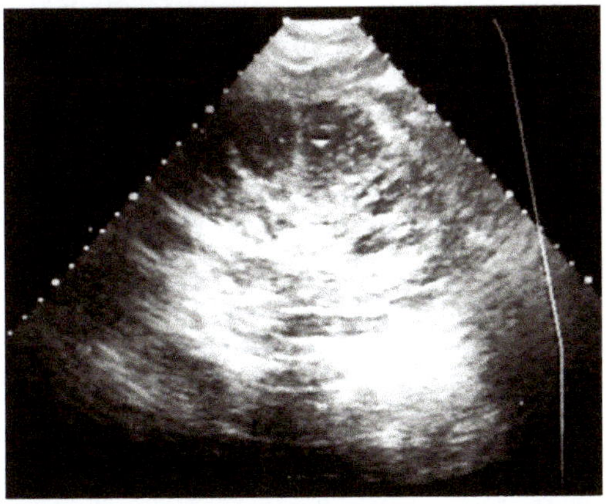

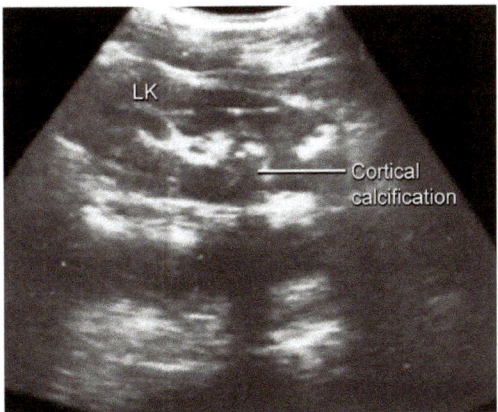

Fig. 8.4.1: Pyonephrosis—stone is seen in renal pelvis with pelvicalyceal hydronephrosis with evidence of debris and air inside it.

Fig. 8.5.1: Renal calculus: Dense echogenic focus with distal acoustic shadowing is seen in the renal cortex suggestive of old tubercular involvement. A calculus is also seen in lower pole. (LK: left kidney)

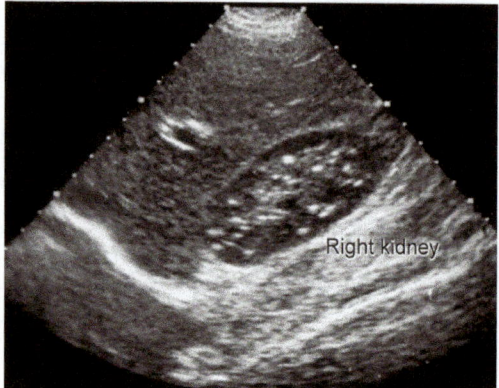

Fig. 8.5.2: Nephrocalcinosis—stippled calcification is seen in the region of the renal pyramid.

- Parenchymal calcification in TB, schistosomiasis, nephrocalcinosis
- Metastatic deposits may sometimes be hyperechoic
- Small RCC.

8.6 DIFFERENTIAL DIAGNOSIS OF DILATED PELVICALYCEAL SYSTEM AND URETER

- Stricture at infundibulum, pelviureteric junction, ureter, this could be due to tumor, calculus or infection **(Figs. 8.6.1A and B)**
- Extrinsic vascular compression occurs most commonly at right upper pole calyx known as Fraley syndrome
  Similar compression on ureter may occur due to retrocaval ureter or even a large aortic aneurysm
- Hydrocalycosismegacalyx, boggy pelvis and megaureter are congenital conditions leading to isolated dilatation of the involved parts. Megacalyx = >12 up to 20-25 **(Fig. 8.6.2)**
- Retroperitoneal fibrosis—leads to medial deviation and partial obstruction of ureter at L4/5 level
- Calculus disease—all calculi whether radiopaque or not are seen as hyperechoic structures

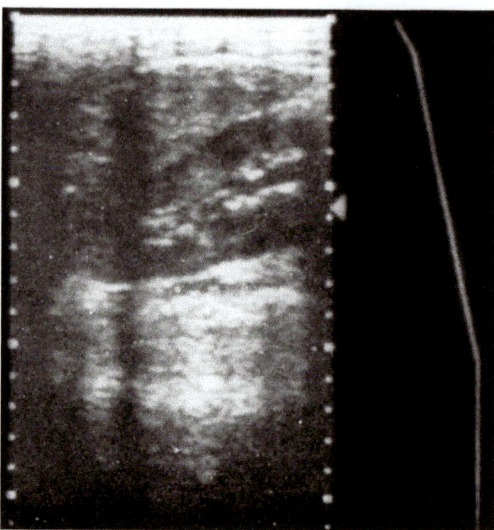

Fig. 8.6.1A: A mild hydronephrosis—minimal splitting of the pelvicalyceal system is noted.

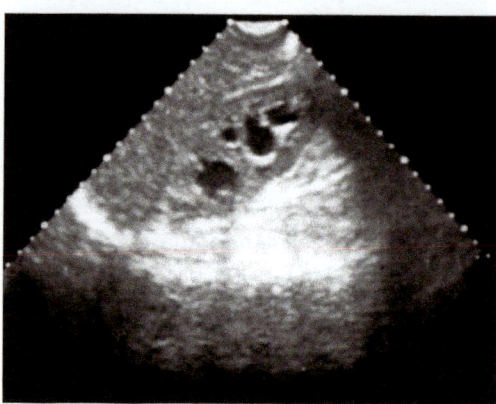

Fig. 8.6.1B: Moderate hydronephrosis.

- Postobstructive atrophy due to volume lose and negative force leads to dilated PCS or calyx **(Figs. 8.6.3 to 8.6.11)**
- Blood clot in the lumen
- Sloughed papilla in the lumen
- Edema of walls
- Trauma
- Retroperitoneal masses
- Transitional cell carcinoma **(Fig. 8.6.12)**
- Vesicoureteric reflux
- Postpartum up to 6 months
- Following urinary tract infection.

Renal

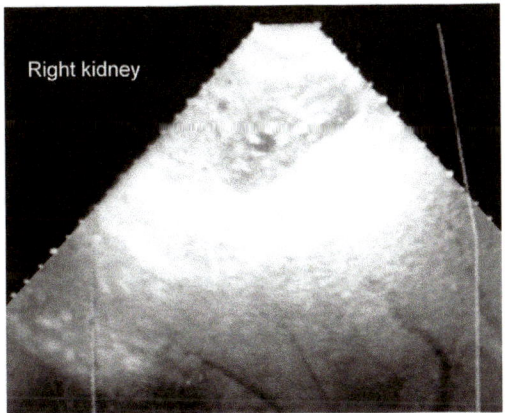

Fig. 8.6.2: Focal caliectasis seen in upper pole of right kidney, old case of TB kidney.

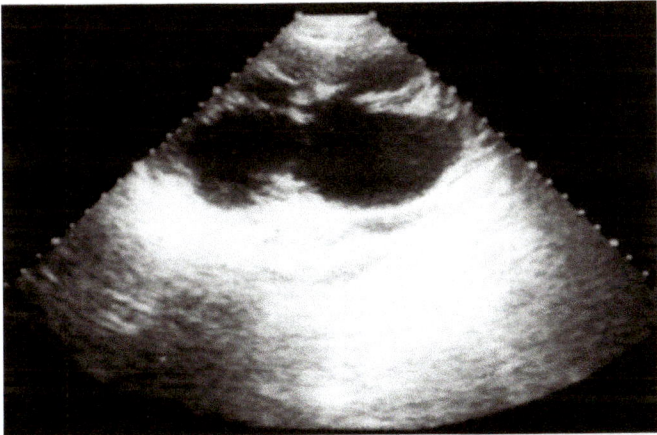

Fig. 8.6.3: PUJ obstruction—longitudinal scan showing gross pelvic dilatation and dilated calyces due to pelviureteric obstruction.

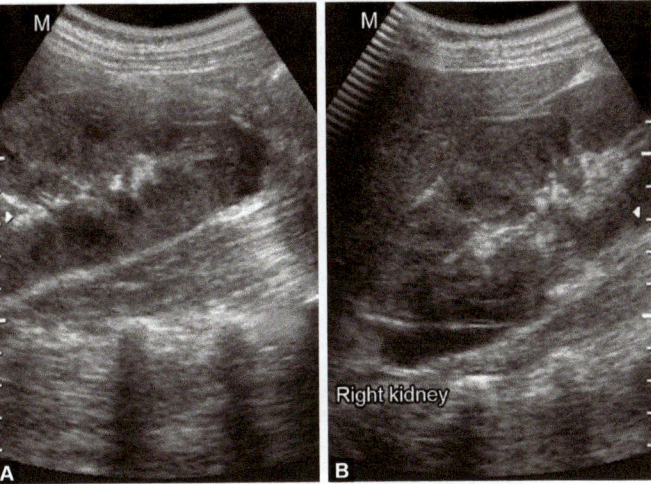

Figs. 8.6.4A and B: US scans show acute pyelonephritis with collection near the superior pole.

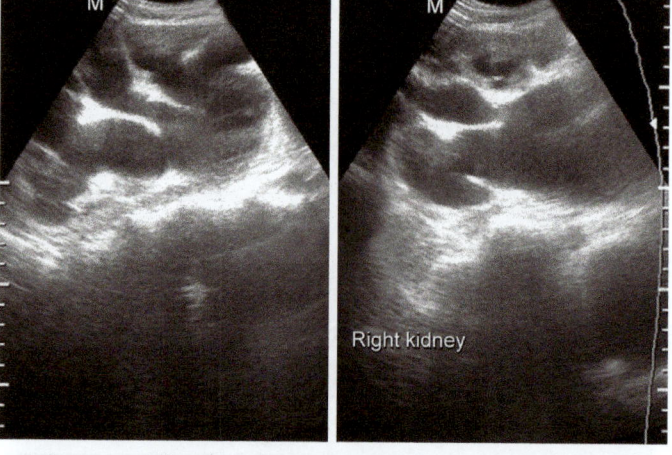

Fig. 8.6.5: US scans show gross dilatation of pelvicalyceal system with parenchymal thinning. (M: mass)

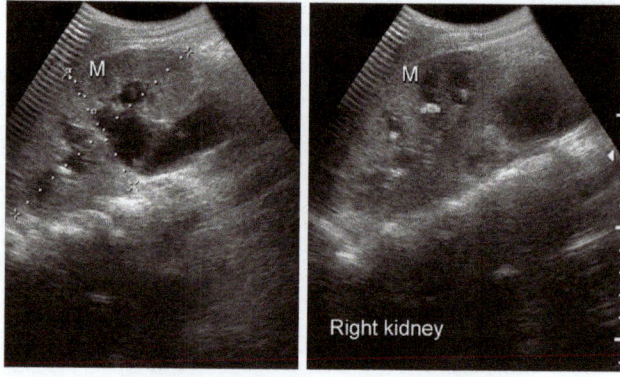

Fig. 8.6.6: US scans show hydronephrosis with multiple caliceal calculus and signs of obstructive uropathy. (M: mass)

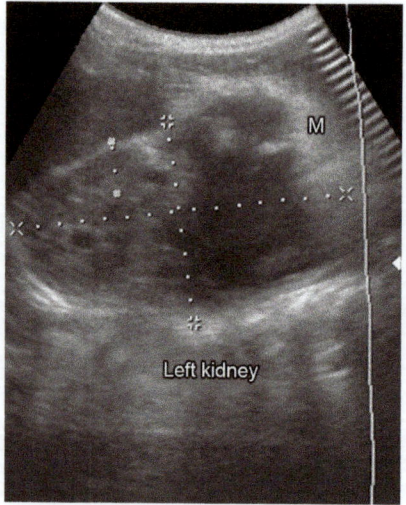

Fig. 8.6.7: US scan shows abscess at the inferior pole of left kidney. (M: mass)

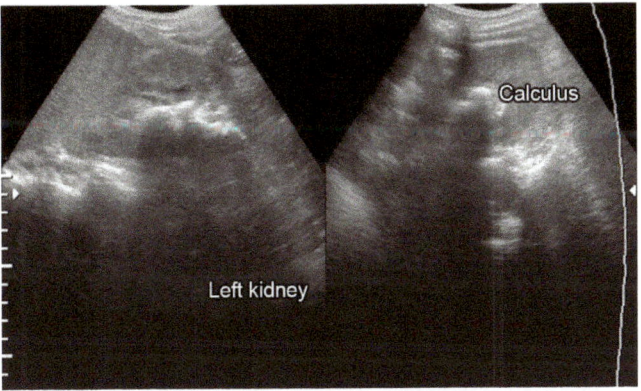

Fig. 8.6.8: US scans show staghorn calculus in left renal pelvis.

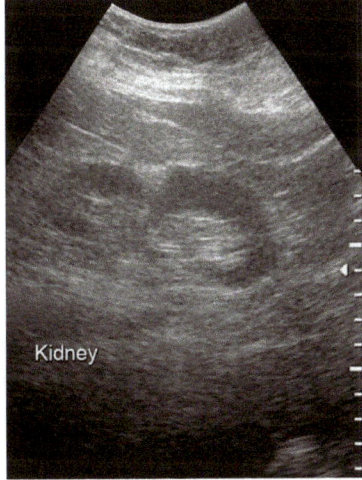

Fig. 8.6.9: US scan shows cortical sac in a case of chronic pyelonephritis.

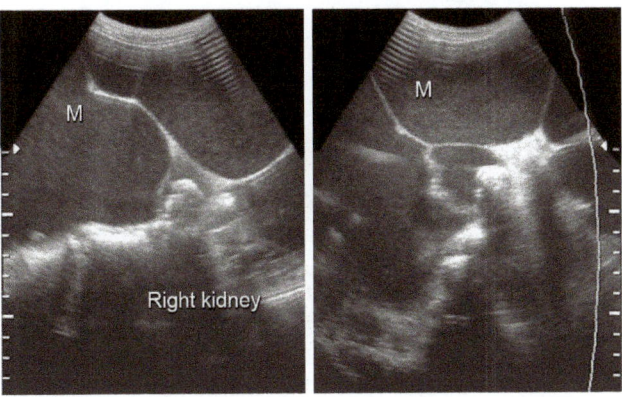

Fig. 8.6.10: US scans show pyonephrosis secondary to obstructing renal calculi. (M: mass)

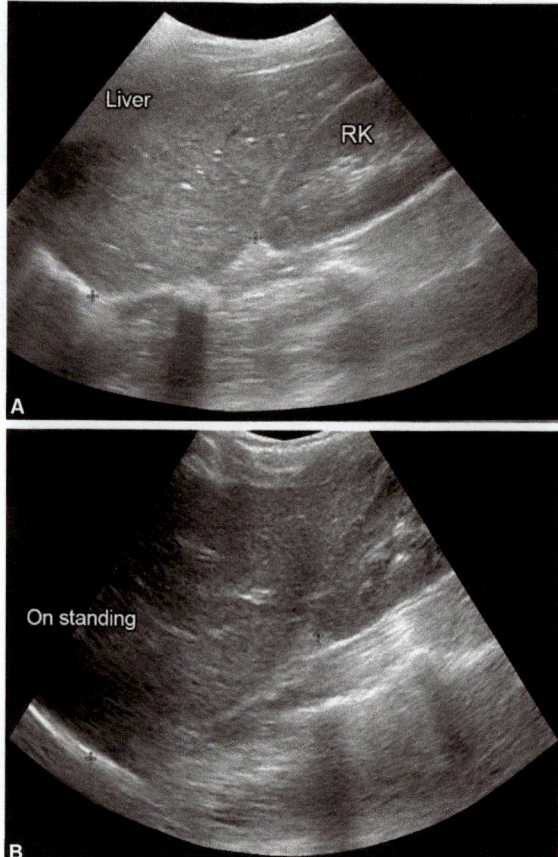

Figs. 8.6.11A and B: Sagittal image of at RUQ showing distance between liver and upper pole of right kidney in supine position and standing position. The distance increased in standing position suggesting mobile kidney. (RK: right kidney)

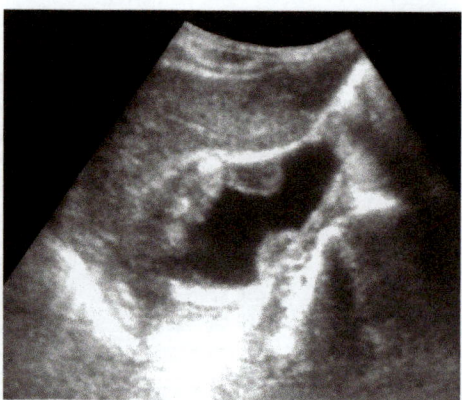

Fig. 8.6.12: Multicentric transitional cell carcinoma (TCC)—multiple hypoechoic masses seen in the renal pelvis.

Renal Tuberculosis—Sonographic Classification (Xuefang Rue et al, 2008)

Type-1: Neprectasia type
Type-2: Hydrops type
Type-3: Empyema type
Type-4: Inflammatory and atrophy type
Type-5: Calcification type
Type-6: Mixed type

Normal renal indices

Index	Range
Pulsality index (PI)	0.7–1.4
Resistance index (RI)	0.56–0.7
Peak systolic velocity (PSV)	60–140 cm/sec (<180)
Renal artery/aorta ratio (RAR)	<3.5
Acceleration time	0.04–0.05 sec
Acceleration index	2.5–3.8 m/sec

CHAPTER 9

Urinary Bladder

9.1 DIFFERENTIAL DIAGNOSIS OF BLADDER WALL THICKENING

Diffuse thickening: (>3 mm when distended and >5 mm when not distended)
- Acute cystitis (**Figs. 9.1.1 and 9.1.2**)
- Bladder outlet obstruction
- Neurogenic bladder
- Schistosomiasis
- Tuberculosis
- Radiation cystitis
- Malakoplakia
- Cyclophosphamide cystitis.

Focal Thickening/Masses
- Nephrogenic adenoma
- Transitional cell papilloma
- Transitional cell carcinoma (**Figs. 9.1.3 to 9.1.5**)
- Squamous cell carcinoma

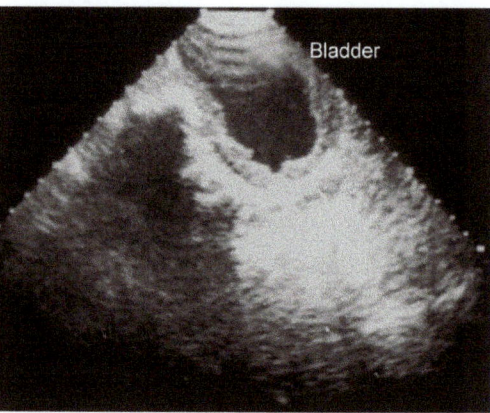

Fig. 9.1.2: Cystitis—the walls of urinary bladder are irregularly thickened.

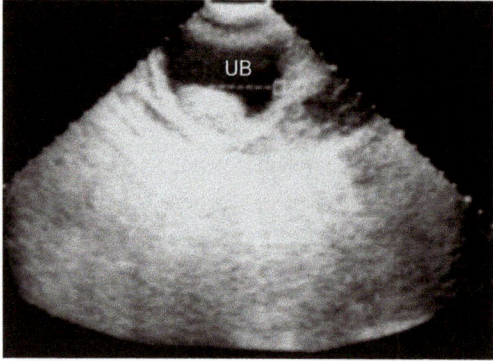

Fig. 9.1.1: Clot in urinary bladder is seen as a large echogenic lesion in relation to the posterior wall of urinary bladder (UB).

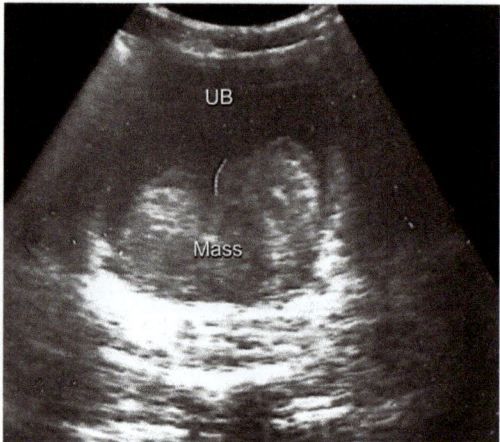

Fig. 9.1.3: Transitional cell carcinoma—a polypoidal mass is seen to arise from post-wall of urinary bladder urinary bladder (UB).

- Adenocarcinoma
- Leiomyoma/Leiomyosarcoma
- Rhabdomyosarcoma
- Hemangioma **(Fig. 9.1.6)**
- Paraganglioma
- Sarcoma botryoides **(Figs. 9.1.7A and B)**
- *Invasion by pelvic malignancies:*
  - Females more than males
  - Most commonly *Escherichia coli*

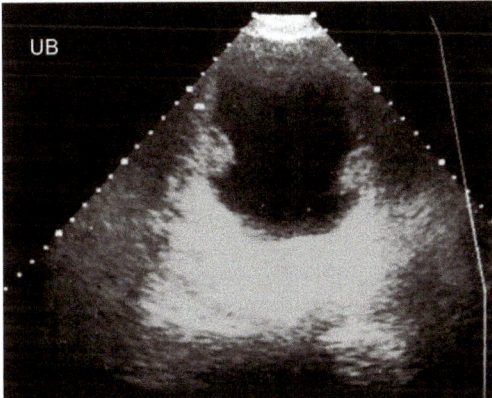

Fig. 9.1.4: Multifocal carcinoma—transverse scan of urinary bladder (UB) showing nodular growth at two different regions.

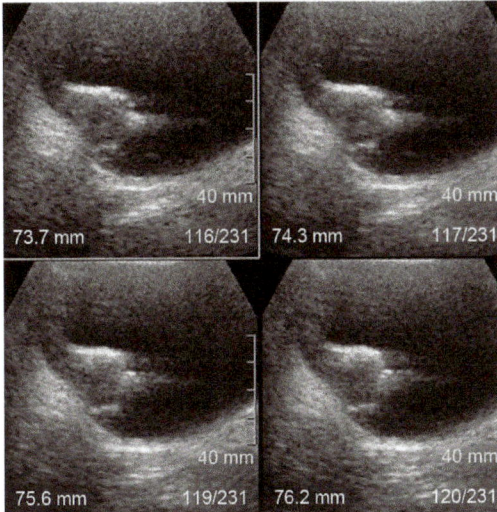

Fig. 9.1.5: 3D US scans show transitional cell carcinoma of urinary bladder with calcification.

- Gas in the lumen and in the wall is seen in emphysematous cystitis. This occurs in immunocompromised patients.

Schistosomiasis

- A disease of submucosa and lamina propria leading to mucosal ulcerations and malignancies in late phases
- Diffuse, irregular wall thickening associated with lumpy, sometimes polypoidal granulomas and strakey curvilinear calcification is the hallmark
- Eventually, the bladder becomes small and fibrotic.

Tuberculosis

- A process that descends from upper tract and so the earliest changes are seen at ureteral orifices whereby they spread centrifugally
- Diffuse but lumpy thickening with calcification in late stages is seen
- Small fibrosed bladder is the terminal event.

Cyclophosphamide Cystitis

- *Acute*: Edematous, hyperemic, ulcerated mucosa with intraluminal clots
- *Chronic*: Small fibrose bladder
- Malignancy.

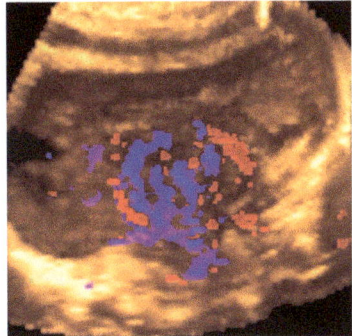

Fig. 9.1.6: 3D color Doppler US scan shows hemangiomatous lesion in urinary bladder.

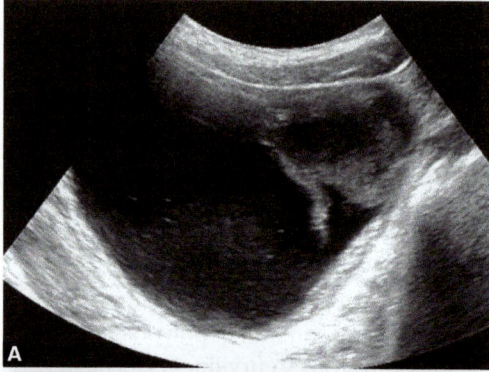

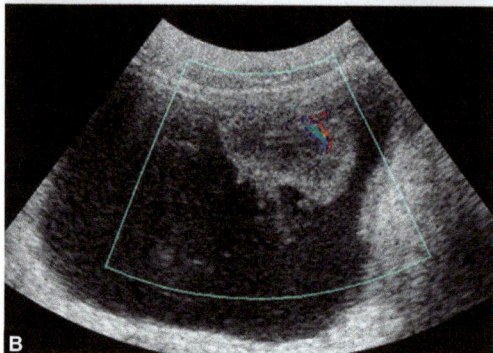

Figs. 9.1.7A and B: Sarcoma botryoides urinary bladder (UB)—polypoidal mass from anterior wall of UB having vascularity.

Malakoplakia

- An uncommon granulomatous response to UTI, especially to that caused by *E. coli*
- Females; 5th–6th decades
- Associated with diabetes, alcoholism, liver disease, mycobacterial infection, sarcoidosis and post-transplant
- 3–5 cm, solitary/multiple mural-based masses with mural thickening.

Radiation Cystitis

- *Acute*: It is like any other diffuse cystitis
- *Chronic*: It occurs on an average after four years
- No specific feature is seen.

Cystitis Cystica and Cystitis Glandularis

- Occur due to chronic cystitis causing cystic change and later on glandular change in Brunn's nest (urothelial cell rest in submucosa)
- Difficult to differentiate from malignancy and may lead to adenocarcinoma
- Cyst (intramural) and solid papillary masses with wall thickening may be seen.

Bladder Outlet Obstruction

Urinary retention with markedly increased post void residual urine on ultrasound.

Neurogenic Bladder

Generally, a markedly contracted or distended urinary bladder with multiple diverticula.

Endometriosis

- Most common site for endometriotic deposits in urinary tract is bladder
- Serosal deposits protruding into lumen or even intraluminal deposits may be seen.

Paraganglioma

- Trigone is the most common location followed by dome and lateral walls
- Lesion is vascular.

Hemangioma

- Dome and posterolateral walls
- *Two types of appearance:*
  - A rounded, well-defined, hyperechoic solid mass in lumen showing in vascularity in Doppler
  - Diffuse wall thickening with hypoechoic spaces and calcification.

Adenocarcinoma

- Has to be differentiated from adenocarcinoma elsewhere infiltrating
- Associated stone/calcification is a feature.

Squamous Cell Carcinoma

Large, solid, infiltrative lesion.

Transitional Cell Carcinoma

- Men, 6th–7th decades, trigone/posterolateral walls
- About 70% superficial, rest are invasive
- USG is 95% sensitive in its detection
- Presents as a focal nonmobile mass/wall thickening.

9.2 DIFFERENTIAL DIAGNOSIS OF BLADDER CONTOUR AND CALIBER ABNORMALITY

Symmetric Narrowing

- Pelvic lipomatosis
- Pelvic hematoma
- Lymphoma
- Iliopsoas hypertrophy
- Narrow bony pelvis
- Nonlymphomatous lymphadenopathy
- Lymphocele/lymphangioma
- Iliac artery aneurysm
- Iliac vein varices
- Seminal vesicle cysts.

Asymmetric Narrowing/Contour

- Diverticulum
- Fistula
- *Hernia:*
  - In all above conditions the dome is tapering while the base is rounded due to external compression
  - Mucosa is uniformly normal
- Bladder outlet obstruction (**Figs. 9.2.1 to 9.2.4**).

Pelvic Lipomatosis

- Black, males
- Proliferation of fat in pelvic organs seen as echogenic tissue compressing the bladder symmetrically

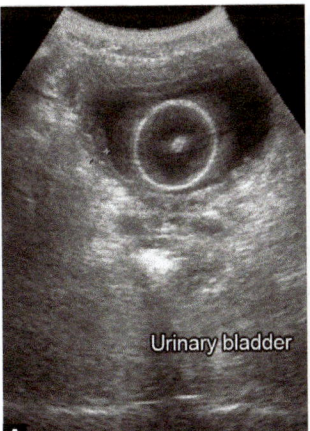 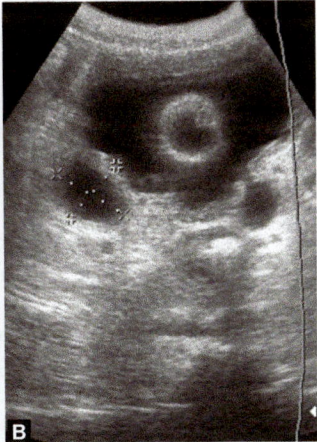

Figs. 9.2.1A and B: US scans show bladder wall hypertrophy with vesical diverticula in a case of bladder outlet obstruction.

Differential Diagnosis in Ultrasound

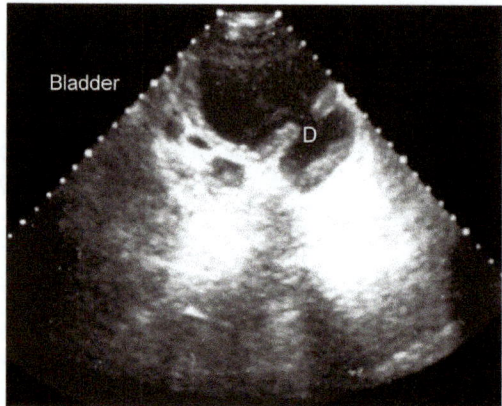

Fig. 9.2.2: Narrow neck diverticulum as seen from the posterior wall of urinary bladder with evidence of debris inside. (D: diverticular)

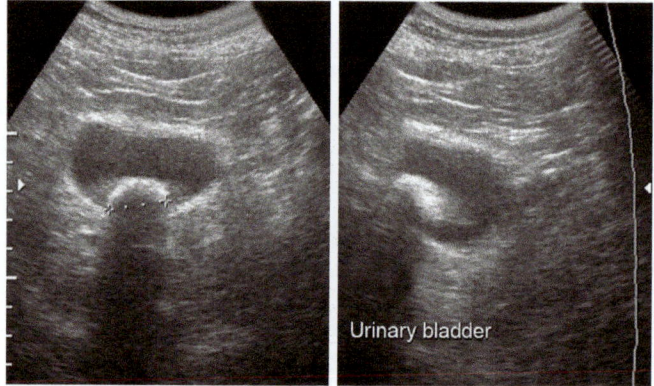

Fig. 9.2.3: US scans show vesical calculus.

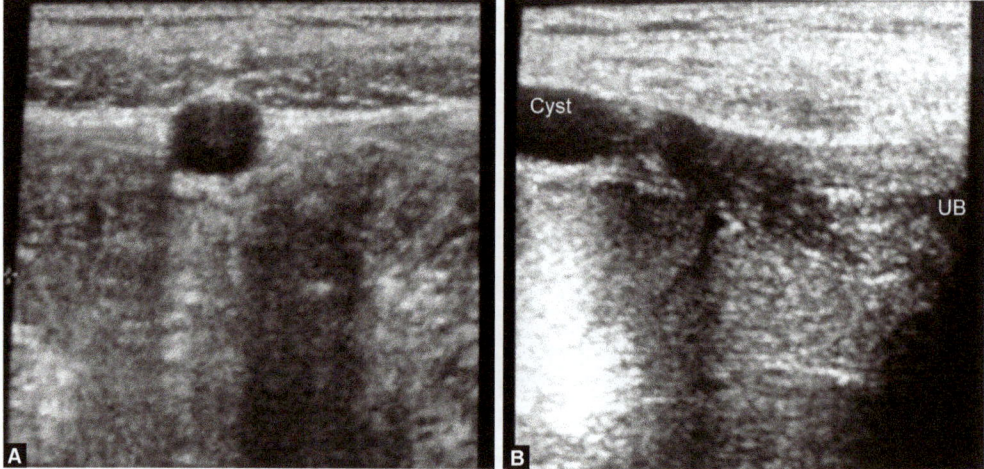

Figs. 9.2.4A and B: (A) TS and (B) LS of midline at infraumbilical level showing urachal cyst—urachus seen as hypoechoic band extending from superior aspect of urinary bladder (UB) to umbilicus in relation to anterior abdominal wall with a cyst in it. (TS: transverse section; LS: longitudinal section)

- A pear-shaped/tear drop bladder ureter and elongated rectosigmoid.

Pelvic Hematoma

- History of blunt abdominal trauma is important
- Less echogenicity of extravesical tissue is the only factor that differentiates it.

Lymphoma

Involving pelvic nodes cause symmetric narrowing.

Iliopsoas Hypertrophy

- Young athletic individual
- The deviation of midureter clinches the diagnosis.

CHAPTER 10

Adrenal Gland

10.1 BILATERAL LARGE ADRENAL GLAND

- Lymphoma
- Hyperplasia
- Hemorrhage.

Infections

- Tuberculosis
- Histoplasmosis
- Immunodeficiency states
- Pheochromocytoma (10%)
- Adenomas (10%)
- Metastasis
- Wolman's disease.

Lymphoma

Non-Hodgkin's is the most common cell type.

On sonography, they appear as bilateral enlarged adrenal with discrete or conglomerate hypoechoic masses. Masses may be so hypoechoic as to stimulate cysts. The medulla cannot be differentiated from the cortex as in any other infiltration process.

Hyperplasia

Congenital adrenal hyperplasia is an autosomal recessive condition clinically presenting with features of visualization or salt loss depending upon the hormone which is deficit. Both adrenals are enlarged but the differentiation of medulla and cortex is preserved.

Hemorrhage: Adrenal hemorrhage may be spontaneous or post-traumatic. Sonographic appearance of acute hemorrhage is a bright echogenic mass in the adrenal bed, which becomes smaller and anechoic with time. Patients with bilateral hemorrhage are at increased risk for development of acute adrenal insufficiency.

Infections: Tuberculosis may cause bilateral diffuse, inhomogeneous enlargement of adrenals. Punctate calcification may also be seen. Infection of adrenal glands is seen in association with AIDS and organ transplantation. Common offending organisms are fungi, mycobacteria, cytomegalovirus (CMV), herpes, toxoplasmosis, etc. On ultrasound, bilateral adrenal glands show, heterogeneously hypoechoic masses. On formation of abscesses gas may be demonstrated in the lesion.

Pheochromocytoma

They are usually solitary but in 10% cases they are bilateral.

Sonographically most are large and well-marginated. Either homogeneous or heterogeneous (because of necrosis and hemorrhage) solid masses.

Metastasis (Fig. 10.1.1)

The most common primary tumors to give rise to adrenal metastasis are lung, breast, melanoma, kidney, thyroid and colon cancers.

May be unilateral or bilateral.

Adrenal Gland

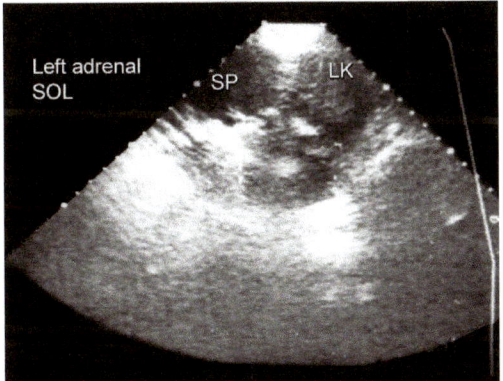

Fig. 10.1.1: Metastases—a hypoechoic mass with irregular outline is seen in the region of left adrenal in a case of bronchogenic carcinoma. (SOL: space-occupying lesion; LK: left kidney; SP: spleen)

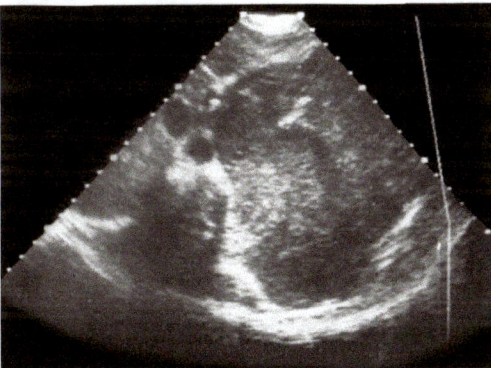

Fig. 10.1.2: A large predominantly hypoechoic well-defined left adrenal mass lesion seen with evidence of calcification in it.

On ultrasound appears as solid masses round to oval hypoechoic lesions. They may show inhomogeneity due to necrosis, hemorrhage and calcification **(Fig. 10.1.2)**.

Wolman's Disease

This is a rare autosomal recessive lipid storage disease. Infants less than 6 months of age show marked hepatosplenomegaly and massive bilateral adrenal gland enlargement.

10.2 UNILATERAL ADRENAL MASSES

- Pheochromocytoma
- Lymphoma
- Adenoma **(Fig. 10.2.1)**
- Neuroblastoma
- Myelolipoma
- Hemorrhage
- Adenocarcinoma
- Metastasis.

Adenoma

Adrenal adenoma may be hyperfunctioning or non-hyperfunctioning. Hyperfunctioning adenomas give rise to Cushing's syndrome or Conn's disease.

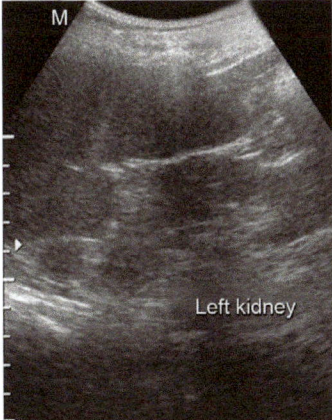 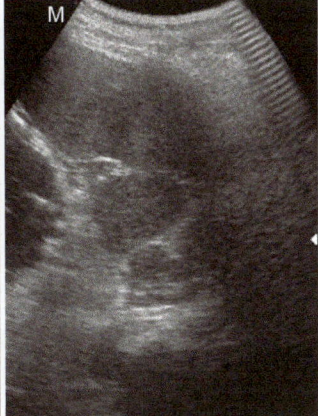

Fig. 10.2.1: US scans show adrenal adenoma. (M: mass)

On sonography they appear as solid, small, round and well-defined lesions. Right upper quadrant retroperitoneal fat reflection is displaced posteriorly by hepatic or subhepatic masses while kidney and adrenal masses displace it anteriorly.

Neuroblastoma (Fig. 10.2.2)

The second most common abdominal tumor of childhood. Thirty percent occurring in children <5 years. On ultrasound, they are seen as on poorly defined and heterogeneous lesion with areas of calcification, hemorrhage and necrosis. The lesion often crosses the midline and causes displacement and compression of ipsilateral kidney without otherwise distorting the internal renal architecture. They also tend to spread early and widely spreads around aorta, celiac and SMA arteries.

Pheochromocytomas

Pheochromocytomas (**Figs. 10.2.3 and 10.2.4**) are hyperfunctioning tumor-secreting norepinephrine and epinephrine and showing features of episodic hypertension, palpitation with tachycardia, headache. Sonography demonstrates large, well-marginated and heterogeneous (due to necrosis and hemorrhage) solid lesions. About 10% lesions may demonstrate calcification.

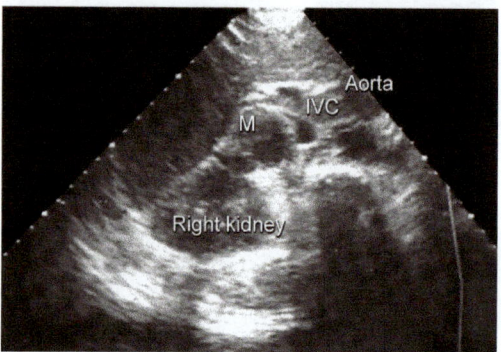

Fig. 10.2.3: Pheochromocytoma—a hypoechoic rounded well-defined lesion with uniform echogenicity is seen in the right adrenal gland. (IVC: inferior vena cava; M: mass)

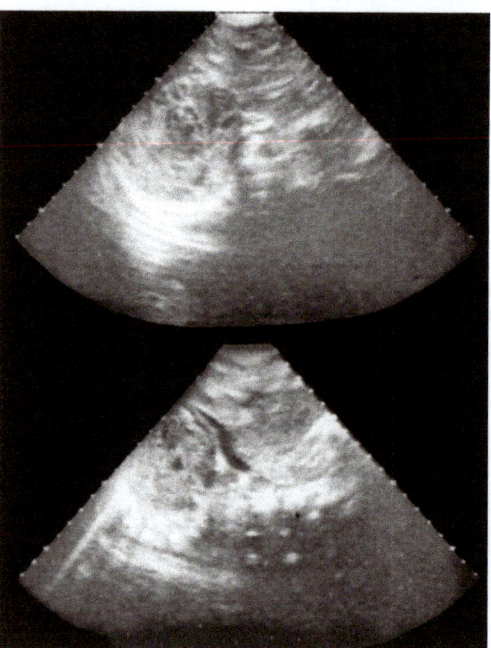

Fig. 10.2.2: Longitudinal and transverse scan of abdomen of a 6-month-old child with marked heterogenicity and areas of high reflectivity within it—neuroblastoma.

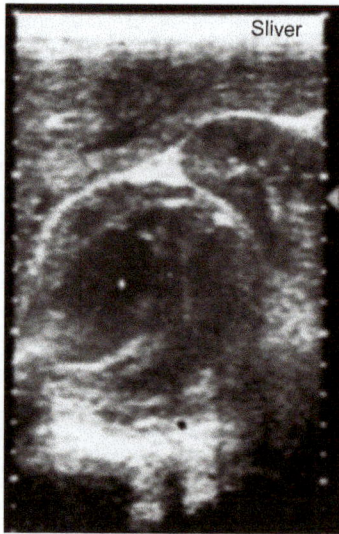

Fig. 10.2.4: A solid heterogeneous mass with a well-defined echogenic capsule and cystic areas of necrosis—pheochromocytoma.

Myelolipoma

Adrenal myelolipomas are rare benign nonhyperfunctioning tumors composed of fat and bone marrow elements.

On sonography, an echogenic mass with apparent diaphragmatic discursion is diagnostic of the condition. Tumor may appear isoechoic if composed predominantly of myeloid element.

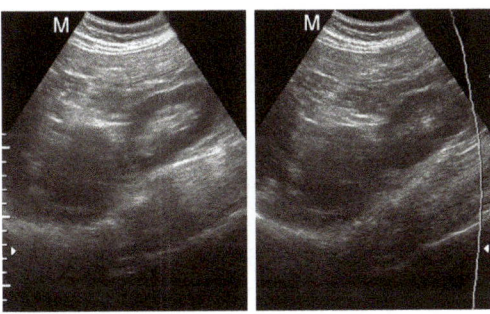

Fig. 10.3.1: US scans show evidence of large pheochromocytoma of adrenal gland. (M: mass)

Adrenocarcinomas

Adrenocarcinomas are malignant tumors. They may arise from any of the layers of adrenal cortex.

Hyperfunctioning tumors are small and homogeneous in echo pattern, similar to renal cortex.

The nonhyperfunctioning tumors are larger and heterogeneous with central areas of necrosis and hemorrhage. All lesions tend to be well-defined with a lobulated border. Calcification may be seen in 20% cases. A surrounding thin echogenic vascular capsule is a specific feature of adrenal cortical carcinoma.

10.3 LARGE SOLID ADRENAL MASSES

- Cortical carcinoma
- Pheochromocytoma
- Neuroblastoma **(Figs. 10.3.1 and 10.3.2)**
- Ganglioneuroma
- Myelolipoma
- Metastasis
- Hemangiomas may become large in size. They have nonspecific US features with cystic, solid or complex appearances. Phleboliths may be seen within the lesions—inflammation/infection—tuberculosis, abscess.

Ganglioneuroma is a rare benign adrenal neoplasm. It is slow-growing and clinically

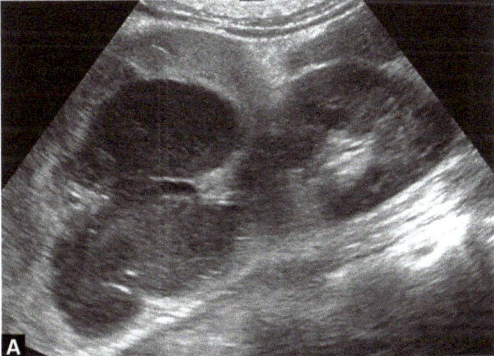

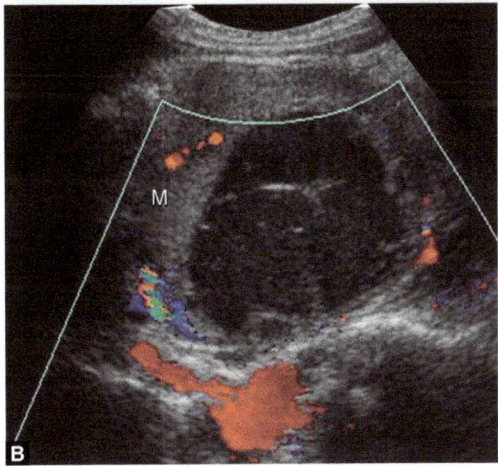

Figs. 10.3.2A and B: Heterogeneous mass with internal septa and vascularity in left adrenal gland. (M: mass)

silent until pressure symptoms are evident. Sonographically, they appear homogeneously solid and change shape rather than displacing adjacent organs.

10.4 CYSTIC ADRENAL MASSES

Adrenal Cyst

- Rare benign lesion, found incidentally
- Typically unilateral but bilateral in 15% of cases
- Most common in 3rd to 4th decades and show a female preponderance.

Sonographically, they are round or oval with a thin smooth wall. Good through-transmission is present but often internal debris is noted.

According to their origin they are classified as:

- *Endothelial*: Most common variety and include angiomatous, lymphangiectatic and hamartomatous lesions
- *Pseudocysts*: Secondary to hemorrhage into a normal adrenal gland, i.e. old hemorrhage or tumor-cystic adenoma—neuroblastoma
- *Epithelial cysts*
- *Parasitic*: Echinococcal cyst.

10.5 ADRENAL PSEUDOMASSES

Structures that may simulate adrenal masses include:

- Thickened diaphragmatic crura
- Accessory spleen
- Gastric fundus
- Gastric diverticulum
- Renal vein
- Retrocrural and retroperitoneal lymphadenopathy
- Upper pole renal cysts and renal tumors
- Pancreatic tumors
- Hypertrophied caudate lobe of liver
- Fluid-filled colon interposed between stomach and kidney.

10.6 ADRENAL CALCIFICATIONS

- Inflammatory—tuberculosis and histoplasmosis
- Addison's disease
- Pheochromocytoma
- Carcinoma
- Ganglioneuroma.

CHAPTER 11

Peritoneal and Mesenteric Masses

11.1 ROUND SOLID MASSES IN MESENTERY

- Metastasis
- Lymphoma
- Leiomyosarcoma
- *Metastasis* from colon and ovary. Metastasis due to intraperitoneal seedlings are seen in primary mucinous tumors of ovary, appendix, colon and breast
- *Lymphoma:* Lymphoma may present as an endoexoenteric mass with a solid mass in the mesentery and adjacent small bowel mass
- *Leiomyosarcoma:* Of small bowel is most commonly seen in ileum. The large extrinsic component of the lesion is seen as a well-defined solid mesenteric mass with areas of necrosis
- Neural tumors
- Lipoma
- Fibrous histiocytoma
- Hemangioma
- Desmoid tumors

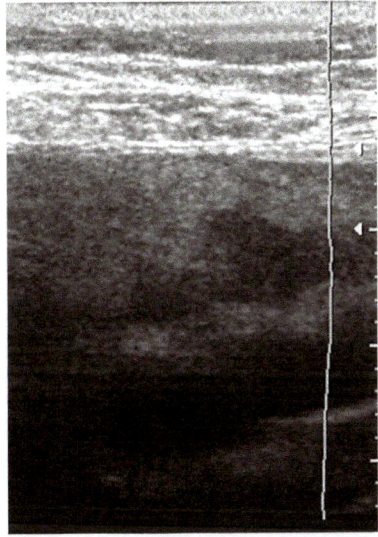

Fig. 11.1.2: US scan shows mesenteric thickening.

- *Mesenteritis:* Various conditions such as Crohn's, tuberculosis (**Figs. 11.1.1 and 11.1.2**) trauma, surgery and pancreatitis may cause inflammation and thickening of the mesentery which on US may appear as a focal echopoor mass. This may also be seen as a part of retroperitoneal fibrosis.

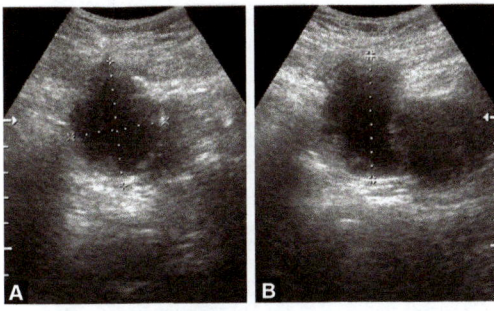

Figs. 11.1.1A and B: US scans show chronic tubercular peritoneal collection in the pelvis.

11.2 ILL-DEFINED MASS

Metastasis: Direct extension from adjacent neoplasm (ovary uterus, pancreas) may infiltrate the mesentery.

Lymphoma: Infiltrating small bowel lymphoma is plaque like involvement of the bowel wall and may be associated with desmoplastic reaction involving the mesentery.

The mesenteric lymph node involvement may be seen as an ill-defined component mass engulfing and encasing adjacent normal loops.

Carcinoid

- *Lymphoma*: Infiltrating small bowel lymphoma is plaque-like involvement of the bowel wall and may be associated with desmoplastic reaction involving the mesentery. The mesenteric lymph node involvement may be seen as ill-defined confluent mass engulfing and encasing adjacent bowel loops.
- Fibromatosis.
- Chronic or retractile mesenteritis, fibrosing mesenteritis: Retractile mesenteritis also called as chronic fibrosing mesenteritis or mesenteric hypodystrophy is a rare condition of unknown etiology causing fibrofatty thickening of the small bowel mesentery. On ultrasound, it may be seen as a nonspecific ill-defined (hypoechoic or heterogeneous) lesion at the root of the mesentery extending till the bowel border.
- Lipodystrophy.
- Peritoneal mesothelioma.
- Fibrotic reaction of carcinoid.
- Desmoid tumors.

Liposarcoma

Diffuse Infiltrative Lipomatosis

- Tuberculosis (**Figs. 11.2.1 to 11.2.11**)
- Diverticulitis
- Pancreatitis.

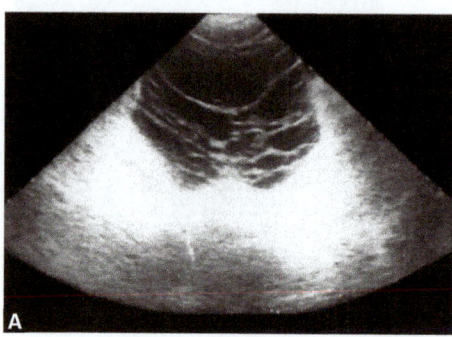
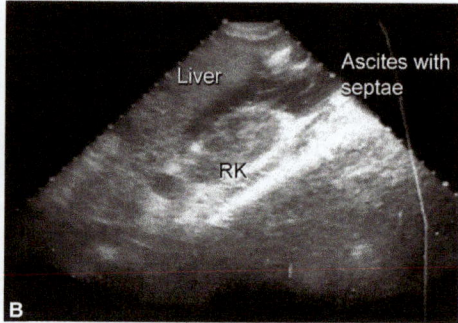

Figs. 11.2.1A and B: Ascites with multiple thick internal septae seen in (A) pelvis and (B) hepatorenal pouch. (RK: right kidney)

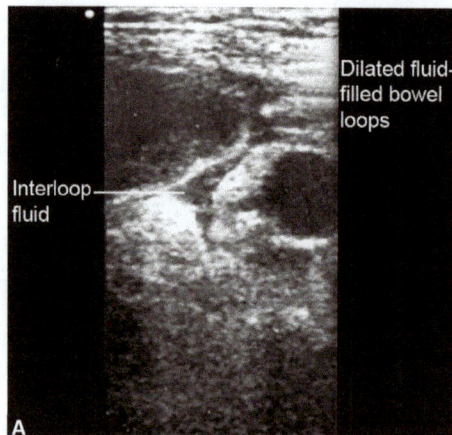
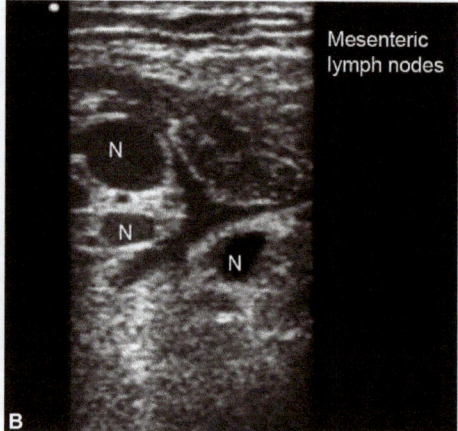

Figs. 11.2.2A and B: (A) Abdominal tuberculosis: Interloop fluid between loops; (B) Abdominal tuberculosis: Multiple hypoechoic well-defined lesion seen in the mesentery suggestive of lymph nodes. (N: node)

Peritoneal and Mesenteric Masses

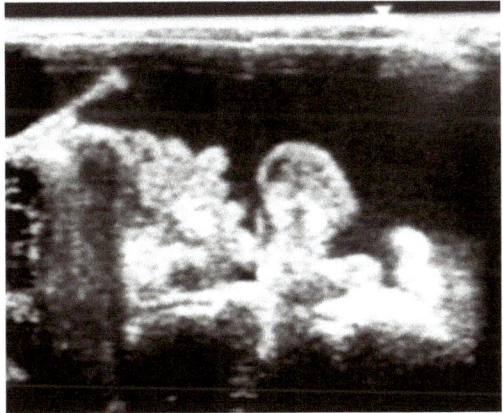

Fig. 11.2.3: Ascites outlining bowel loops.

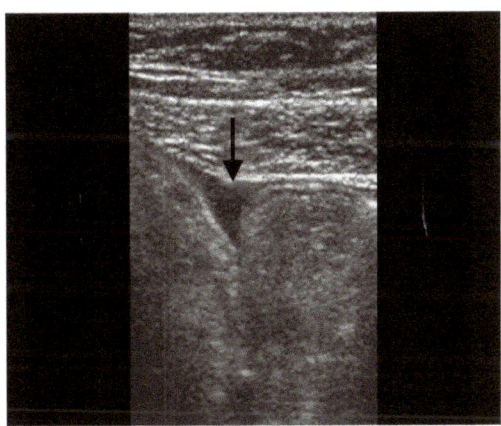

Fig. 11.2.6: Interbowel loop fluid (black arrow).

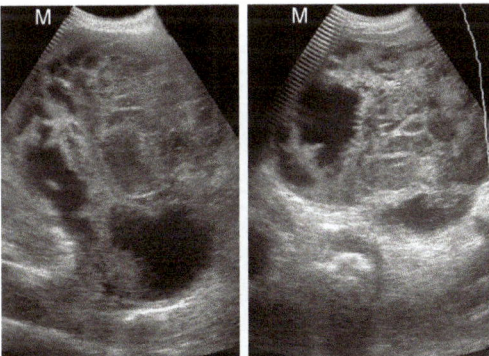

Fig. 11.2.4: US scans show evidence of omental sarcoma. (M: mass)

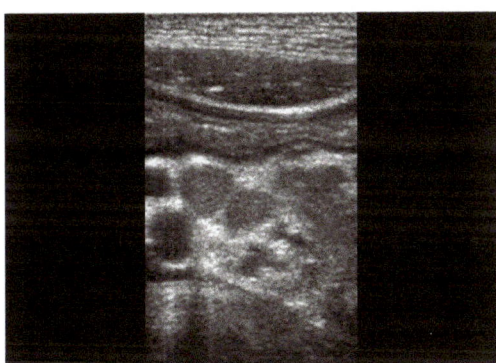

Fig. 11.2.7: Enlarged mesenteric lymph nodes.

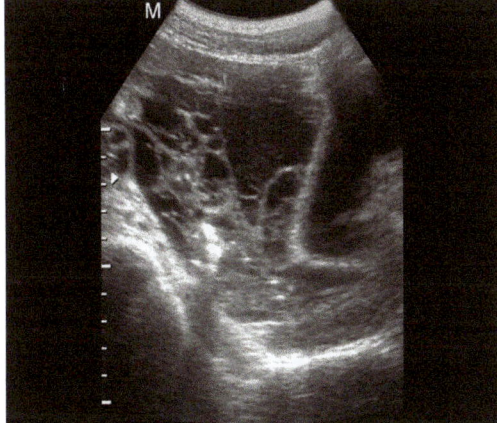

Fig. 11.2.5: US scan shows septate collection in perforation peritonitis. (M: mass)

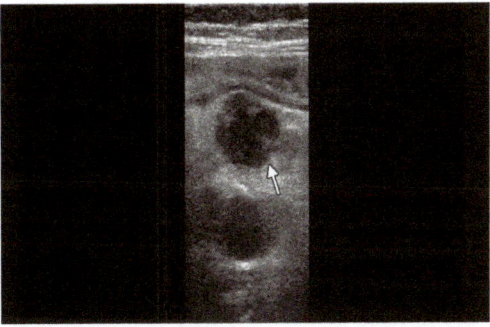

Fig. 11.2.8: Necrotic mesenteric lymph nodes (arrow) showing posterior acoustic enhancement—case of tubercular peritonitis.

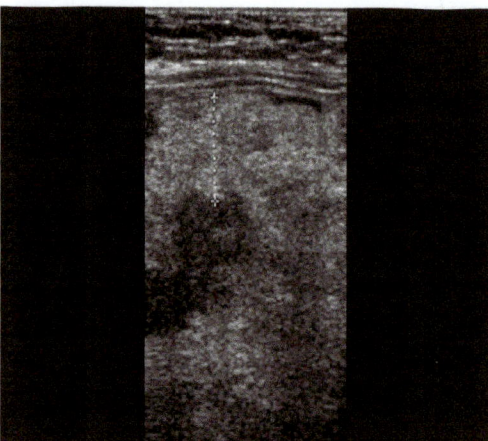

Fig. 11.2.9: Tubercular peritonitis—thickened omentum (in calipers).

11.3 LOCULATED CYSTIC PERITONEAL MASSES

- *Mesenteric*: Lymphangioma, mesenteric cyst, mesenteric hematoma
- Pseudomyxoma peritonei
- Intra-abdominal abscess
- Lymphocele
- Meconium peritonitis
- Peritoneal tuberculosis
- Omental cyst
- Cystic mesothelioma
- Cystic spindle-shaped tumors
- Paracardiac pseudocyst
- Intraperitoneal hydatid (**Figs. 11.3.1 and 11.3.2**).

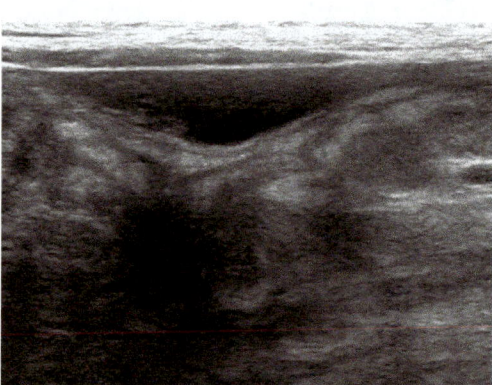

Fig. 11.2.10: Transabdominal ultrasound image showing the collection in the peritoneal cavity with internal septae suggestive of loculated ascites.

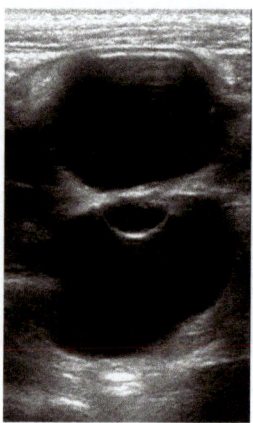

Fig. 11.3.1: Two hydatid cysts in peritoneal cavity—lower one shows daughter cyst.

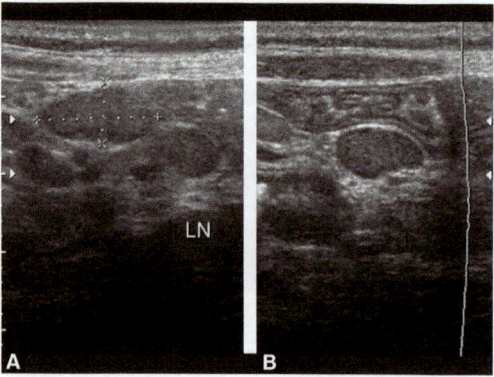

Figs. 11.2.11A and B: US scans show mesenteric adenopathy in a case of Koch's abdomen. (LN: lymph nodes)

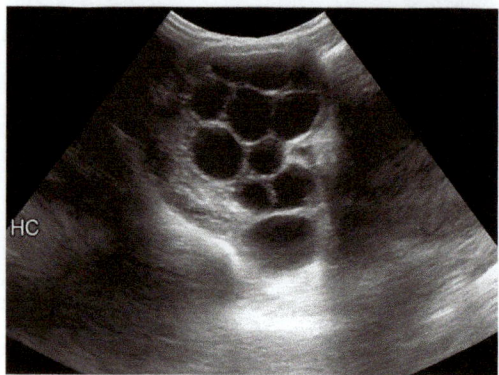

Fig. 11.3.2: Hydatid cyst in right iliac fossa. (HC: hydatid cysts)

11.4 SOLID PERITONEAL LESIONS

- Mesothelioma
- Carcinomatosis
- Pseudomyxoma peritonei
- Leiomyomatosis peritoneal disseminate.

Mesenteric Cyst (Figs. 11.4.1 and 11.4.2)

- Usually found in the root of the mesentery
- Sonographically, it appears as unilocular cystic lesion.

That may be septated, rarely a fat-fluid level may be seen. When differentiation from solid peritoneal lesions and mesenteric cystic teratoma becomes difficult.

- Desmoid tumors
- Occurs most commonly in abdominal wall
- Occurs in mesentery also
- Mesenteric dermoids are hypoechoic masses with area of mesenteric shadowing due to fibrous tissue.

Mesenteric lymphangioma are multiseptated lesions, which can attain large size and change shape. They have minimal noneffect on the adjacent bowel and no displacement of the mesenteric vessels is seen.

Intraperitoneal Abscess

These develop usually following surgery, bowel perforation, trauma, pancreatitis or in patients with decreased immune response. The majority develop in the upper and down and on the right side.

A loculated fluid collection containing gas bubbles (echogenic foci with reverberation artifacts) is strongly suggestive of an abscess. Ultrasound may reveal this typical appearance or it may be seen as an ovoid or irregularly-shaped collection with debris, debris-fluid level **(Figs. 11.4.3 and 11.4.4)** or septations. A complex appearance with solid and cystic components can also be seen. Some abscess may simulate as echogenic solid mass.

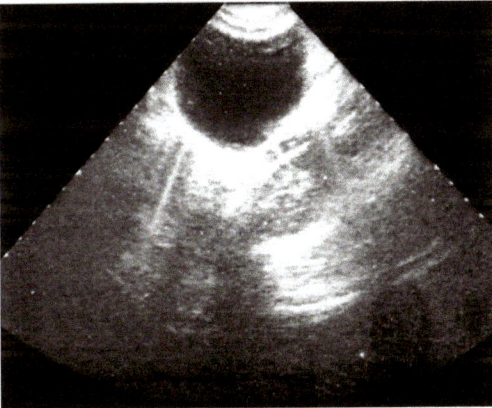

Fig. 11.4.1: Mesenteric cyst—a large cystic anechoic space-occupying lesion (SOL) with thin wall seen displacing the bowel loops.

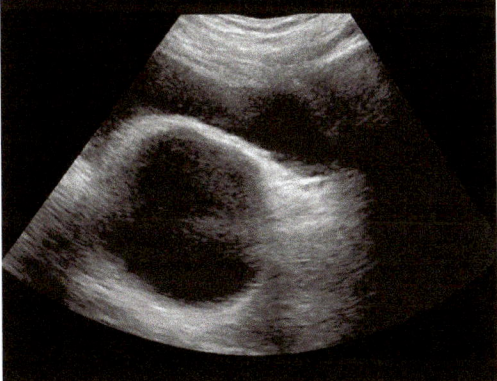

Fig. 11.4.2: Hypoechoic cystic lesion in peritoneal cavity suggestive of mesenteric cyst.

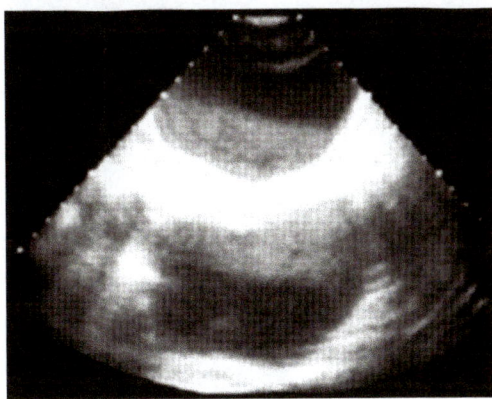

Fig. 11.4.3: Pelvic abscess—fluid debris level is seen inside it.

Lymphocele

Surgery or trauma causes disruption of lymphatic vessels resulting in lymph collection. They are most commonly seen in pelvis or intraperitoneal recesses **(Fig. 11.4.5)**.

They usually appear as anechoic collection of variable size. Large collections can cause significant pressure symptoms. Complicated lymphocele contains debris or septae.

Meconium Peritonitis

Antenatal bowel perforation spill meconium into the peritoneal cavity which incites a foreign body reaction results in formation of a cystic or complex mass having echogenic walls.

Intestinal stenosis/atresia and meconium ileus are the common causes.

Occurs most commonly in the abdominal wall, but also in the mesentery. Mesenteric-dermoid tumors are hypoechoic masses with areas of acoustic shadowing due to fibrotic tissue.

Lymphoma

- Most common primary mesenteric malignancy
- Isolated enlarged lymph nodes measuring more than 1.5 cm in diameter are seen around the celiac axis
- SMA and in the porta hepatis
- Often hypoechoic
- Lobulated mass encasing the mesenteric vessels that manifests as linear echoes within the mass-referred to as "Sandwich" sign
- May present as an exophytic mass in bowel wall with a solid mass in the mesentery.

Mesothelioma

- Is a sarcoma arising from the serous membrane
- Closely related to asbestos exposure
- Thickening of the omentum forming an omental mantle or cake is evident on US. This appearance is also seen in tuberculosis or peritoneal carcinomatosis
- Minimal ascites
- Liver metastasis pleural plaques and effusion, small nodules may be identified on peritoneal surface or in the mesenteric fat.

Cystic Mesothelioma

Very rare neoplasm of the peritoneum. It has no association with asbestos exposure.

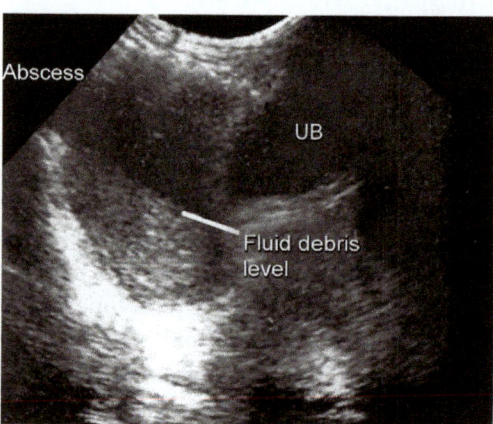

Fig. 11.4.4: Fluid-debris level seen inside a collection in the pelvis. (UB: urinary bladder)

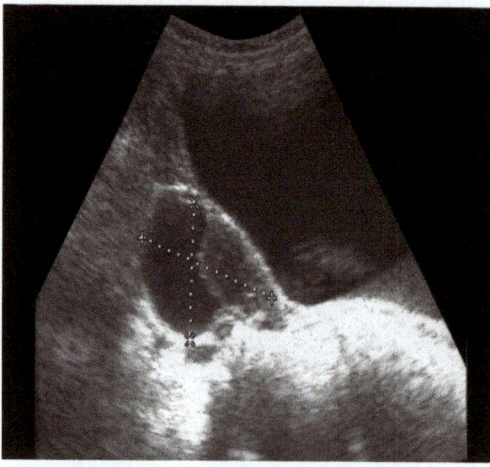

Fig. 11.4.5: Pelvic abscess (in calipers).

Peritoneal tuberculosis may be caused by direct spread of bowel tuberculosis or by hematogenous dissemination of a lung lesion. On sonography a loculated fluid collection with septae and debris may be seen. Associated features are mesenteric lymphadenopathy, omental case, bowel thickening and ascites.

Omental Cyst

On ultrasound, this appears as a well-defined, rounded, anechoic lesion present close to the bowel wall. This resembles a mesenteric cyst which is present in the root of the mesentery.

Pancreatic Pseudocyst (Figs. 11.4.6A and B)

Pancreatic pseudocysts are collection of pancreatic fluid with a high amylase content surrounded by a fibrosis wall. These develop in 50% of patients 2 to 3 weeks after an attack of acute pancreatitis. On US, they appear as a well-defined, walled-off anechoic collection most commonly seen in the lesser sac. Few dependent debris may be evident. Septae and echoes develop within it following infection. Other features or complications of pancreatitis may also be evident.

Metastasis

Metastasis to the peritoneum and mesentery usually arises due to intraperitoneal readings from a variety of sources most common being carcinoma of ovary and GIT and breast.

On ultrasound thickened sheet-like greater omentum (secondary to infiltration by metastasis cells) appear as "omental mantle or cake". In the presence of ascites, small nodules attached to the peritoneal surface are seen clearly.

Enlarged isolated mesenteric lymph nodes or conglomerated hypoechoic lymph node may be evident masses **(Figs. 11.4.7A and B)**.

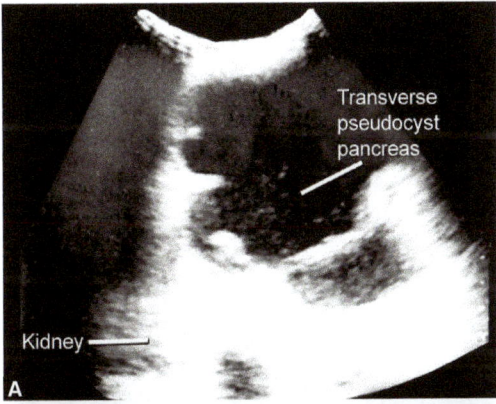
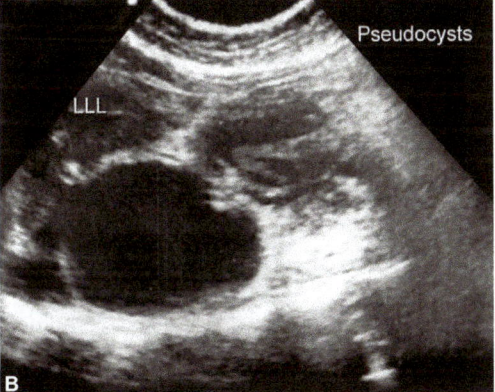

Figs. 11.4.6A and B: (A) Pseudocyst pancreas—a large multiloculated collection seen in lesser sac with evidence of debris in it; (B) A large pseudocyst seen in lesser sac posterior to left lobe of liver (LLL). Another pseudocyst is seen adjacent to it with evidence of internal septae.

Pseudomyxoma Peritonei (Figs. 11.4.8A and B)

Characterized by mucinous peritoneal implants and gelatinous ascites.

Most often caused by secondary metastasis from mucin- producing adenocarcinoma of ovary, appendix, colon and rectum. Hypoechoic to strongly echogenic nodular masses distributed throughout the peritoneal cavity. These deposits characteristically scalloping the adjacent liver surface.

Leiomyomatosis peritonealis disseminated: This condition occurs in pregnant or women

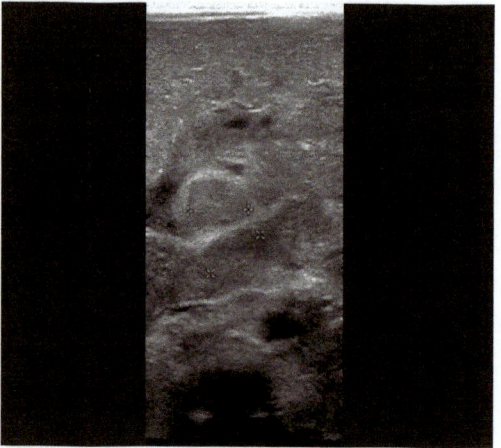

Fig. 11.4.7A: Multiple enlarged mesenteric lymph nodes.

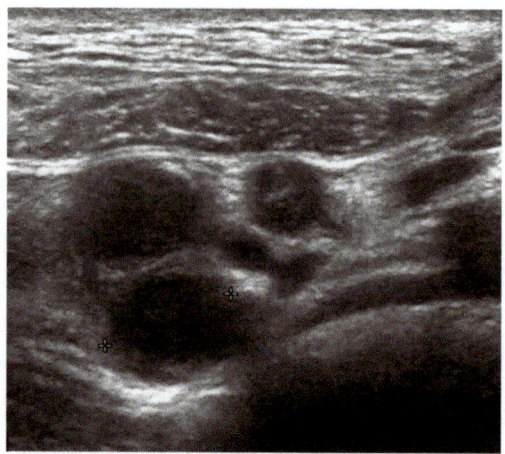

Fig. 11.4.7B: Ultrasound image showing multiple enlarged multiple mesenteric lymph nodes.

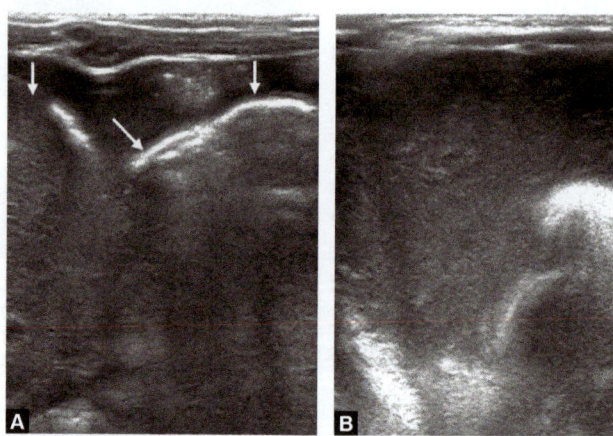

Figs. 11.4.8A and B: Meconium peritonitis in an infant—calcification (arrows) on bowel wall surface with meconium-filled peritoneal cavity.

of childbearing age group. Disseminated solid benign leiomyoma are seen a solid peritoneal masses. Ascites is usually not present.

Diffuse infiltrative lipomatosis: This rare disease entity affects young people is characterized by overgrowth of fat in the retroperitoneum. On US, an echogenic mass is evident which cannot be differentiated from liposarcoma.

Peritoneal Inclusion Cyst

- It is also called multilocular peritoneal inclusion cyst or benign cystic mesothelioma
- Uncommon benign primary peritoneal tumor that has no relation with the malignant mesothelioma
- Occurs in premenopausal women with prior gynecological surgery or infection that results in peritoneal scarring. The hormonally active ovaries secrete fluid that becomes loculated in the pelvis
- *The imaging features are nonspecific except that it has to be located in the pelvis:*
  - Multicystic pelvic mass
  - Peritoneal surfaces of uterus, bladder
  - May extend into upper abdomen.

CHAPTER 12

Scrotum

12.1 DIFFERENTIAL DIAGNOSIS OF ACUTE SCROTUM

Causes

- Testicular torsion
- Epididymitis with or without orchitis
- Torsion of testicular appendages
- Testicular trauma
- Acute hydrocele (**Fig. 12.1.1**)
- Incarcerated hernia
- Idiopathic scrotal edema
- Henoch-Schönlein purpura
- Scrotal fat necrosis
- Familial Mediterranean fever
- Abdominal pathology.

Testicular Torsion

- Normal size and appearance early
- Hypoechoic after 4-6 hours due to edema
- Heterogeneous after 24 hours due to hemorrhage infarction known as missed torsion
- Hypoechoic epididymis
- Reactive hydrocele
- Skin thickening
- Enlarged twisted spermatic cord.

Epididymitis with or without Orchitis

- The part affected is bulky, heterogeneous and hypoechoic (**Figs. 12.1.2 to 12.1.4**)
- Associated reactive hydrocele, skin-thickening

- Increased/normal color flow is the point of differentiation from torsion (**Figs. 12.1.5 and 12.1.6**)
- Infarction and abscess are the complications.

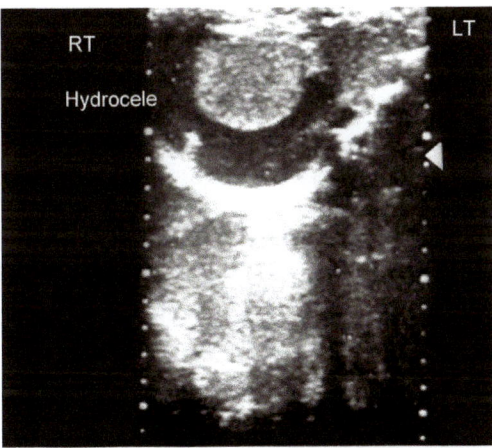

Fig. 12.1.1: Transverse section of right scrotal sac showing hydrocele. (RT: right; LT: left)

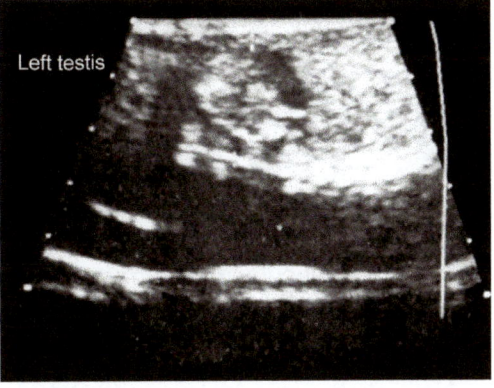

Fig. 12.1.2A: Epididymis is swollen with a collection adjacent to it with internal echoes—epididymitis with scrotal abscess.

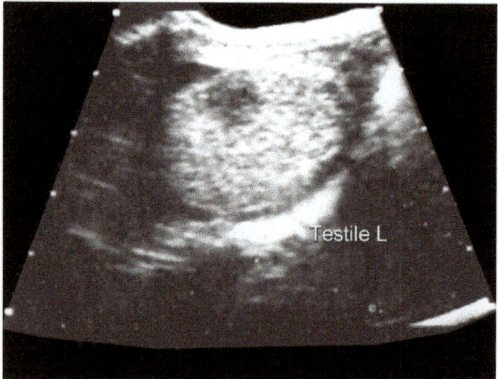

Fig. 12.1.2B: Epididymis is swollen and shows a hypoechoic lesion in testis. FNAC confirmed tubercular epididymo-orchitis.

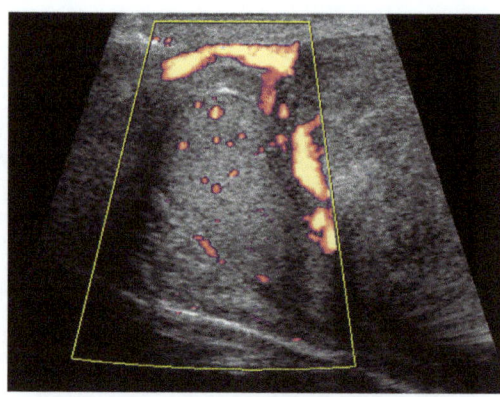

Fig. 12.1.5: Power Doppler US scan shows vascular extratesticular mass.

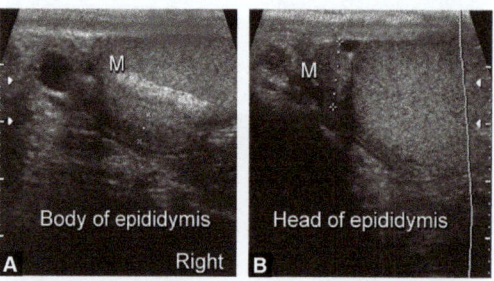

Figs. 12.1.3A and B: US scans show cystic lesion in head of epididymis. (M: mass)

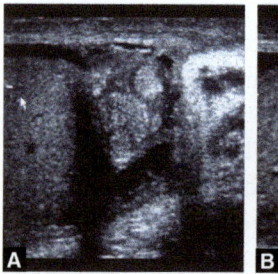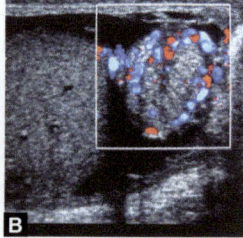

Figs. 12.1.6A and B: Epididymitis—thickened epididymis showing increased vascularity.

Testicular Trauma

- Pathologies that occur are hematoma, fracture, rupture
- A ruptured testis is ill-defined, hypoechoic, heterogeneous with loss of normal contour and ruptured tunica. Seminiferous tubules may be extruded
- Fracture may or may not be seen as a hypoechoic line
- Hematoma is seen as a mass of variable appearance according to age.

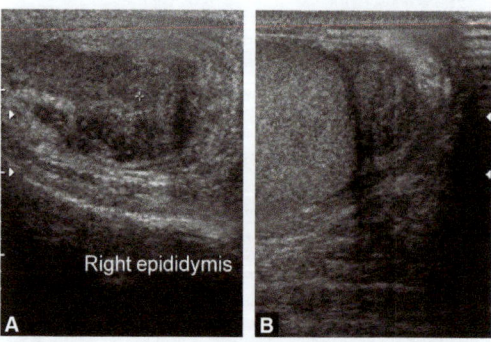

Figs. 12.1.4A and B: US scans show chronic epididymitis.

Torsion of Testicular Appendage (Fig. 12.1.7)

- Variable sized, ovoid to round, mobile hypoechoic mass with hyperechoic rim
- Decreased internal and increased external vascularity.

Idiopathic Scrotal Edema

- Between 5 and 11 years of age
- Pain, swelling, erythema
- Thickened scrotal wall with normal testes and epididymis
- Increase/normal color flow in wall.

Scrotum

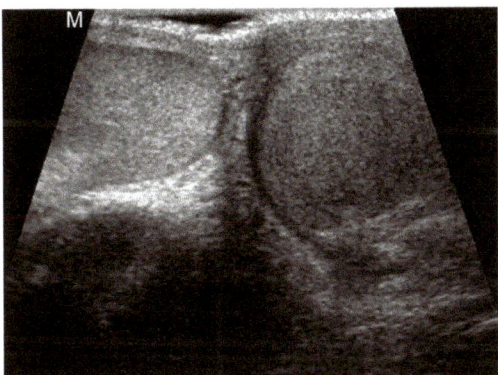

Fig. 12.1.7: US scan shows torsion of left testis. (M: mass)

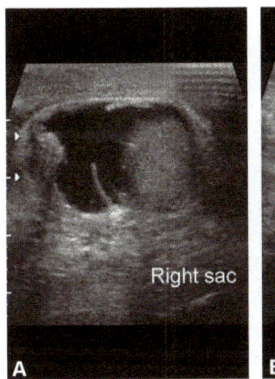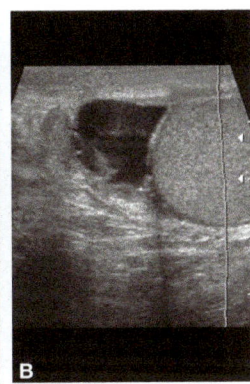

Figs. 12.2.1A and B: US scans show tubercular collection in scrotal sac.

Henoch-Schönlein Purpura

- Diffusely swollen scrotum and its contents with normal color flow/increased flow
- Resolves completely and spontaneously.

Abdominal Pathology

- Especially in neonates with patent processus vaginalis
- Conditions that can cause secondary symptoms in scrotum are adrenal hemorrhage, delayed spleen rupture of battered baby, hepatic laceration, Crohn's disease, acute appendicitis, appendix perforation
- Scrotal vein thrombosis due to catheterization of femoral vein during cardiac catheterization is an unusual cause.

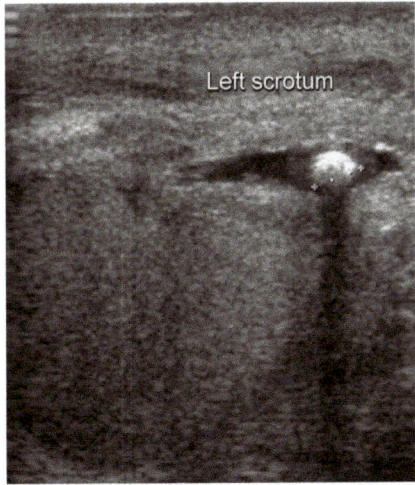

Fig. 12.2.2: US scan shows scrotolith.

12.2 DIFFERENTIAL DIAGNOSIS OF SCROTAL CALCIFICATION

Testicular Calcifications

- *Infective:* Granuloma, tuberculosis **(Figs. 12.2.1 and 12.2.2)**, filariasis, sarcoidosis
- *Vascular:* Infarcts, vascular malformation arterial wall
- Testicular microlithiasis
- *Neoplasms:* Burnt out germ cell tumor, large sertoli cell tumors, teratoma/teratocarcinoma gonadoblastoma **(Figs. 12.2.3 and 12.2.4)**.

Extratesticular Calcifications

- Chronic epididymitis
- Scrotal pearls
- Schistosomiasis
- Hematomas
- Meconium peritonitis.

Testicular Microlithiasis
(Figs. 12.2.5 and 12.2.6)

- Calcified specks within seminiferous tubules
- Corpora-amylacea-like bodies formed

152 Differential Diagnosis in Ultrasound

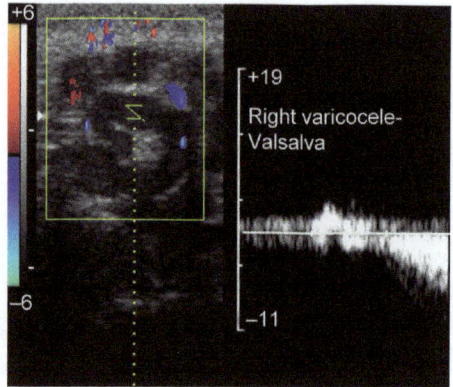

Fig. 12.2.3: US scans show reversal of flow in varicocele.

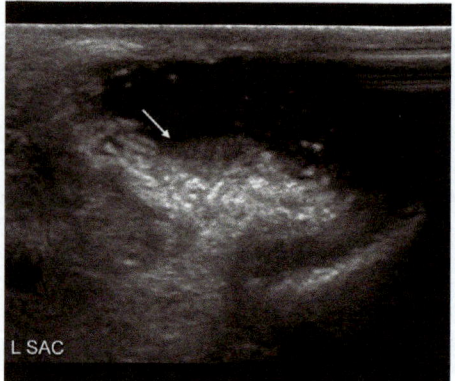

Fig. 12.2.6: Calcification in scrotal sac. (L SAC: left sac)

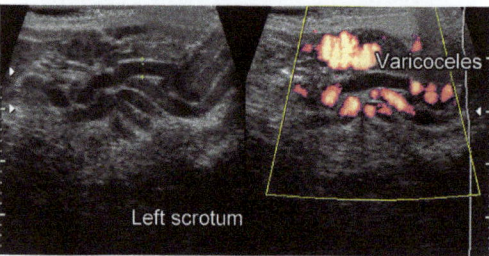

Fig. 12.2.4: US and color Doppler scans show varicoceles.

- Bilateral
- Follow-up 6 monthly with tumor marker evaluation is a must.

Isolated Microlithiasis

Fewer than fine simple calcification.

Scrotal Pearls

- Parts of tunica break loose when inflamed or even from a tarted appendix testes/epididymis
- Lie between two layers of tunica with associated hydrocele
- Consists of hydroxyapatite core with fibrinoid material deposited around it.

Sarcoidosis

- Epididymal involvement more than testicular
- Recurrent painless inflammation, enlargement.

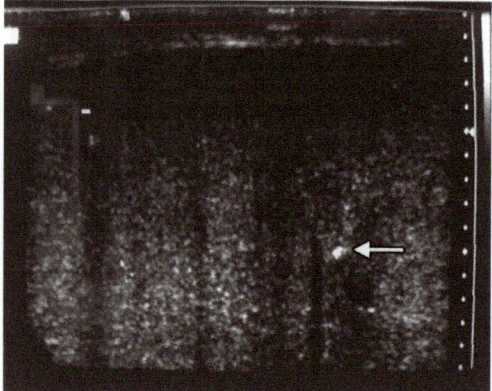

Fig. 12.2.5: Testicular calcification (arrow).

- Associated with cryptorchidism, Klinefelter's syndrome, tumors, pseudohermaphroditism
- Echogenic specks with comet tail artefact and no shadow

12.3 DIFFERENTIAL DIAGNOSIS OF SCROTAL GAS

- *Infection by gas forming bacteria:*
  - Associated calcification, fluid, thickened wall/tunica
  - Testes is bulky and hypoechoic

Scrotum

- Heterogeneous echotexture
- Flow increased
• *Hernia of bowel loops, if processus vaginalis is patent:* Intrascrotal peristalsis is confirmatory
• Trauma/intervention
• Pneumoperitoneum with patent PV.

12.4 DIFFERENTIAL DIAGNOSIS OF SCROTAL MASSES

Intratesticular

• *Secondary:* Metastasis, lymphoma, leukemia
• *Primary:* Malignant **(Fig. 12.4.1)**.

Germ Cell Tumors

- More common in testis when it is in ectopic position **(Figs. 12.4.2 and 12.4.3)**
- About 90–95% mostly malignant.
- *Tumors of one histologic type:*
  - *Seminoma:*
    - Classical
    - Spermatocytic
  - *Embryonal cell carcinoma—adult type:*
    - Infantile type
    - Endodermal sinus tumor (yolk sac tumor)
  - *Teratoma—mature:*
    - Immature

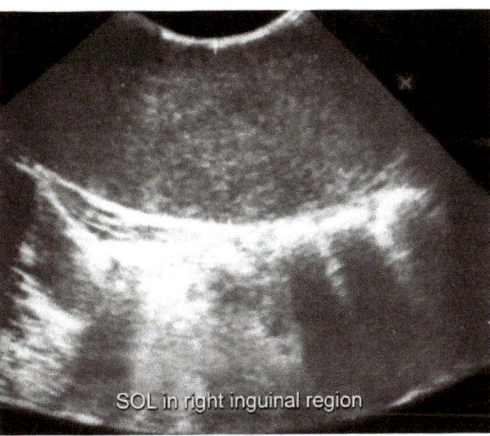

Fig. 12.4.2A(i): Well-defined round homogeneous echotexture space-occupying lesion (SOL) seen in the right inguinal region.

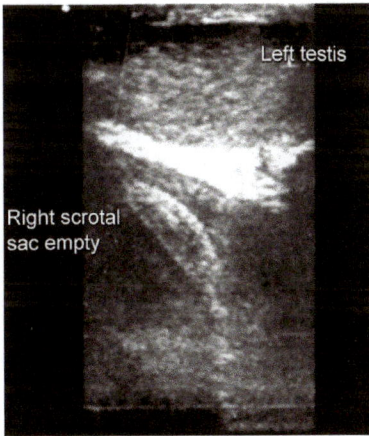

Fig. 12.4.2A(ii): The right scrotal sac is empty and left testis is normal in position.

   - With malignant transformation
   - Choriocarcinoma.
• *Tumors of more than one histologic type:*
   - Teratocarcinoma (teratoma with embryonal cell carcinoma)
   - Any other combination.

Gonadal Stromal Tumor

- About 3–6%, mostly benign
- Leydig cell tumor
- Sertoli's cell tumor

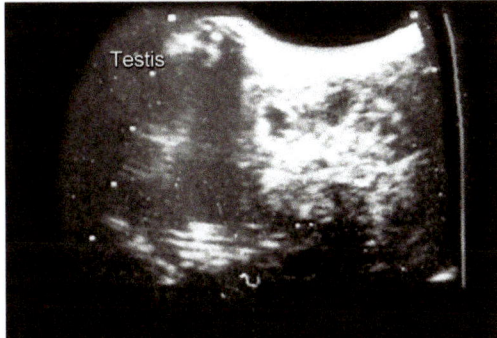

Fig. 12.4.1: Testicular malignancy—right testis is replaced by a solid mass of heterogeneous echotexture with few hypoechoic, anechoic and hyperechoic areas.

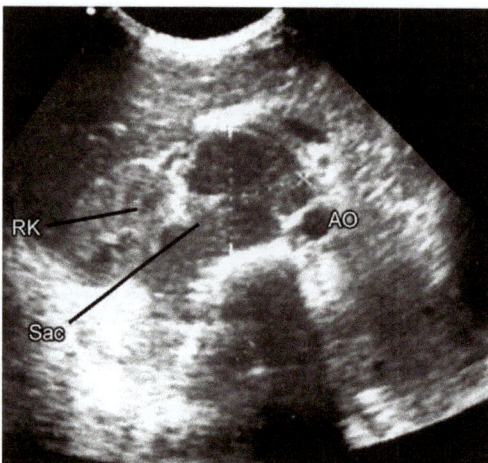

Fig. 12.4.2A(iii): There are para-aortic lymph nodes. Excision biopsy from the lesion revealed seminoma testis. (RK: right kidney; AO: aorta)

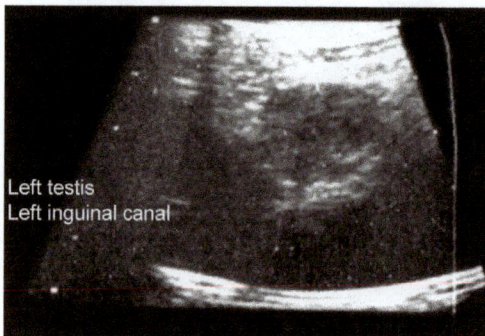

Fig. 12.4.2B: Left ectopic testis lying in the inguinal canal.

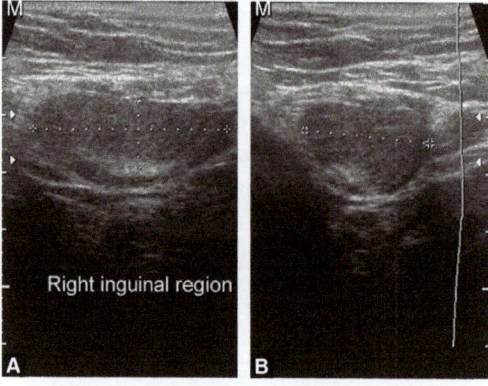

Figs. 12.4.3A and B: US scans show undescended testis in inguinal canal. (M: mass)

- Granulosa cell tumor
- Theca cell tumor
- Tumors of primitive gonadal stroma
- Mixed.

Benign

- Simple cyst
- Epidermoid cyst
- Cystic dysplasia
- Abscess
- Tubular ectasia
- Tunica albuginea cyst
- Adrenal rests
- Sarcoidosis
- Infarcts
- Calcification.

Extratesticular

- Varicocele **(Figs. 12.4.4A and B)**
- Inguinoscrotal hernia
- Hemato-/Pyo-/hydrocele **(Figs. 12.4.5 and 12.4.7)**
- Epididymal lesions
- *Tumors:* Benign—adenomatoid and cystadenoma, cholesterol granuloma, soft tissue tumors **(Fig. 12.4.6)**.

Malignant: Soft tissue tumors, lymphoma, metastasis.

Extratesticular Male Genital Tract Calcification

- Diabetes mellitus
- Chronic infection—tuberculosis, schistosomiasis
- Ejaculatory duct calculi
- Chronic prostastitis
- Calcified corpora amylacea.

Scrotum

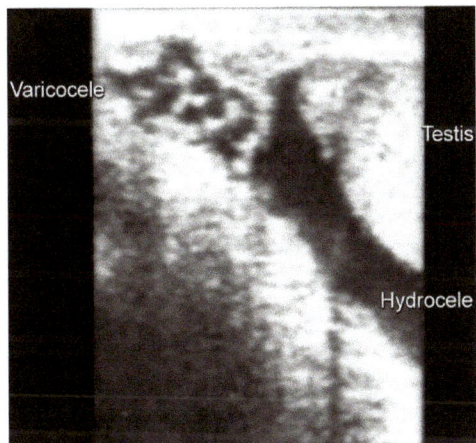

Fig. 12.4.4A: Varicocele—multiple anechoic tubular channels are seen in both the scrotal sacs.

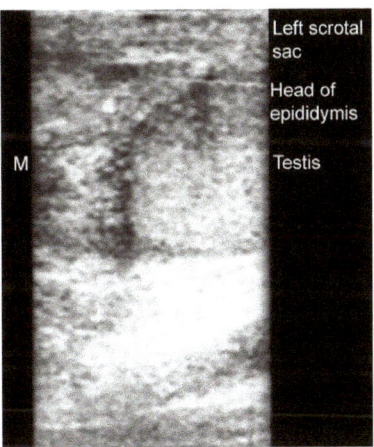

Fig. 12.4.6: A heterogeneous predominantly echogenic SOL is seen in the left scrotal sac superior to testis in a case of left inguinal hernia. (M: mass)

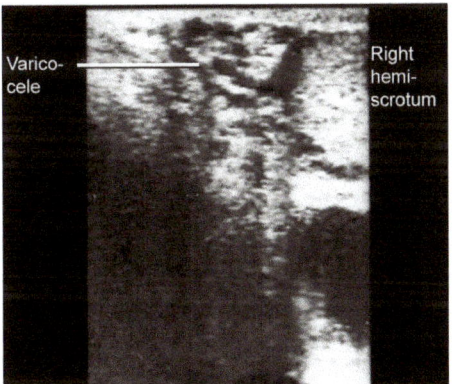

Fig. 12.4.4B: Hydrocele is seen on the left side.

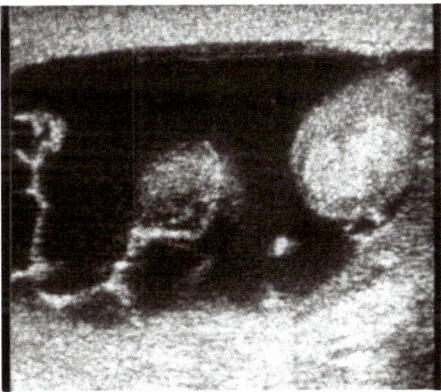

Fig. 12.4.7: Fluid with thick septations in scrotal sac—pyocele.

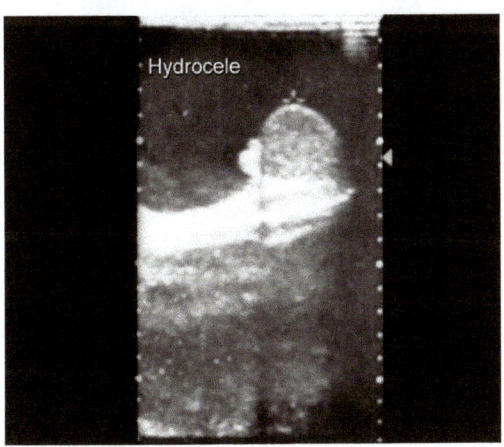

Fig. 12.4.5: Gross hydrocele.

GENERAL POINTS

- Most extratesticular masses are benign while intratesticular masses should be considered malignant unless proved otherwise
- Most benign lesions are uniformly echogenic while all echogenic lesions should not be considered benign blindly
- Most malignancies are hypoechoic to normal testes unless complicated by calcification, necrosis, hemorrhage and fatty change.

CHAPTER 13

Testis and Epididymis

13.1 DIFFERENTIAL DIAGNOSIS OF CYSTIC TESTICULAR LESIONS

Benign Cysts

- Simple cyst **(Fig. 13.1.1)**
- Tubular ectasia
- Cystic dysplasia
- Abscess
- Tunica albuginea cyst
- Epidermoid cyst
- Infarction **(Figs. 13.1.2A to C)**.

Malignant Cystic Lesions

- Teratocarcinoma
- Yolk sac tumor

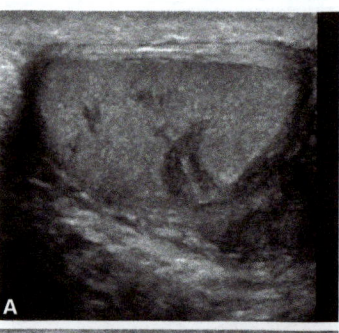
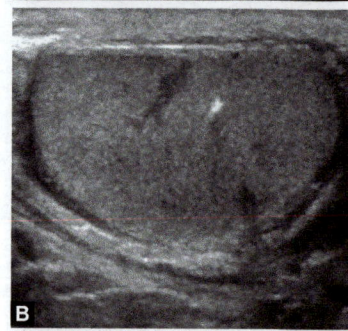
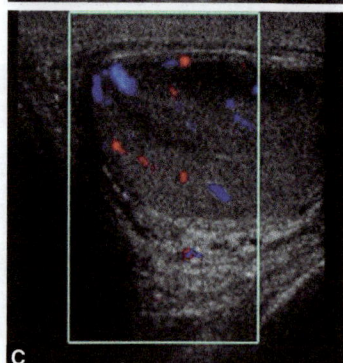
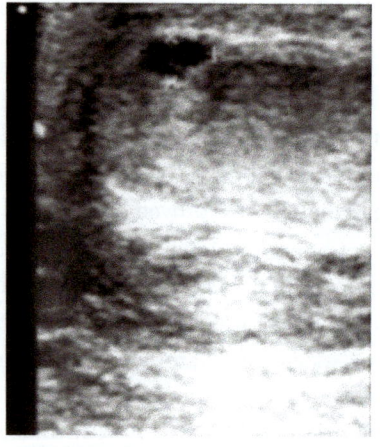

Fig. 13.1.1: Testicular cyst—a small well-defined anechoic area seen in the left testis.

Figs. 13.1.2A to C: Wedge-shaped hypoechoic lesion in the posterior wall of right testis and focus of calcification showing no flow on color Doppler examination suggesting testicular infarct.

- Hemorrhage and necrosis in any mass
- Tubular obstruction because of any tumor
- Lymphoma.

Cysts in Testis are Discovered Incidentally in 8–10% of Population

Tunica Albuginea Cysts

- About 2-5 mm, located on anterior/lateral aspect
- Simple cystic in nature
- 5th to 6th decades, asymptomatic
- Solitary/multiple, unilocular/multilocular.

Tubular Ectasia

- Tubular ectasia of rete testis can occur due to malignant/inflammatory traumatic obstruction of the epididymis
- Seen as multiple abnormal, tortuous channels in the region of mediastinum showing no color flow
- Usually bilateral, may be associated with ipsilateral spermatocele formation.

Cystic Dysplasia

- Congenital noncommunication between tubules and rete testes/efferent ductules
- Infant and young children
- Associated with renal agenesis/dysplasia
- Multiple interconnecting simple cysts in area of rete testis extending into adjacent parenchyma, causing it atrophy.

Epidermoid Cyst

- Benign tumor of germ cell origin
- About 1% of all testicular tumors
- 2nd to 4th decades of life
- Lying below tunica albuginea
- Are basically teratomas showing monomorphic, monodermal differentiation along the lines of ectodermal cell differentiation

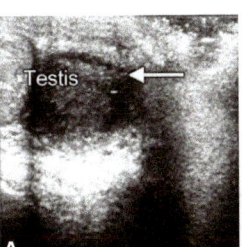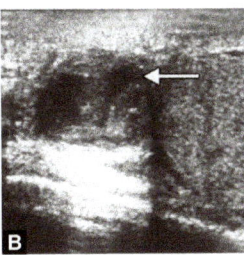

Figs. 13.1.3A and B: Epididymal abscesses—heterogeneously hypoechoic lesions (arrows) with posterior acoustic enhancement in bilateral epididymis in tubercular epididymo-orchitis.

- Present as testicular enlargement or a painless solitary nodule
- Well-defined, solid, hypoechoic mass which may have internal echoes and has an echogenic capsule.

Abscess (Figs. 13.1.3A and B)

- Looks like an abscess elsewhere and differentiation from malignancy especially in AIDS patients is sometimes very difficult
- May occur as a complication of epididymo-orchitis, missed testicular torsion, primary pyogenic arthritis and gangrenous/infected tumor
- Infections that may cause it are mumps, smallpox, scarlet fever, influenza, typhoid, sinusitis, osteomyelitis, appendicitis
- May lead to pyocele formation if it rupture through tunica vaginalis or a fistula from skin.

Malignancies are considered in next topic.

13.2 PEDIATRIC TESTICULAR MASSES

- Mostly malignant
- Two peaks, i.e. 2½ years and adolescent
- Incidence increases 30–50 times in a dysplastic gonad like undescended testes, male pseudohermaphroditism, true hermaphroditism, testicular feminization syndrome

- The malignancies seen most commonly in dysplastic gonads are seminoma and gonadoblastoma due to absence of hormonal effects
- All tumors have a nonspecific USG appearance, i.e. focal/diffuse, increase/decrease echogenicity or even isoechogenicity, the size of testes may/may not increase the contour may be smooth or lobulated
- Because most lesions are isoechoic therefore altered vascularity by color Doppler is an important indicator
- Orchitis which shows similar features seldom occurs without epididymitis and is always associated with constitutional symptoms
- Simple cyst though rare may be seen
- Endodermal sinus tumor—1-2 years age + hernia + hydrocele + lung secondaries minus retroperitoneal lymph nodes
- Embryonal cell carcinoma—adolescent + lung metastasis + retroperitoneal lymphadenopathy.

GERM CELL TUMORS

Seminoma

Age

4th to 5th decades, rare prepuberty.

Nature

- Less aggressive than others
- Confined within tunica
- Only 25% metastasize at presentation
- Most favorable prognosis
- Metachronous/synchronous germ cell tumor occurs in 1–25% cases
- Increased incidence in a cryptorchid testes and even in a contralateral normal testes.

Ultrasonography

- Well-defined/ill-defined
- Hypoechoic/very hypoechoic
- Homogeneous
- No cyst/calcification.

Embryonal Cell Carcinoma

Age

2nd to 3rd decades, uncommon prepubertal.

Nature

- Usually in combination with others
- Aggressive, poorly radio/chemosensitive
- Visceral metastasis seen.

Ultrasonography

- Inhomogeneous
- Poorly marginated
- Distorts the contour, invades tunica
- Cystic area/calcification may be seen.

Endodermal Sinus/Yolk Sac Tumor

Age

- Less than two years
- Most common germ cell tumor in infants
- 60% of testicular tumor in infants.

Nature

- Infantile form of above
- Increased serum alpha-fetoprotein (AFP) in 95%.

Ultrasonography

Same as above.

Teratoma

Age

Infancy and early childhood.

Nature

- Second peak in third decade
- Second most common testicular tumor

- One-third metastasize via lymphatics
- Prognosis however is fair
- In young mostly mature nonaggressive.

Ultrasonography

Well-defined, markedly inhomogeneous with solid, cystic areas and calcification.

Choriocarcinoma

Age

Second/third decade of life.

Nature

- Rarest type, rarely occurs in pure form
- Highly malignant
- Metastasize early by hematogenous and lymphatic routes
- Symptoms referable to metastatic sites are common presenting feature like cerebrovascular accident, hemoptysis
- Gynecomastia due to increased human chorionic gonadotropin (hCG).

Ultrasonography

Mixed echogenicity, ill-defined lesion.

Mixed Germ Cell Tumor

- Second most common testicular malignancy after seminoma
- Most common combination is one of teratoma and embryonal cell carcinoma known as teratocarcinoma.

Differentiating features of germ cell tumors

Sl. No.	Features	Seminoma tumors	Nonseminomatous tumors
1.	Age group	4th to 5th decade	2nd to 3rd decade
2.	Incidence	More common	Less common
3.	Behavior	Less aggressive	More aggressive

Contd...

Contd...

4.	Ultrasound appearance	Homogeneous hypoechoic	Inhomogeneous heteroechoic
5.	Calcification	Uncommon	Common

STROMAL TUMORS

- Usually constitute of multiple cell types
- A combination with germ cell tumors also known as gonadoblastoma, occurs predominantly in males with cryptorchidism, hypospadias and female internal secondary organ
- Most common stromal tumor is Leydig cell tumor which presents at about 20–50 years of age as a case of painless unilateral testicular enlargement or mass
- Above is associated with impotence, loss of libido or precocious virilization, gynecomastia
- Above is a small, solid, hypoechoic mass with few cystic areas.

OCCULT PRIMARY TUMORS

Due to high metabolic rate and vascular compromise large tumors regress on their own leaving only a fibrocalcific scar, and such are known as burned out tumors.

TESTICULAR METASTASIS

- Most common testicular tumor in men over sixty years of age
- Most common bilateral testicular tumor especially malignant lymphomatous deposits
- Poor prognosis
- Homogeneously hypoechoic, extending to adjacent areas and increased vascularity
- Nonlymphomatous deposits though rare come from lung, prostate, kidney, stomach, colon, pancreas, melanoma and neuroblastoma.

13.3 DIFFERENTIAL DIAGNOSIS OF EPIDIDYMAL LESIONS

Epididymal Cysts (Fig. 13.3.1)

- Dilated epididymal tubules
- Result from prior epididymitis or trauma
- Appear as simple cystic lesion.

Spermatocele (Fig. 13.3.2)

- Commoner but radiological indistinguishable from epididymal cyst
- Their location is almost always in head as against cyst that may occur in any part of epididymis
- The contents are slightly more echogenic and granular due to presence of fat, lymphocytes and spermatozoa as compared to cyst that have a simple serous content.

Sperm Granuloma

Results after vasectomy due to extravasation of seminiferous fluid into epididymis.

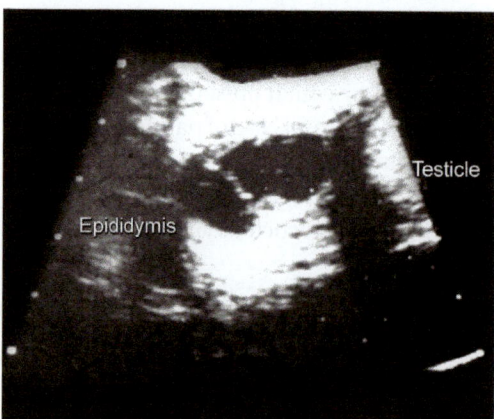

Fig. 13.3.1: Anechoic simple cyst with a thin septa seen in the region of head of the epididymis. Note the absence of internal echoes.

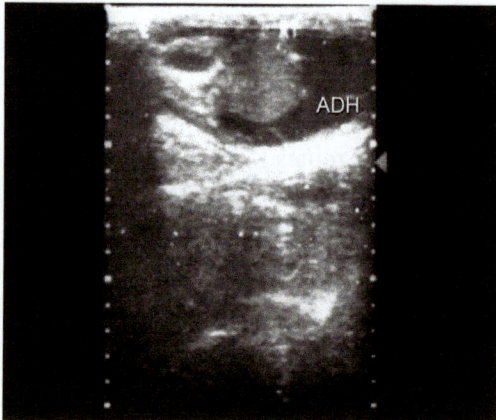

Fig. 13.3.3: Hydrocele with epididymitis (tubercular)—the epididymis is swollen and shows a hypoechoic area in it. Hydrocele shows multiple strands in it.

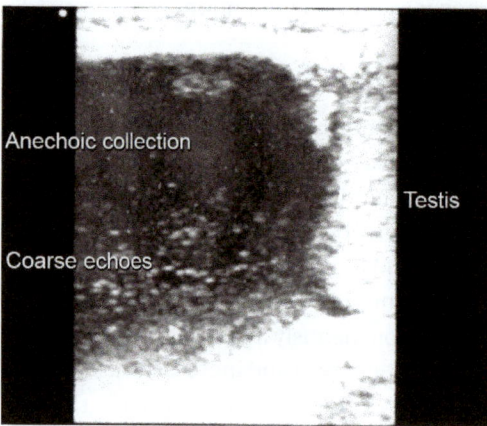

Fig. 13.3.2: A large anechoic collection with coarse internal echoes superior to left testis—spermatocele.

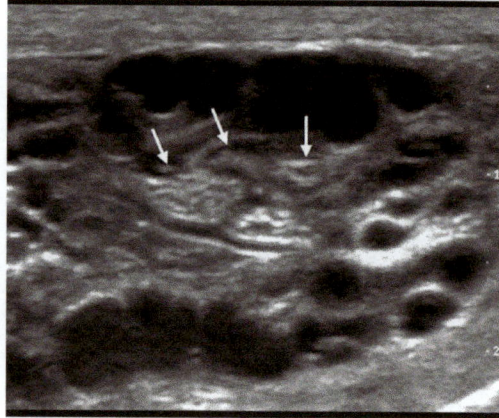

Fig. 13.3.4: Filarial worm (marked by arrows) in the epididymis (continuous movement of the worm was seen in real time).

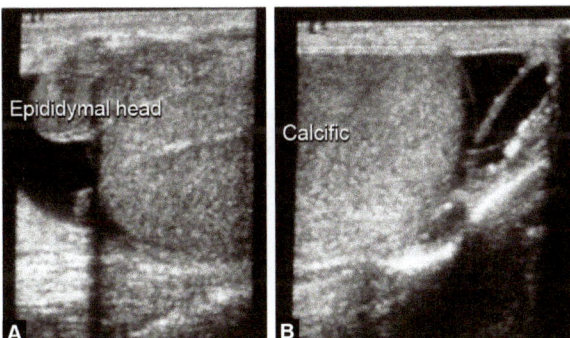

Figs. 13.3.5A and B: Tubercular epididymitis—thickened epididymis with multiple calcific foci.

Post-vasectomy Changes

Enlargement of epididymis associated with heterogeneity of echotexture and formation of cysts and granuloma.

Chronic Epididymitis (*see* Figs. 13.3.3 to 13.3.5)

- Few complex cystic lesions associated with thickened tunica and calcifications are the features
- Associated changes in the testes may also be seen.

CHAPTER 14

Prostate

14.1 DIFFERENTIAL DIAGNOSIS OF PROSTATIC CYST

Congenital

- Müllerian remnant cyst
- Utricle cyst.

Acquired

- Ejaculatory duct obstruction due to stone/operation
- Cystic change in tumors
- Retention cysts
- Benign prostatic hypertrophy (**Figs. 14.1.1A to C**).

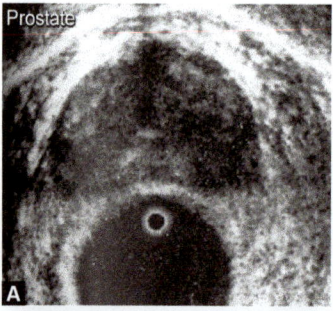
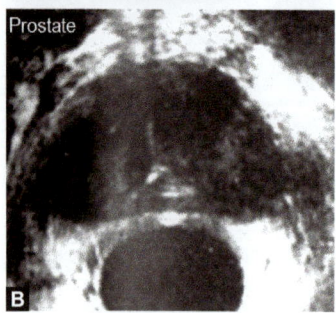

Figs. 14.1.1A and B

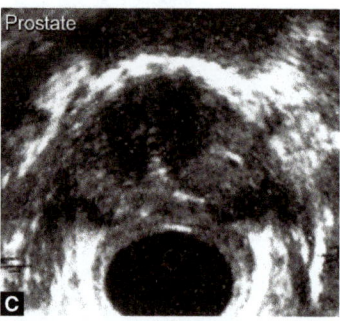

Figs. 14.1.1A to C: Benign prostatic hypertrophy.

14.2 MÜLLERIAN CYST

Müllerian cyst	Utricle cyst (Fig. 14.2.1)
1. Large in size	Small in size
2. Lateral/paramedian	Median
3. Has no sperms in it	Sperms present
4. No other associations	Associated with renal anomalies

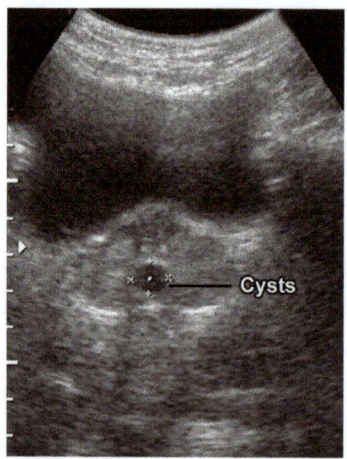

Fig. 14.2.1: US scan shows midline cyst in prostate.

Prostate

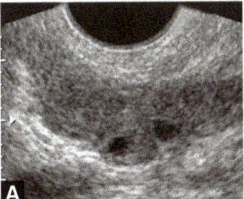 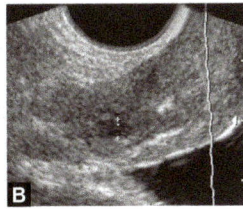

Figs. 14.3.1A and B: US scans show bilateral ejaculatory duct dilatation.

14.3 EJACULATORY DUCT CYST

- Small **(Figs. 14.3.1A and B)**
- Represent a diverticula or dilated obstructed duct
- Associated with infertility, perineal pain and low sperm count.

14.4 SEMINAL VESICLE CYST

- Result of Wolffian duct abnormality **(Figs. 14.4.1A and B)**

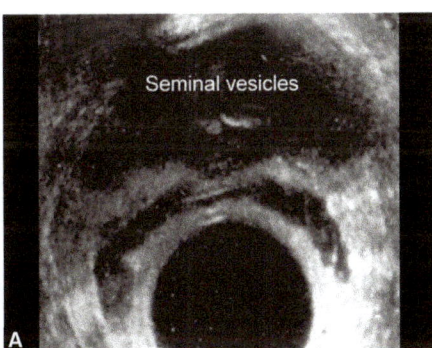

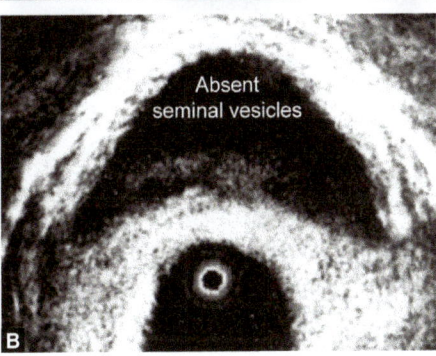

Figs. 14.4.1A and B: (A) Normal seminal vesicles; (B) Absent seminal vesicles.

- May be associated with ipsilateral renal agenesis, and ectopic ureter and vas deferens agenesis congenital
- Usually large, unilateral, solitary
- Associated with infection, invasive bladder tumor, and ejaculatory duct obstruction.

14.5 HYPOECHOIC LESIONS

- Adenocarcinoma (35%) **(Figs 14.5.1 to 14.5.3)**

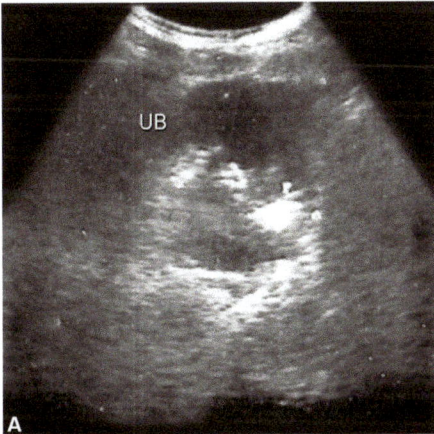

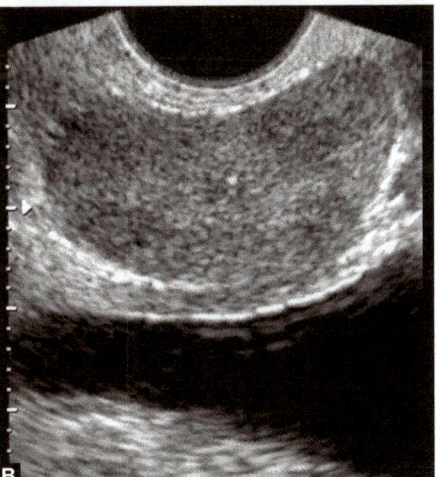

Figs. 14.5.1A and B: Carcinoma prostate: (A) Transverse scan of prostate shows a predominantly hypoechoic enlarged prostate with a focus of calcification invading the bladder base: the interface between prostate and bladder base is lost; (B) US scan shows granulomatous prostatitis. (UB: urinary bladder)

- Benign prostatic hyperplasia (18%)—rarely may originate in peripheral zone **(Fig. 14.5.4)**
- *Normal prostate tissue (18%):*
  - Cluster of prostate retention cysts
  - Prominent ejaculatory ducts

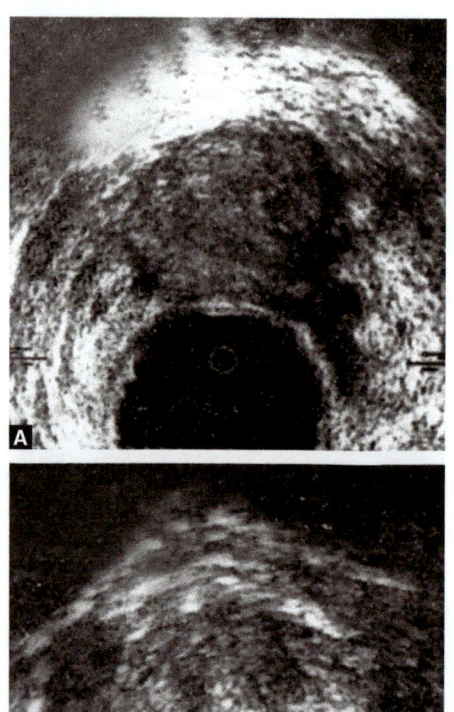

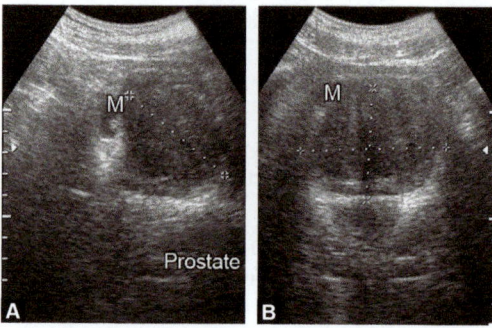

Figs. 14.5.4A and B: US scans show enlargement of median lobe in a patient of benign prostatic hyperplasia (BPH). (M: mass)

Figs. 14.5.2A and B: (A) Carcinoma prostate: Peripheral zone capsular invasion; (B) Carcinoma prostate: Peripheral zone capsular invasion.

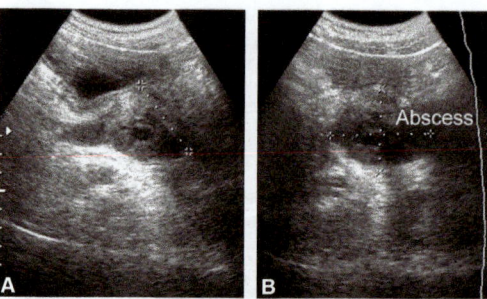

Figs. 14.5.5A and B: US scans show prostatic abscess.

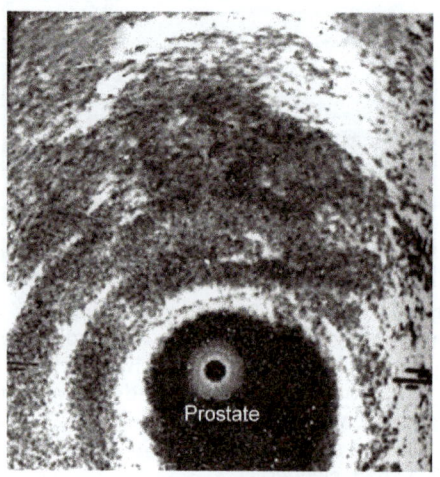

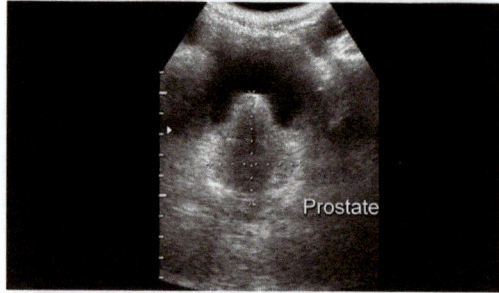

Fig. 14.5.3: Advanced carcinoma of prostate.

Fig. 14.5.6: US scan shows enlarged median lobe projecting into the neck of urinary bladder in a patient of BPH with bladder outlet obstruction.

Prostate

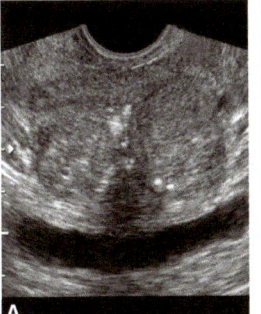
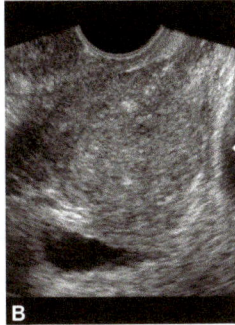

Figs. 14.5.7A and B: US scans show BPH with prostatic calcification.

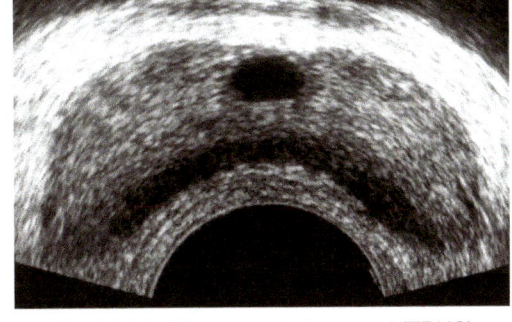

Fig. 14.5.8: Transrectal ultrasound (TRUS) showing simple prostate cyst.

- Acute/chronic prostatitis (14%) **(Figs. 14.5.5 to 14.5.8)**
- Granulomatous prostatitis (10.80%)—most common due to Calmette-Guérin Bacillus
- *Atrophy (10%):*
  - Occurs in (70%) of young healthy men
  - May be confused from carcinoma
- Prostatic dysplasia (6%).

14.6 PROSTATIC CALCIFICATION

- Calcified corpora amylacea—calcified proteinaceous material which may accumulate and cause prostatic duct obstruction in benign prostatic hyperplasia
- Tuberculosis
- Chronic prostatitis.

CHAPTER 15

Breast

Breast ultrasound (**Figs. 15.1.1 to 15.1.3**) is an important adjunct to screen-film mammography in the evaluation of breast disease.

The indication of sonography includes:
- To differentiate solid from cystic lesions
- To differentiate palpable masses in women who are pregnant and lactating
- As a primary modality for imaging of breast in women of less than 30 years of age

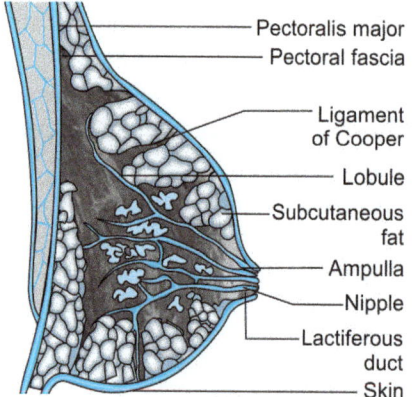

Fig. 15.1.1: Line diagram showing normal breast anatomy.

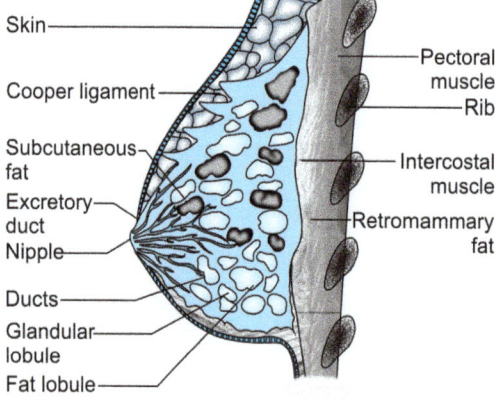

Fig. 15.1.2: Line illustration showing normal breast anatomy with detail breast parenchyma as seen on ultrasound.

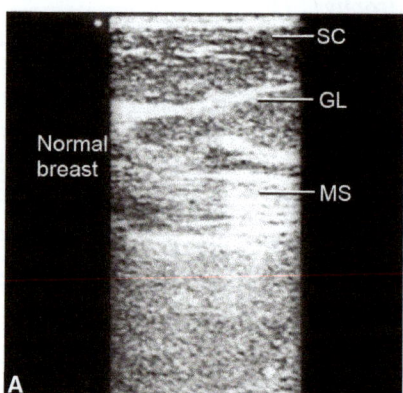

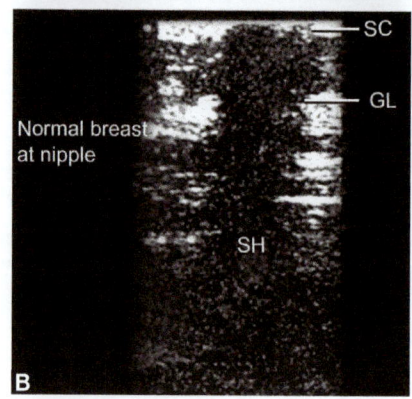

Figs. 15.1.3A and B: Ultrasound of breast shows normal anatomy. (SC: subcutaneous; GL: glandular lobule; MS: muscle; SH: shadowing)

- To evaluate asymmetric density on mammogram
- To provide guidance for interventional procedures such as cysts, aspiration, fine needle aspiration, biopsy, etc.

15.1 CYSTIC LESIONS

- *Simple cysts* **(Figs. 15.1.4 and 15.1.5)**—typical appearance is:
  - Round or oval in shape
  - Well-defined
  - Smooth thin wall
  - Echo-free mass
  - Distal enhancement
  - Through transmission
  - If sonographic criteria of a simple cyst are not met, it is classified as a complicated cyst wherein cyst aspiration is warranted.
- *Infected cysts:*
  - With fine mobile internal echoes, thick walls and surrounding edema
  - Color Doppler flow imaging (CDFI)—increased low resistance vascularity surrounding the lesion.
- *Intracystic papilloma:* Typically, polypoidal mass is noted within the cyst with demonstrable vascularity in color Doppler.
- *Intracystic carcinomas:* Complicated cyst with wall irregularity.
  Often the aspirated contents are blood stained and it reappears quickly.
- *Oil cysts:* Frequently seen in postoperative breasts
- *Breast abscess* **(Figs. 15.1.6 to 15.1.8)**: Seen as anechoic or echo poor area with diffusely increased echogenicity of the breast tissue and surrounding prominent vascularity.
- *Sebaceous cysts:* Can be echo-free or contain some reflective material and even calcification.
- *Hydatid cyst* **(Fig. 15.1.9):** Variable appearance on ultrasound (US) as elsewhere in the body, simple cystic appearance, is rare.

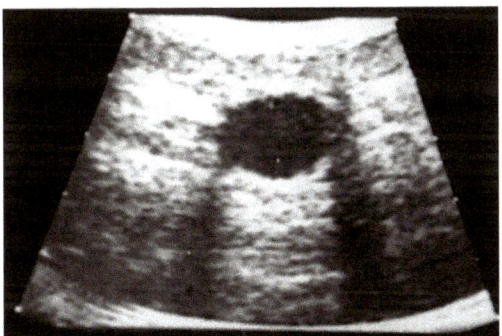

Fig. 15.1.4: A well-defined rounded cystic space-occupying lesion (SOL) with scattered internal echoes with posterior acoustic enhancement.

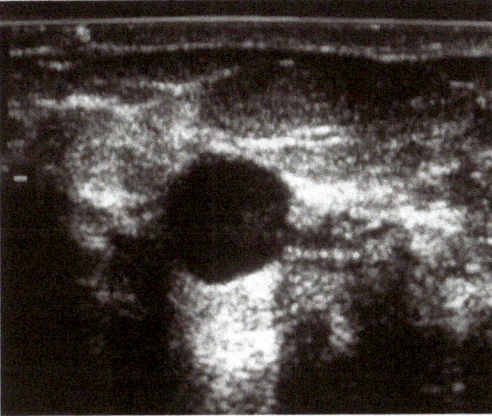

Fig. 15.1.5: Simple cyst in breast.

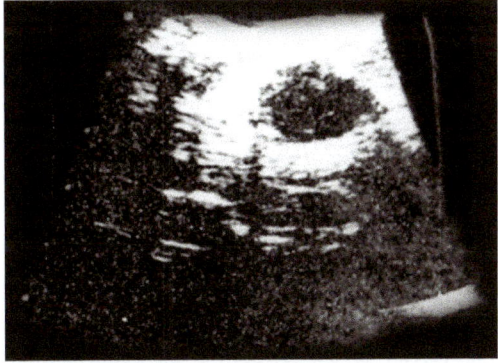

Fig. 15.1.6: Chronic abscess—right breast: US shows a well-defined hypoechoic mass with internal echoes and postedge enhancement.

- *Filarial cyst:* A moving filarial worm (filarial dance) is a rare specific finding on realtime US.
- *Lymphocele:* Usually in postoperative cases.
- Breast prosthesis.

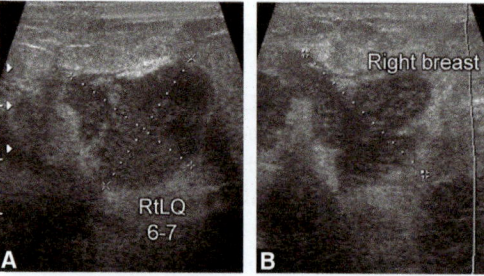

Figs. 15.1.7A and B: US scans show breast abscess. (RtLQ: right lower quadrant)

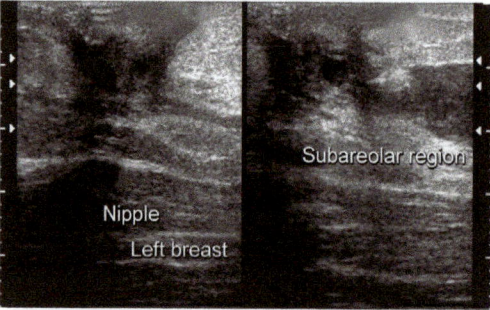

Fig. 15.1.8: US scans show breast abscess in subareolar region draining through nipple.

- *Galactocele:* It is a milk-filled retention cyst during pregnancy lactation, in newborn and infants.

  On US appears as single/multiloculated cystic lesion which is easily compressible.
  - Anechoic or hypoechoic (depending upon type of milk).

15.2 HYPERECHOIC LESIONS

- Lipomas have echogenicity similar to the subcutaneous fat
- Hemangioma
- *Hamartoma*: US features depend on the amount of fatty, glandular or fibrous tissue
- *Abscess*: Typically, reveals reflective zone in the inflamed area and surrounding high vascularity **(Fig. 15.2.1)**
- Ruptured breast prosthesis with granuloma
- Carcinomas larger than 2 cm especially colloid carcinoma
- Mastitis
- *Hematoma*: Acute
- Angiosarcoma.

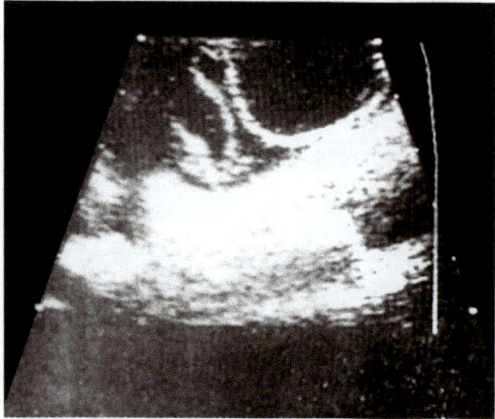

Fig. 15.1.9: Ultrasonography of left breast showing an anechoic lesion with collapsed membranes and septations—hydatid cyst.

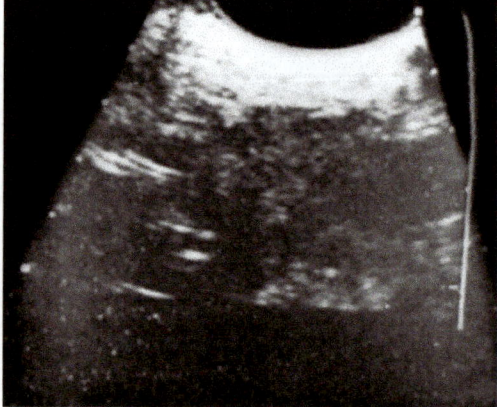

Fig. 15.2.1: Breast abscess—space-occupying lesion with ill-defined margins with internal echoes in outer quadrants of left breast. Superficial fat is thickened and echogenic.

15.3 HYPOECHOIC LESIONS

A. Benign Lesions

- *Fibroadenoma (Figs 15.3.1 to 15.3.3):*
  - Giant fibroadenoma
  - Juvenile fibroadenoma
- *Pseudoangiomatous stromal hyperplasia (PASH):* Seen in perimenopausal women
- Fat necrosis
- Old hematoma
- Sclerosing adenosis
- Radial scar
- Intramammary lymph node
- Scar granuloma.

B. Malignant Lesions

Principal US features are:
- Mass (nidus)
- Surrounding reflective zone (halo)

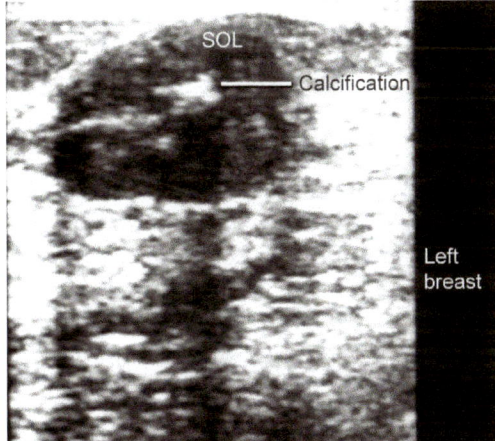

Fig. 15.3.1: Benign breast neoplasm—a well-defined homogeneously hypoechoic space-occupying lesion (SOL) with a dense focus of calcification.

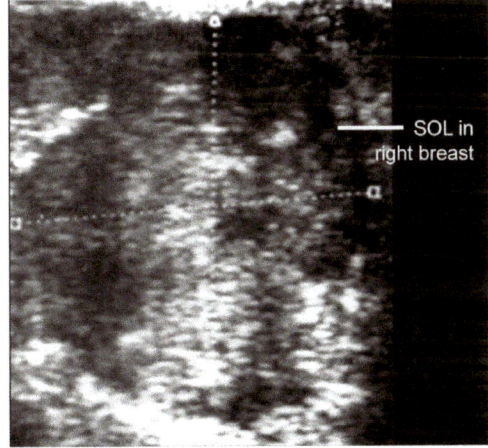

Fig. 15.3.3: Giant fibroadenoma large mass occupying most of breast with well-defined margin and slightly heterogeneous echotexture. (SOL: space-occupying lesion)

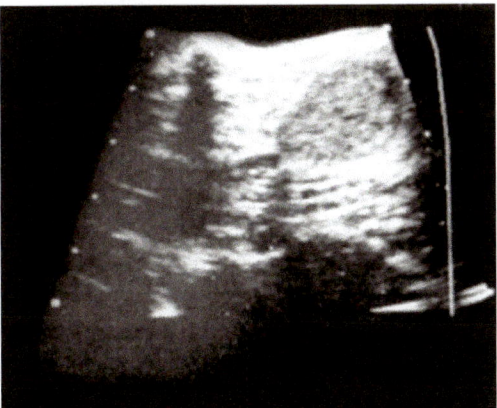

Fig. 15.3.2: Fibroadenoma—well-defined space-occupying lesion (SOL) of homogeneous echotexture as a mobile lump in right upper outer quadrant.

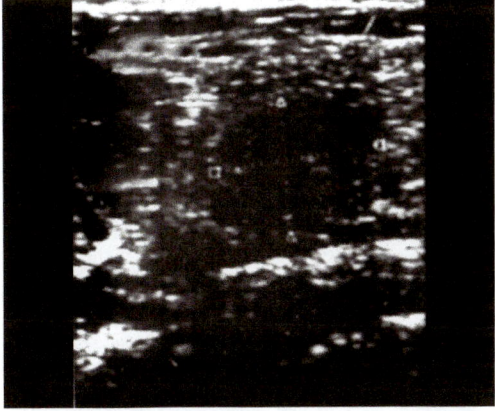

Fig. 15.3.4: Hypoechoic space-occupying lesion (SOL) with ill-defined lateral margins fine-needle aspiration cytology (FNAC) confirmed infiltrating duct carcinoma.

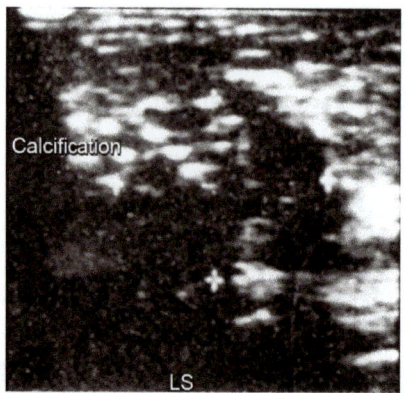

Fig. 15.3.5: Infiltrating duct carcinoma—mass calcification in breast carcinoma. (LS: longitudinal section)

- *Retrotumoral attenuation (shadow):*
  - Invasive ductal carcinoma
  - Medullary carcinoma **(Figs. 15.3.4 and 15.3.5)**
  - Sarcomas
  - Metastasis
  - Lymphoma
  - Recurrent tumors.

15.4 DUCTAL DILATATION

- Duct ectasia—on US **(Figs. 15.4.1 and 15.4.2)** this entity is diagnosed when the duct caliber exceeds 3 mm

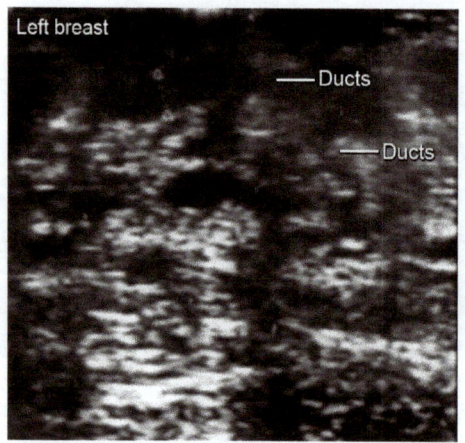

Fig. 15.4.1: Dilated ducts are seen in left breast.

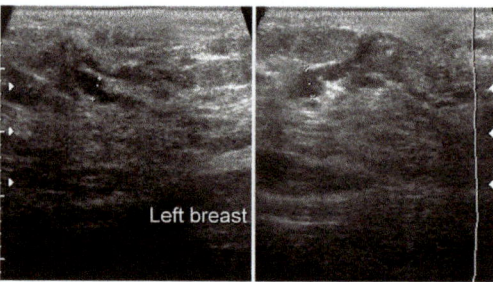

Fig. 15.4.2: US scans show ductal ectasia in breast.

- Plasma cell mastitis. Minimal ductal dilatation with thick reflective walls
- Intraductal papilloma can occasionally be identified in the subareolar ducts; smaller and peripherally located lesions are not revealed on US
- *Ductal carcinoma in situ (DCIS):* Sonography does not contribute to the detection of DCIS. It may reveal larger microcalcification as relatively strong echoes or dilated hypoechoic ductal structures
- Late pregnancy and lactating breasts.

15.5 BENIGN VS MALIGNANT

Type	Benign	Malignant
Shape	Oval/ellipsoid	Variable
Alignment	Wider than deep. Aligned parallel to tissue planes	Deeper than wide
Margins	Smooth/thin echogenic, pseudocapsule with 2–3 gentle lobulations	Irregular or spiculated Echogenic 'halo'
Echotexture	Variable to intense hyperechogenicity	Markedly hypoechoic
Homogeneity	Uniform	Absent
Shadowing	Present	Absent

Contd...

Contd...

Posterior enhancement	Minimal	Marked
Other signs	Coarse calcification macrolobulation, well-defined	Fine/stippled calcification, microlobulation, infiltration across tissue planes

15.6 MASTITIS

Mastitis **(Figs. 15.6.1A and B)** is a diffuse inflammation of the breast or a part of it. It can be infectious (usually Staphylococcus) and noninfections (after irradiation). On US, there is an increased reflectivity of the subcutaneous fat, skin thickening which later on can progress to abscess formation. CDFI reveals increased vascularity.

Plasma cell mastitis results in focal or more generalized attenuation with disruption of the tissue planes in the breast and thickened duct walls.

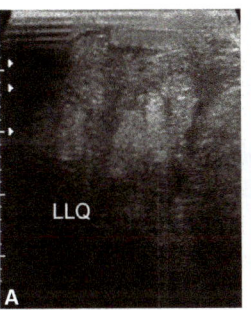 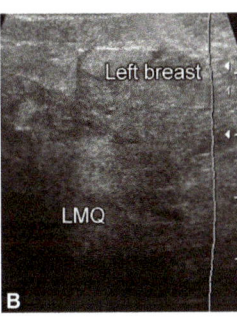

Figs. 15.6.1A and B: US scans show acute mastitis. (LLQ: left lower quadrant; LMQ: lower medial quadrant)

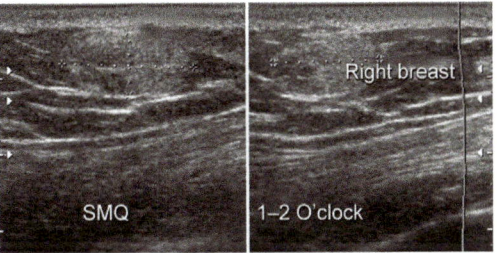

Fig. 15.6.2: US scans show lipoma in breast. (SMQ: superior medial quadrant)

Vascular Abnormalities

Can occur in the form of solid masses as hemangiomas or cystic lesions as venous malformations.

Mondor's Disease

Mondor's disease is a thrombosed subcutaneous vein, clinically presenting as phlebitis and retraction of the skin along the track of the vein which can be easily demonstrated on ultrasound.

Lipomas (Fig. 15.6.2)

Lipomas are common benign findings which on US appear as well-delineated compressible masses with an echotexture similar to normal fat. Some lipomas have fibrous reaction due to which they are more reflective than the surrounding fat.

Sclerosing Lesions

On US, they are sharply delineated hypoechoic lesions which may show round attenuation. Examples in this category are—medial scar or sclerosing adenosis.

Hamartoma or Fibroadenolipomas

Hamartoma of breast are composed of mixture of fatty, glandular and fibrous tissue in varying amounts but fat is the permanent constituent.

Breast Prosthesis

Mammography is difficult in these cases which makes ultrasound and MRI a much popular choice for evaluating such patients. The breast tissue is located superficially to the prosthesis and therefore easily visualized.

Prosthesis is seen as an echopoor structure which is commonly superficially with significant reverberation artefacts and outer double envelope or sometimes a fibrous capsule larger fluid collections with wrinkles of the disrupted envelope suggest ruptured prosthesis.

Gynecomastia

Refers to the condition characterized by unilateral (73%) enlargement of the glandular tissue of the breast in males which could be due to hormonal imbalance or drug induced changes. Sonographically, it can be seen as an oval-shaped, well-circumscribed mass or a diffuse reflective area similar to the parenchyma of an adult mature female breast.

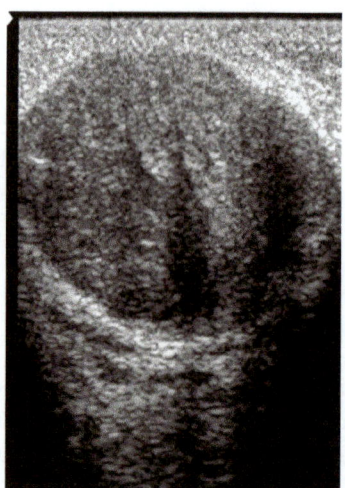

Fig. 15.7.1: US scan shows fibroadenoma.

15.7 BENIGN LESIONS

Cysts

- Quite common
- One quarter of the patients aged 35–50 years
- Almost invariably, multiple and bilateral
- Calcification is infrequent, however thin peripheral eggshell may be seen
- US shows—A well-defined echo-free mass with distal enhancement, round when tense and through transmission.

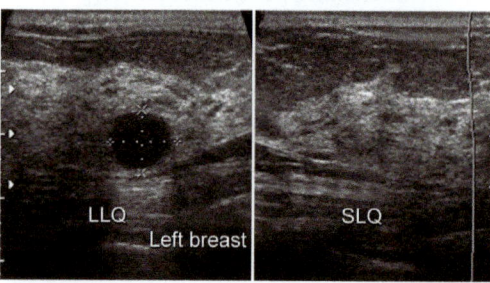

Fig. 15.7.2: US scans show fibrocystic disease of breast. (LLQ: left lower quadrant; SLQ: superior lower quadrant)

Variants

- Fluid level if few thickened internal contents
- Solid lesion if complete filling by thick contents in these cases, aspiration under US guidance clarifies the diagnosis
- Infected cysts reveal fine internal echoes, thick walls and surrounding edema. On CDFI, there is an increased low resistance vascularity around the infected cyst
- Intracystic papillomas are more common than the intracystic carcinomas. On US, seen as a polypoid mass within the cyst with demonstrable vascularity on color Doppler
- Intracystic carcinomas are rare but synchronous occurrence is common. Often the aspiration contents from such a lesion is blood stained. The US sensitivity for cysts is almost 100%.

Fibroadenoma
(Figs. 15.7.1 to 15.7.3)

It is the commonest benign tumor of breast which is thought to arise from adenosis.

- These are frequently multiple and bilateral and rarely exceed 30 mm in diameter

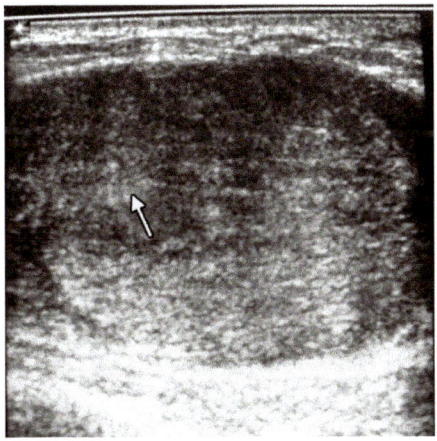

Fig. 15.7.3: Fibroadenoma breast—well-marginated hypoechoic lesion with posterior acoustic enhancement.

- They generally are seen in young females
- On US, it is demonstrated as a hypoechoic solid, well-defined, round or oval-shaped, slightly lobulated mass with uniform internal echotexture. Its long axis less along the tissue planes of the breast.

Coarse calcifications in it are brightly reflective on US, lesion is mobile and compressible:
- Fibroadenomas classically cause displacement of the glandular tissue rather than disruption and do not have a halo around the lesion
    - Giant fibroadenoma is the term used for large lesion of 4 cm or more and tends to appear more in younger patients and can be more vascular
    - Juvenile fibroadenoma are formed in adolescents, they grow rapidly. Lesions are poorly reflective and because of the volume it may cause acoustic enhancement. These lesions are usually highly vascular, probably corresponding to their rapid growth.

Phylloides Tumor

It is uncommon, also known as 'cystosarcoma phylloides' and may appear at any age.

- On US, they are well-circumscribed mass, with an oval, rounded or lobulated shape and without a halo. Slit-like fluid-filled spaces when seen are diagnostic. Necrosis and hemorrhage in larger tumors may give inhomogenous echotexture.

Pseudoangiomatous Stromal Hyperplasia (PASH)

The PASH is a rare benign lesion in perimenopausal women seen as a solid, well-defined poorly reflective mass similar to fibroadenoma.

Papilloma

- Usually occurs in the retroareolar region and found in 35–55 years age group
- Clinically, there is serous or serosanguineous nipple discharge
- Papillomas can be intraductal, intracystic or solid-like masses.

Fat Necrosis

It is usually post-traumatic. On US, seen as markedly attenuating poorly defined echopoor masses with fluid spaces. CDFI helps in differentiating it from the carcinoma.

Oil Cysts

These are frequently seen in postoperative breasts. US features depend on the density of the content and amount of calcification of the cyst wall.

15.8 MALIGNANT LESIONS

Invasive ductal carcinoma **(Figs. 15.8.1 to 15.8.3)** accounts for 80% of the breast carcinomas. The principal US features of a breast carcinoma are a mass, a surrounding reflective zone and retrotumoral attenuation along with often findings such as disruption of the tissue planes, skin thickening, architectural distortion and microcalcification.

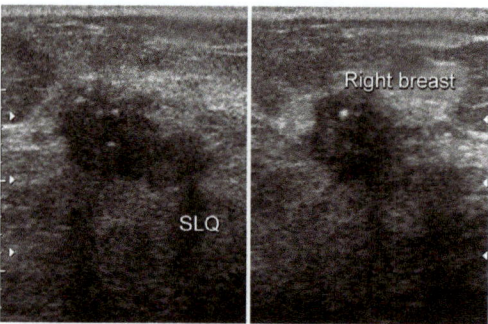

Fig. 15.8.1: US scans show breast carcinoma with microcalcifications. (SLQ: superior lower quadrant)

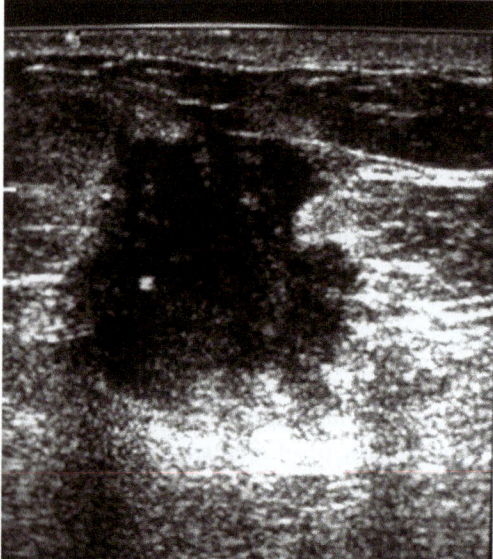

Fig. 15.8.2: Breast carcinoma—hypoechoic lesion having lobulated irregular margins, a tiny calcific foci and is taller than wider.

The tumor mass is poorly reflective with ill-defined margins and heterogeneous echotexture, if tumor is of longer size due to areas of necrosis.

Medullary carcinomas are typically well-defined though not as sharply marginated as a typical fibroadenoma.

About 83-97% of carcinomas >2 cm in diameter are attenuating which is deep to the center of the carcinoma.

Intraductal spread can sometimes be demonstrated on US.

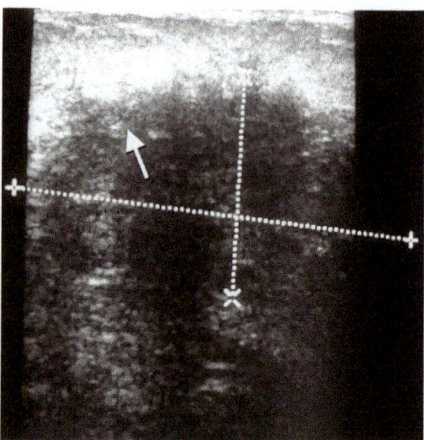

Fig. 15.8.3: Carcinoma breast—ill-defined hypoechoic lesion with angulated margins and causing posterior acoustic shadowing.

Colloid carcinomas appear on US as a well-defined lobulated mass which are highly reflective similar to the subcutaneous fat and more echogenic than other tumors.

Diffuse carcinoma—gives rise to two appearances: First is in which the breast is largely replaced by poorly reflective tissue without any posterior attenuation. In these cases, fine-needle aspiration cytology (FNAC) is required for the diagnosis. Second diffuse change occurs when there is either widespread involvement of lymphatics by cancer or following axillary dissection in which case there is breast edema. CDFI may show diffuse hyperemia.

Metastasis

Though rare but common primaries are opposite breast, lung, kidney, gastrointestinal tract (GIT), melanoma or hematological malignancies. The lesions are often multiple, hypoechoic, rounded and grow faster.

Lymphoma

Accounts for only 0.5% of all breast malignancies. Their appearances are described: first is a discrete, solitary or multiple nodular form which are hypoechoic and secont, it is a diffuse hypoechoic enlargement of breast tissue with enlarged lymph nodes.

Local Recurrence

Usually occurs after mastectomy or conservative surgery. Sometimes lesion occurs even after 10 years of surgery. Lesion is often in skin or subcutaneous tissue which are seen on US as ill-defined hypoechoic lesions with high vascularity.

Fibrosis scar which is sometimes difficult to differentiate from the recurrent tumor is usually echogenic without a demonstrable mass or nidus and vascularity on CDFI.

Fifty percent of all breast cancers arise in upper outer quadrant since it contains more glandular tissue than any other section of the breast. The next commonest site is retroareolar region (18%) on which ducts from the entire breast converge.

- Scar granulomas seen as hypoechoic small nodules with/without distal acoustic shadowing
- *Silicon granulomas:*
  - US shows a hyperechoic masses with marked acoustic attenuation if calcified—a thin crescentic hyperechoic rim is seen to the transducer
  - Characteristically the acoustic shadow gives a snow strom appearance (shadow if within lesion) contains clearly identifiable echoes that decrease with depth
- *Hydatid:*
  - Cyst with dependent echoes
  - Multiseptated, cyst within cyst
  - Complex cyst
  - Calcified cyst seen as curvilinear hyperechoic scar with acoustic shadowing
- *Hamartoma/adenofibrolipoma:*
  - Abnormal collection of normal parenchymal tissues found within the breast.

- Asymptomatic, detected on mammography.
- Soft palpable lesions.

Ultrasound shows however typically smooth margin, hypoechoic lesion having hyperechoic septa, pseudocapsule best appreciated distally, lesion is compressible.

Hematoma

- History of trauma, either accidental or iatrogenic, is usually present
- US findings depend on the stage of hematoma.

Acute Hematoma

- Area of increased echogenicity with indistinct outline
- Area of decreased echogenicity
- Uncharacteristic architectural distortion.

With increasing age it becomes more sharply demarcated from the surrounding tissues. It appears hypoechoic, cystic with/without echogenic components.

Sarcomas

Sonographically they present as hypoechoic nodular lesion with smooth or indistinct contour. Depending upon the tissue type tumor is soft and compressible (liposarcoma and angiosarcoma) or firm (fibrous histiocytomas and fibrosarcomas).

Central necrosis usually reveals an 'irregular hypoechoic center'. Angiosarcoma can be hyperechoic sonography, hyperechogenicity representing hemorrhage.

Late Pregnancy and Lactation

Overall echogenicity decreases, echopattern is homogeneous and the distented lectiferous ducts are seen as tubular extremely hypoechoic or anechoic structures cysts up to 7 mm in diameter.

CHAPTER 16

Musculoskeletal System

16.1 HYPERECHOIC FOCI WITHIN THE SYNOVIUM

- Crystal deposition (uric acid–calcium precipitates)
- Infection (due to cellular elements and fibrin)
- Corticosteroids (especially following recent injection)
- Bony fragments (in neuropathic joints)
- Rarely in normal joint—probably related to nitrogen.

16.2 CYSTIC MASS IN POPLITEAL FOSSA

- *Popliteal cyst/Baker's cyst:*
  - Caused by abnormal distension of gastrocnemio-semimembranosus bursa
  - Communicates with knee joint through a slit at the posteromedial aspect of the joint capsule
  - Large cysts dissecting into the calf or ruptured cysts produce a swollen painful limb that mimics thrombophlebitis
- *Aneurysms, especially popliteal artery:*
  - Pulsatile cystic masses with outpouching or dilatation of an artery **(Fig. 16.2.1)**
  - CFI will settle the diagnosis
  - Seen in midline or laterally
- *Neurilemmomas:*
  - Seen laterally
  - Pathology establishes the diagnosis

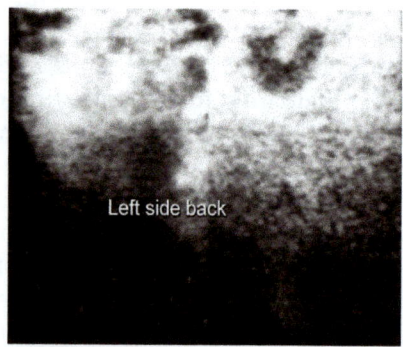

Fig. 16.2.1: US scan showing dilated vascular channels suggestive of hemangioma.

- *Ganglion cysts:*
  - Most commonly seen at the wrist
  - Usually midline
  - Oval fluid collection adjacent to the joint space or tender
  - Chronic cyst or cysts with viscous material may have internal echoes
- Adventitial cystic disease of popliteal artery
- Cystic appearing sarcomas, e.g. synovial sarcomas, myxoid liposarcoma.

16.3 HIP JOINT EFFUSION IN ADULTS

Causes

- Septic arthritis
- Avascular necrosis
- Inflammatory and noninflammatory arthritis
- Hemorrhage, e.g. hemophilia and other bleeding disorders

- Tumors as pigmented villonodular synovitis and synovial osteochondromatosis.

16.4 PROLIFERATIVE SYNOVITIS

- Rheumatoid arthritis
- Septic arthritis (a) acute: bacterial, (b) subacute: tuberculosis, fungal, etc.
- Crystal-induced arthropathies
- Amyloid arthropathy
- Pigmented villonodular synovitis
- Synovial osteochondromatosis
- Hemophilic arthropathy.

16.5 TENDON TEARS

Signs of partial tear	Complete tear
Discontinuity of some fibers (Figs. 16.5.1A and B)	Discontinuity of all fibers
Acute tear appears as retracted tendon	Nonvisualization of hypoechoic defect in tendon (Figs. 16.5.2 and 16.5.3)
Hematoma, usually very small	Hematoma, usually small
	Bone fragment in case of bone avulsion

Partial tear needs to be differentiated from focal tendinitis.

Signs of Tendinitis

- Thickening of the tendon
- Decreased echogenicity
- Blurred margins
- Increased vascularity on CFI
- Calcification in chronic cases.

USG Findings in Proliferative Synovitis

- Hypoechogenicity and thickening of synovial membrane often with irregularity and nodularity

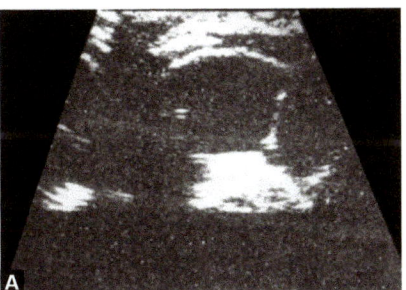
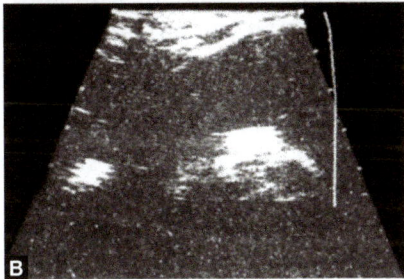

Figs. 16.5.1A and B: Sagittal and transverse scans of right shoulder showing break in continuity of rotator cuff.

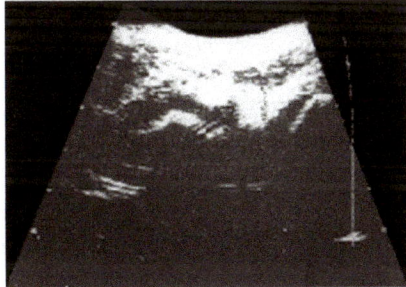

Fig. 16.5.2: US of the right knee showing linear hypoechoic area—tear in posterior horn of lateral meniscus.

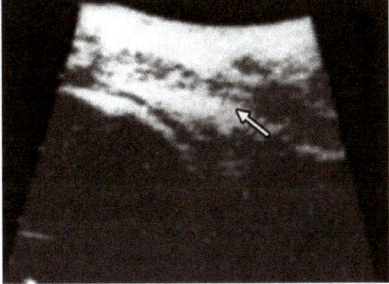

Fig. 16.5.3: US—sagittal view showing hypoechoic area (arrow) within homogenicity of echotexture of posterior horn of medial meniscus suggestive of meniscal tear.

- Hyperechogenicity of fat adjacent to inflamed synovium
- Effusion in joint cavity.

16.6 PEDIATRIC HIP JOINT: AN OVERVIEW

The most important determinant of the outcome of an infected hip is the delay between the onset and treatment. Conventional radiographic examinations are of little help in early diagnosis. Computed tomography and MRI, though informative, are very expensive and not universally available. With ultrasound (US) scanning even small fluids/pus collections of 1–2 mL can be accurately detected. The use of other (invasive) imaging modalities can be minimized as US can be used to demonstrate effusions early in the disease along with the status of the intra-articular compartment, joint capsule, bony surface and adjacent soft tissues. US scanning should be used more commonly to diagnose infective arthritis and no patient should be subjected to arthrotomy or drainage, if US scan has ruled out the presence of a fluid collection. Over the last one decade, sonography of hip has been used in the diagnosis of congenital dislocation, or dysplasia and Perthes' disease. US scan well-demonstrates the soft tissue structures around hip and unossified cartilage without any radiation and pain. Arthrography, though useful, is painful, requires anesthesia and injection of contrast. The sonography can suggest dysplasia/dislocation by presence of rounded deformed head, loss of concavity, inclination of acetabular roof, lateralization, delayed ossification center and percentage of coverage. The sonography in Perthes' disease can define the irregularity of femoral head and rate of deformity of the same. The purpose of writing this overview is to highlight the usefulness of US scanning to diagnose various hip disorders in children accurately and quickly.

With development of high-resolution real time transducers, ultrasound (US) scanning has become the investigation of choice in the initial evaluation of hip joint in children. With US scanning, direct imaging of even the unossified parts is also possible. Presence of synovitis and effusion, development of head of femur, acetabulum and their anatomical inter-relationship can be sonographically assessed without any risk of radiation and contrast.

Joint Effusion and Infective Arthritis

Pain, refusal to bear weight and limping can be due to a wide variety of conditions affecting the hip joint. Clinically, it is difficult many times to differentiate between the intrinsic abnormality and the pseudoflexion deformity of the joint. The plain films are both insensitive and unreliable in their diagnosis. Though computed tomography (CT) may be more informative, US provides an easily available, quick and accurate noninvasive technique to detect intra-articular abnormalities. Extra-articular pathologies like pelvic abscess, appendicitis, iliac lymphadenitis and osteomyelitis can also be diagnosed and differentiated from intra-articular pathology although clinical presentation may be similar.

Technique

The patient is examined in the supine position using 4–7.5 MHz linear/sector real-time transducer. Anterior longitudinal approach along the neck femur is the simple and most useful imaging plane. Both hips are examined in every case.

Normal sonographic anatomy reveals the following:
- Joint capsule is seen as a linear echogenic band-like structure (2 mm thick) anteriorly, along the contour of head and neck. The band extends from acetabular rim to its insertion at intertrochanteric line

Musculoskeletal System

- Anterior synovial recess is seen as a 3 mm wide clear space between capsule and bony surface
- Growth plate
- Surrounding soft tissue, iliopsoas muscle and pelvis.

Abnormal Hip
(Figs. 16.6.1 and 16.6.2)

The affected hip may show collection in anterior synovial recess more than 3 mm width and with an asymmetry of at least 2 mm on both sides. Echo pattern of synovial fluid in septic hip may show hyperechoic character due to high cellular content or bleeding. Tubercular arthritis, transient synovitis and treated septic arthritis may show hypoechoic synovial collection but varied picture is present as hyperechoic character though less common has been observed in transient synovitis and tubercular arthritis. The positive predictivity of US for diagnosing effusion in our experience is over 95%. The capsule may show thickening and anterior bulge. The convex contour suggests raised intra-articular pressure which can interfere with blood supply to head and any delay in institution of therapy can result in irreversible changes. Surgical arthrotomy/US-guided aspiration can now be easily done to relieve the pressure and establish the etiological diagnosis. There has been a marked drop in negative arthrotomy at our institution since the use of sonography in evaluation of hip joint. Minimal collections under conservative management and postoperative cases can be monitored sonographically to follow the course of the disease process.

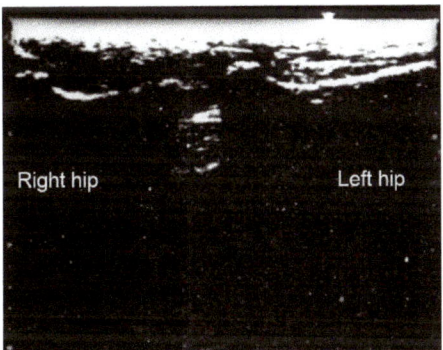

Fig. 16.6.1: Tubercular arthritis—right hip showing increased anterior synovial recess with convex and anechoic collection. Left hip is normal.

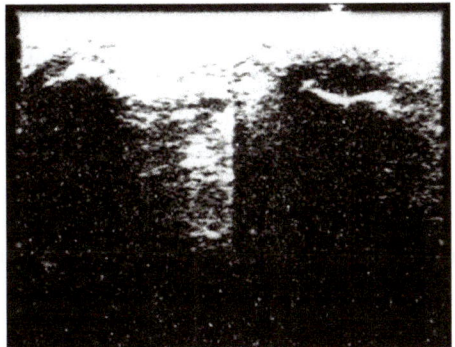

Fig. 16.6.2: Pyogenic arthritis—left hip showing destruction of femoral head. The anterior synovial recess is widened with echogenic collection. Right hip is normal.

Legg-Calvé Perthes Disease (LCP)
(Figs. 16.6.3 and 16.6.4)

Frequent measurements of growth and development of femur head are essential in these patients to monitor the course of the disease. The head should retain its sphericity along with its growth for best functional utility. Many radiographic methods have been developed for this assessment. Precise assessment is not possible with these methods if the child is young and cartilaginous parts are not visible or arthrography is required, which is a painful procedure needing general anesthesia, radiation and injection of contrast.

The US has been used to replace earlier radiographic methods, including arthrography to measure the sphericity of femur head and

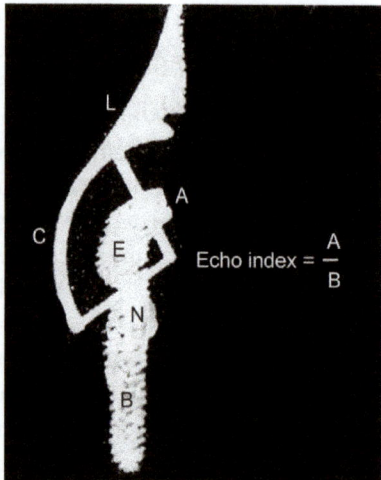

Fig. 16.6.3: Sketch diagram seen in lateral coronal plane with adduction at hip: A—acetabulum, L—labrum, C—capsule, E—epiphysis, N—neck femur, and B—shaft of femur.

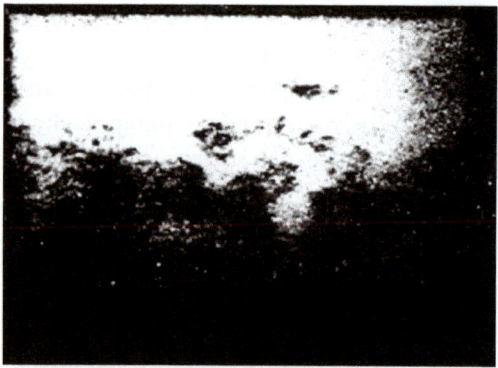

Fig. 16.6.4: Perthes' disease—lateral sonogram demonstrating the flattening head with good cartilaginous covering.

to determine the rate of deformity due to Legg-Calvé-Perthes disease (LCP). US can directly, noninvasively, visualize the bony and cartilaginous parts of the head.

Technique

The patient is examined in supine position with leg abducted at hip by about 35°. This maneuver allows almost lateral 2/3rd of head to be visualized. A 4–7.5 MHz transducer is placed laterally in transverse (axial) and longitudinal (coronal) planes. In the axial plane, the maximum transverse diameter of head is measured. The longitudinal projections show the acetabulum, labrum, capsule, head of femur, epiphysis and growth plate. The maximum height of head from growth plate (A) and maximum width of head (B) at level of growth plate are measured. The ratio of A to B is the Echo Index (EI). The ratio of EI of affected side to normal is defined as Echo Quotient (EQ). The EQ represents the grade of the cartilaginous femur head deformity and this facilitates follow-up correlation in LCP with objective measurements over a prolonged time period. Apart from this, flattening and fragmentation of cartilaginous parts scan also be diagnosed with US scanning. To conclude, US scanning can be used in place of arthrography and radiography to determine the sphericity of femur head in LCP disease.

Congenital Dislocation of Hip

In congenital dislocation of hip, early diagnosis and treatment are essential for proper development. In newborn and infant, the entire proximal femur head and greater trochanter are cartilaginous. Only portions of acetabulum may be ossified. The development of these important unossified structures in hip joint can, therefore, only be assessed indirectly with X-ray radiographs and CT scanning or directly by invasive arthrography.

With improvement in technology of high resolution small parts transducer, sonography can directly visualize both the cartilaginous and bony parts of hip for accurate assessment of its size, shape and symmetry. The radiation-free (US) technique is more reliable than radiography or CT scanning. The US scanning is preferred over arthrography for evaluation of infant hip due to its noninvasive nature.

Table 16.6.1: Classification of hip dysplasia on the basis of ultrasonographic measurements.

Character	Type I (Normal)	Type II (Dysplasia)	Type III (Subluxation)
α-angle	>60°	44–60°	<43°
β-angle	<55°	55–77°	>77°
Percentage	>58°	58–33°	<33°
Coverage	Full	More than 1/3rd covered	Less than 1/3rd covered

With real-time US scanning, dynamic studies are also possible to detect laxity of the ligamentous structures in potentially dislocated hips. Apart from establishing the diagnosis, this technique can be used to monitor the effect of treatment by repetitive studies even when the patient is in spica cast.

The main indications for performing sonography in an abnormal hip, are:
- To determine the position and development of femur head
- To diagnose instability during dynamic studies with lap movements in various positions
- To assess the development of acetabulum, especially the cartilaginous component.

Technique and Normal Anatomy

Both linear and sector transducer from 3–7.5 MHz frequency may be used. Higher frequency is required for neonates and lower frequency for the older patients. The patient is examined in supine position in lateral coronal and transverse planes with the transducer at greater trochanter. The plane of interest should outline the head, neck of femur, iliac bone, acetabulum, greater trochanter and joint capsule.

In lateral coronal approach, the head can be seen within the acetabulum with echogenic bony ileum superiorly. The joint capsule is identified as an echogenic band surrounding the head. The acetabulum labrum is seen as a triangular structure at the edge of bony acetabulum as a hypoechoic structure. Rest of acetabular echoes are seen superiorly and medially with a gap in bony echoes due to posterior limb of triradiate cartilage.

In transverse neutral plane, the cartilaginous head is seen within the acetabulum over the central triradiate cartilage. The triradiate cartilage allows the onward transmission of sound, producing a zone of acoustic shadowing. In transverse flexion projection, the echogenic structures combine to produce a 'U' configuration with vertical limb of triradiate cartilage at its base. Anterior limb of 'U' is due to junction of metaphysis and epiphysis while posterior limb is due to echoes from acetabulum.

The objective assessment of acetabular development can be done by two methods. The first described by Graf (1984) is based on various angles formed by three lines **(Table 16.6.1)**:
1. Baseline (A) which connects the osseous acetabulum convexity to the point where joint capsule and perichondrium unite with iliac bone.
2. The inclination line (a) which connects the osseous convexity to labrum acetabulare.
3. The acetabular roof line (b) connecting the lower edge of ileum to osseous convexity.

Alpha Angle

This is the most important measurement and lies between baseline and acetabular roofline. This angle indicates the formation of acetabular convexity.

Beta Angle

It measures the formation and development of cartilage convexity and lies between inclination line and baseline.

On the basis of these lines and angles, the hip can be classified as follows:

Type I (Normal): α-angle more than 60° and β less than 55°.

Type II (Dysplasia): Includes cases of subluxation which, sometimes, get corrected without treatment (delayed ossification). α angle between 44–60° and β between 55° and 77°.

Type III: The cartilaginous edges pushed outwards and upwards by the laxating femur head. α angle less than 43° and β angle more than 77°. The echo-free cartilaginous head becomes echodense.

Type IV: The femur head is completely dislocated into an empty acetabulum. The deformed cartilaginous edge with flat osseous edge is seen.

A relatively simple method for acetabular assessment by measuring the relative percentage of coverage of the femur head by bony acetabulum has been described. US scanning of the hip joint by lateral approach in coronal view is similar to AP radiograph and has been correlated with radiographic acetabular index. The linear echogenic straight ileum echo is called iliac line, which when extended through the head, normally divides it into two parts. Two lines tangential to femur head at its medial and lateral border and parallel to iliac line are also drawn. The distance between two tangent lines is 'D' and distance between iliac line and medial line is referred to as 'd'. The ratio of D:d × 100 indicates the percentage of femur head coverage by bony acetabulum. When this is correlated with acetabular index measurements made on radiography, a coverage of less than 33% is definitely abnormal and indicates dysplasia, a coverage between 33–58% is the transition zone and coverage of femoral head above 58% is normal. Follow-up of patients on treatment can be made by objective serial measurements of coverage percentage.

Abnormal Hip (Figs. 16.6.5 to 16.6.10)

A small ossific nucleus may be seen as an echogenic focus with the cartilaginous head between 1 and 6 months of age. The ossification

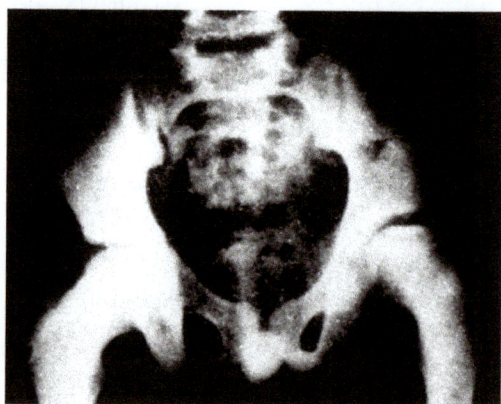

Fig. 16.6.5: AP radiograph of the same patient.

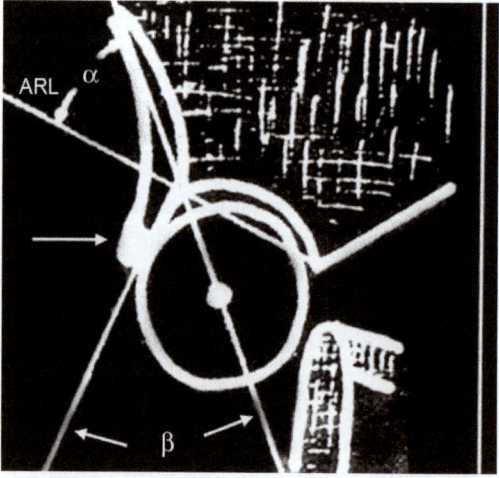

Fig. 16.6.6: Sketch diagrammatic representation of coronal sonography in infant hip—showing baseline (BL), acetabular roofline (ARL) and inclination line (IL), α and β-angles.

Musculoskeletal System

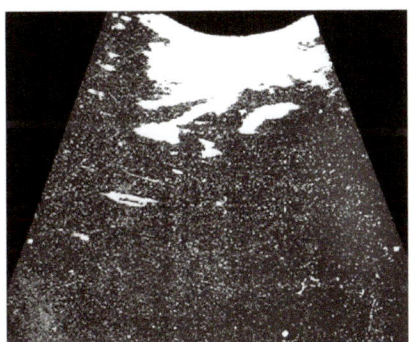

Fig. 16.6.7: Tangential lines along the femur head to measure percentage of coverage.

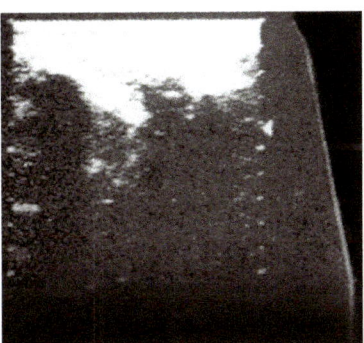

Fig. 16.6.10: Lateral sonogram of right hip showing empty acetabulum suggestive of complete dislocation of head.

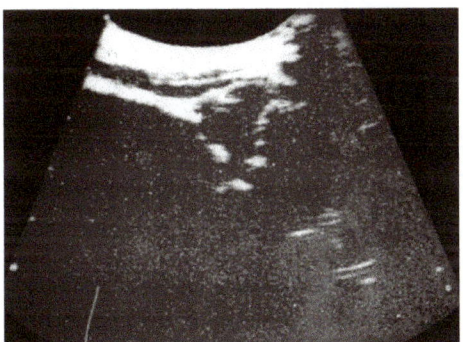

Fig. 16.6.8: Lateral sonogram of left hip showing concentric relationship of head to acetabulum and triradiate cartilage.

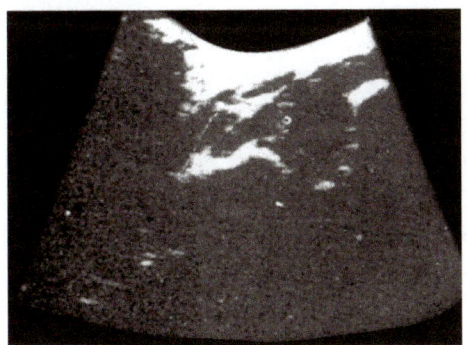

Fig. 16.6.9: Same patient's right hip showing displaced head.

center is sonographically detected earlier compared to X-ray radiography. It is often delayed in congenital dislocation of hip on the affected side.

Apart from angle measurements mentioned earlier, in dislocation the concentric relationship of the femur head to triradiate cartilage will also be seen. Lateral displacement is seen as a gap between the head and acetabular roof. In posterior and superior dislocation, head is often seen against bony ileum, without any gap. In transverse flexion, the 'U' configuration of the head may be laterally positioned limb of 'U'. When there is subluxation, the femur head is often covered by the thickened stretched joint capsule and the posterior part of bony acetabulum is flatter than normal. Children with frank dislocation of hip have a very thick capsule and an abnormally small acetabulum. The head will not be seated within the acetabulum but displaced in surrounding soft tissues. With movement of limb from adduction to extreme abduction, reduction can be seen to occur in an unstable hip.

With advancement of age, US scanning becomes more difficult but is still practical till 2 years of age. The ossification center of more than 10 mm can also interfere with proper evaluation. Caution must be observed in very young infants with dysplasia as many unstable hips may recover spontaneously in 1st week of life.

Finally, with experience, sonographic anatomy and various abnormalities of hip

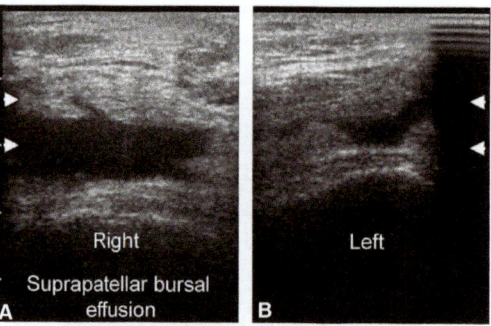

Figs. 16.6.11A and B: US scans show knee joint effusion.

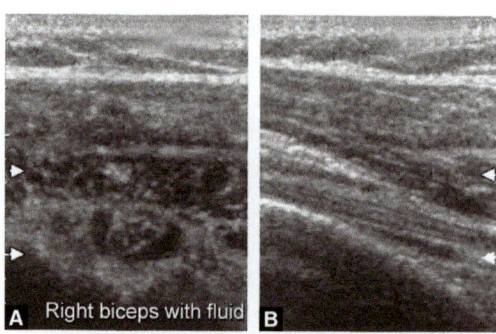

Figs. 16.6.14A and B: US scans show free fluid (arrowheads) in inferior recess of shoulder joint cavity.

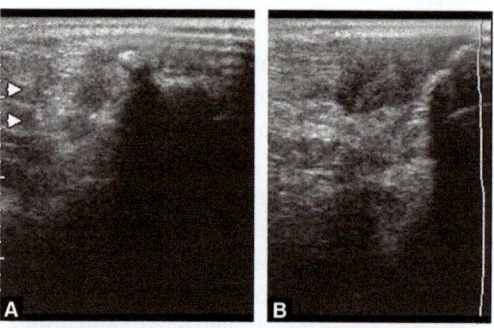

Figs. 16.6.12A and B: US scans show chronic partial rupture of tendo- Achiles (arrowheads).

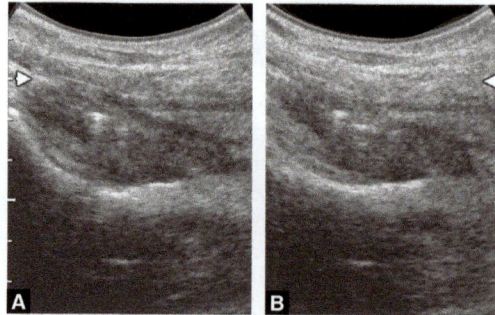

Figs. 16.6.15A and B: US scans show iliopsoas abscess (arrowheads).

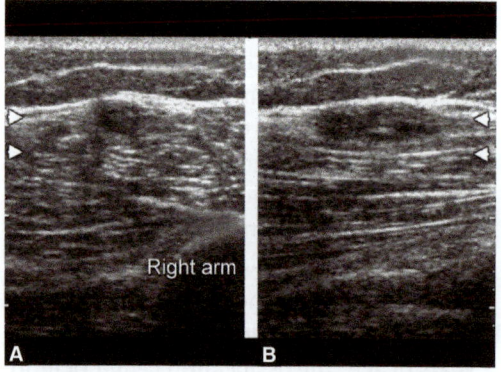

Figs. 16.6.13A and B: US scans show cysticercus cyst in deltoid muscle (arrowheads)

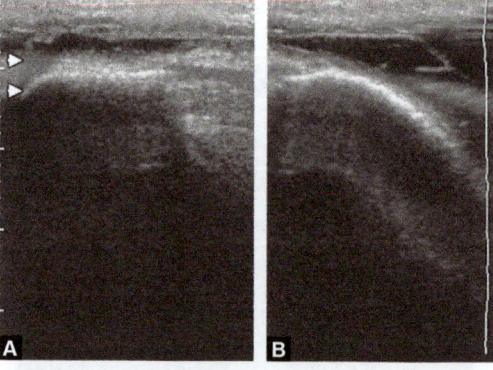

Figs. 16.6.16A and B: US scans show prepatellar collection (arrowheads).

joints can be diagnosed with US scanning. This technique should be extensively used for assessment of the pediatric hip joint.

In addition to the above, high-resolution sonography is very helpful in localizing the other joint, soft tissue and muscle lesion of the body **(Figs. 16.6.11 to 16.6.32)**.

Musculoskeletal System

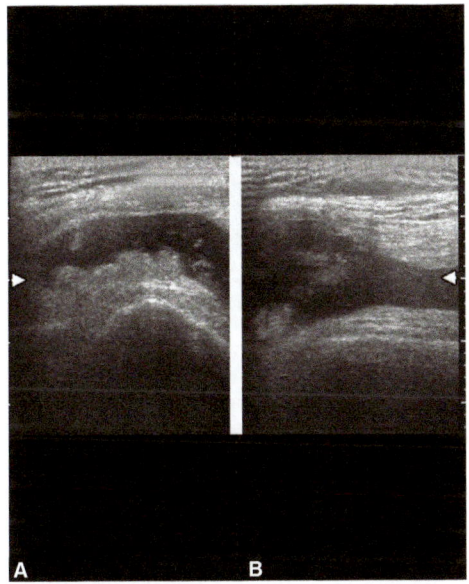

Figs. 16.6.17A and B: US scans show proliferative synovitis in knee joint (arrowheads).

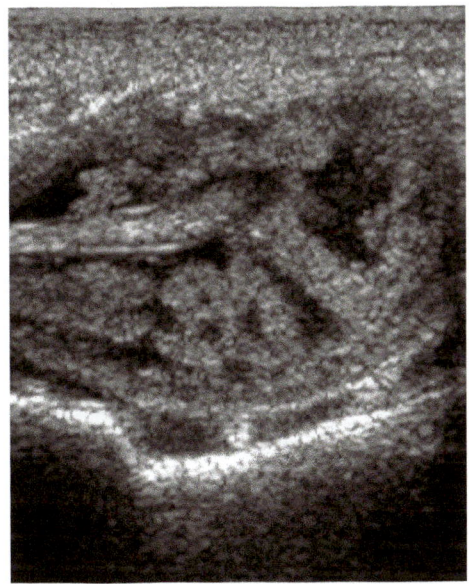

Fig. 16.6.20: US scan shows tenosynovitis.

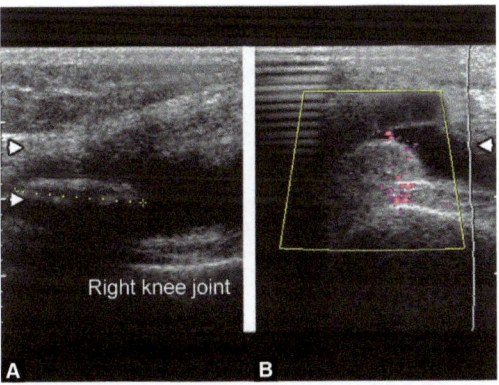

Figs. 16.6.18A and B: US scans show synovitis of knee (arrowhead with asterisk) with loose body (arrowhead).

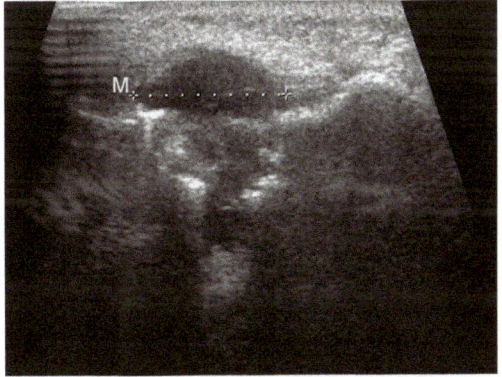

Fig. 16.6.21: US scan shows osteomyelitis of mandible. (M: mass)

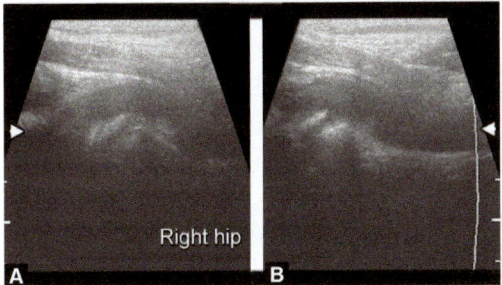

Figs. 16.6.19A and B: US scans show collection in hip joint (arrowheads).

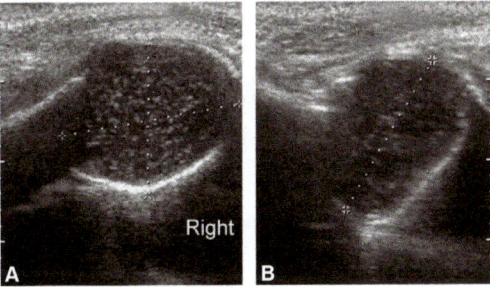

Figs. 16.6.22A and B: US scans show right maxillary cyst (shown by measurement).

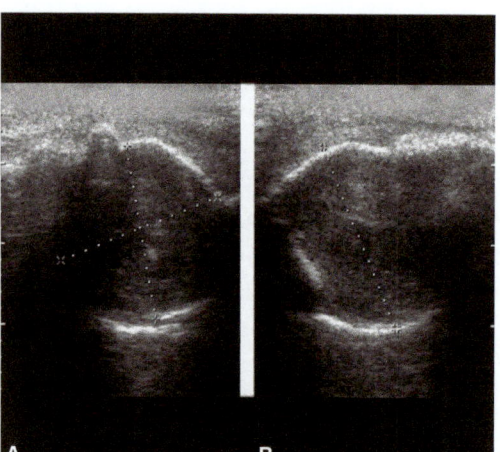

Figs. 16.6.23A and B: US scans show radicular cyst of mandible (shown by measurement).

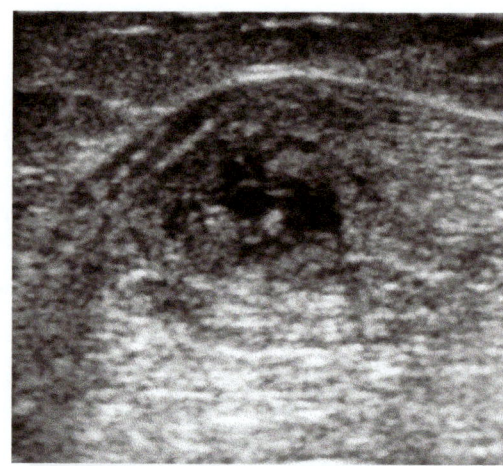

Fig. 16.6.25: Cysticercosis in muscle—cystic lesion with a calcific focus inside it.

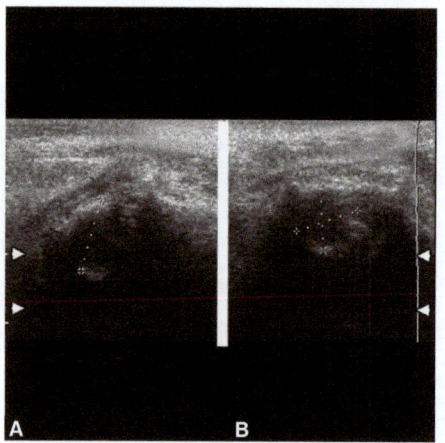

Figs. 16.6.24A and B: US scans show apical cyst of teeth.

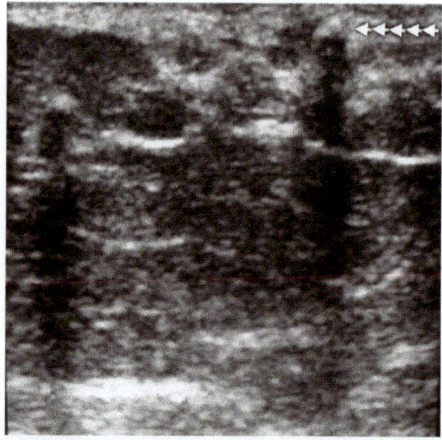

Fig. 16.6.26: Cutaneous venous malformation—multiple dilated vascular channels with calcific foci (arrowheads) inside them.

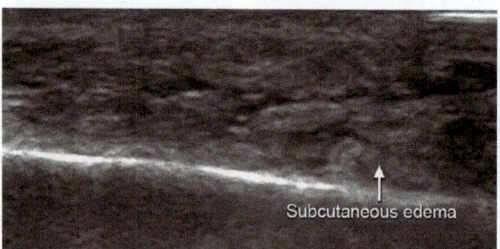

Fig. 16.6.27: Subcutaneous edema in forearm.

Musculoskeletal System

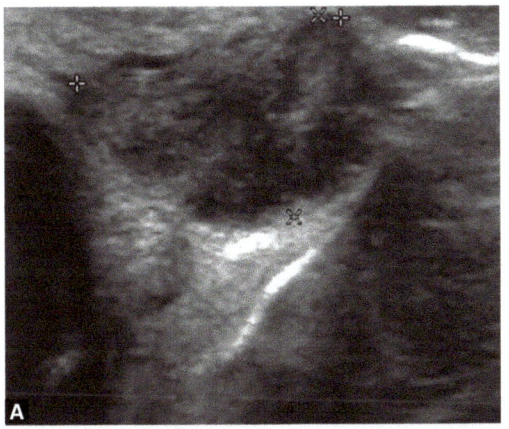

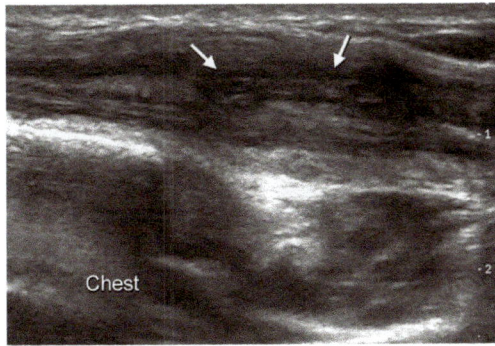

Fig. 16.6.30: Worm (arrows) in chest wall muscle.

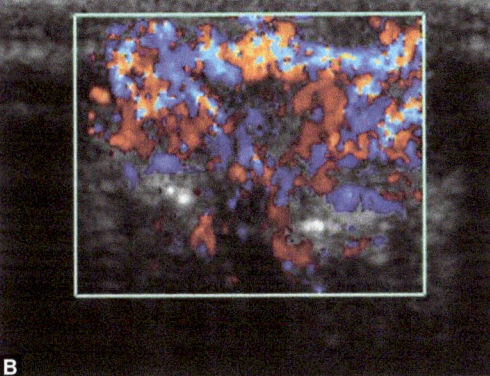

Figs. 16.6.28A and B: Hemangioma at the tip of nose showing vascularity.

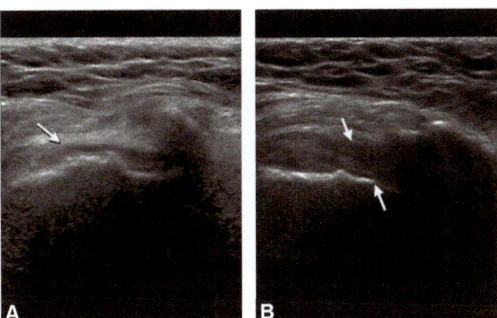

Figs. 16.6.29A and B: Images showing tear at the insertion of supraspinatus tendon (arrows).

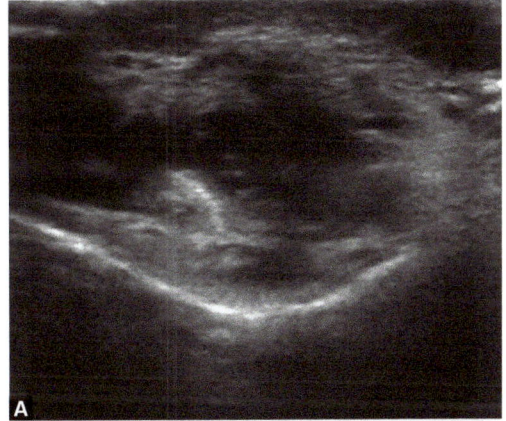

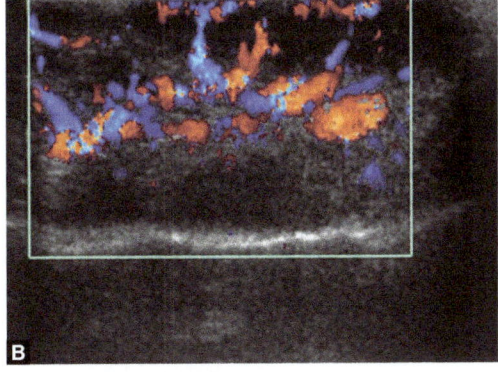

Figs. 16.6.31A and B: Hemangioma in the forearm—heteroechoic mass with multiple channels showing vascularity.

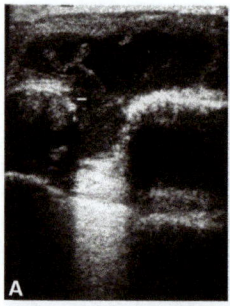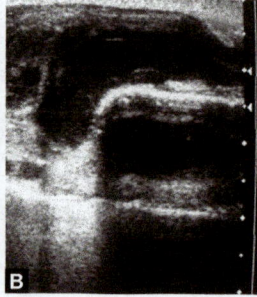

Figs. 16.6.32A and B: Chest wall cold abscess—collection with echoes and septations is seen in the chest wall extending into the intercostal space.

16.7 CAUSES OF ARTICULAR CARTILAGE CALCIFICATION

- Gout
- Calcium pyrophosphate dehydrate deposition disease (CPPD)
- Hyperparathyroidism
- Hemochromatosis
- Alkaptonuria
- Wilson's disease
- Acromegaly.

CAUSES OF SOFT TISSUE NODULE ASSOCIATED ARTHRITIS

- Rheumatoid arthritis
- Gout
- Pigmented villonodular synovitis
- Amyloidosis
- Sarcoidosis.

CHAPTER 17

Orbit

17.1 ANATOMY

The eyeball is a globoid structure with an anterior defect which is filled by part of another globe which forms 1/6th of the total surface area of globe. The posterior part is known as sclera while the anterior part is known as cornea.

Anterior pole is located at the center of cornea while the posterior pole is located at a point on sclera slightly temporal (lateral) to optic nerve exit point, this forms center of posterior part of globe. The line joining the anterior and the posterior poles is the geometric axis of eyeball. The anteroposterior diameter along the geometric axis is 22–27 mm (mean = 24 mm).

The equator is a circumference which encircles the eyeball midway between the two poles and is 69–85 mm in length. The eyeball consists of three layers:
1. Sclera (5/6) + Cornea (1/6)
2. Uvea or uveal tract
3. Retina with optic nerve.

Sclera

Opaque, avascular, tough globoid sheath encasing all other structures of eyeball.

Cornea

- It is a transparent, slightly oval part of large globe which is fitted in the anterior defect in the sclera. Central part of cornea is avascular while the periphery is supplied by the anterior ciliary arteries.
- It is the main reflecting surface of eye with 0.5 mm thick central portion.
- Limbus is the transition between cornea and sclera. It contains the trabecular meshwork all around and the canal of Schlemm for drainage of aqueous humor.
- It can be further divided in five layer:
  1. Epithelium
  2. Bowman's layer
  3. Stroma
  4. Descemet's membrane
  5. Endothelium.

Uveal Tract

- Vascular layer of eyeball consisting from anterior to posterior of iris, ciliary body and choroid. The pupil is a small hole surrounded circumferentially by the irial curtain
- Choroids consist of three vascular layers that nourish the pigmentary and sensory layers of retina. A tough collagenous Bruch's membrane separates the choriocapillaries of choroids from retina. Ciliary body is a piece of fibrovascular tissue anteriorly, while the iris hangs from its surface. It is continuous with the choroid at ora serrata
- Iris is a diaphragm separating anterior chamber of eyeball from posterior chamber. It is attached via ciliary body to and at the scleral spur. Muscular

movement of the iris diaphragm controls the entry of light in the eyeball.

Retina

- Composed of 10 layers extending from ora serrata to optic nerve head
- It is fixed anteriorly at ora serrata and posteriorly at optic nerve head, otherwise it is free separable from choroids.

Lens

A 10 mm × 4 mm crystalline structure situated behind the pupil held in position by zonules. The central fibers of the lens are dense old while peripheral are loosely arranged new forming fibers. Both are contained within the lens capsule.

Globe Overall

- Contains 4.5 mL of thick, gelatinous formed body known as vitreous humor. This is located posterior to lens in the posterior segment
- Anterior hyloid membrane is the flattened vitreous layer which is in close contact to the lens, and on which the lens is somewhat supported
- Posteriorly, the vitreous is attached to retina by loose collagenous fibers while tight attachments are seen at margins of optic disk, ora serrata and ciliary body
- Central part of vitreous contains a gel composed of water (99%), hyaluronic acid while the peripheral part adjacent the retina is thicker and known as cortex
- Anterior to lens in anterior segment, watery aqueous humor is found in this part. The aqueous humor is generated at the ciliary body while drained continuously at trabecular mesh
- Both these structures (i.e. aqueous and vitreous humor) maintains the movement and shape of the globe.

Optic Nerve

- It is the second nerve emanating from the optic chiasma located in the suprasellar cistern
- It has one million nerve fibers arranged in bundles or fasciculus and packed together by fibrous tissue
- *It has four segments:*
  1. Intraocular.
  2. Intraorbital (30 mm) S-shaped.
  3. Intracanalicular (5 mm).
  4. Intracranial (10 mm).

Orbit

- It is a hollow cavity in facial skeleton formed by frontal, maxillary, ethmoid, sphenoid, zygomatic and palatine bones
- It contains the eyeball, extraocular muscle, nerve, vessels, fat and lacrimal apparatus
- Anterior 2/3rd is a four-sided pyramid while posterior 1/3rd is a three-sided pyramid.

17.2 ORBITAL SONOANATOMY AND TECHNIQUE

The technique of orbital sonography better known as B-scan in common clinical practice was first introduced and described by Baum and Greenwood in 1958.

B-scan ultrasonography is supposes to be the most practical method to evaluate the posterior chamber when the light conducting media is hazy and ophthalmological examination is difficult. Because of its direct anatomical depiction, it also acts as a aid to ophthalmological examination. It is also supposed to be the most useful examination prior to iridectomy.

Indications

- Evaluation of intraocular structures when the light conduction media is hazy

- To ascertain the cause of retinal detachment
- Evaluation of intraocular tumors
- Evaluation of vitreous humor
- Evaluation of intraocular and intraorbital foreign bodies
- Evaluation of eyeball in a case of proptosis, especially when painful
- Evaluation of ocular and orbital vascular diseases.

Ultrasound Technique

- In usual practice, a 5-10 MHz (around 7 MHz is the most useful) transducer with small imaging pad is utilized for this purpose. A 'pen type' transducer is most useful
- Patient may be supine or sitting initially but should be examined in both positions
- A perocular (closed lid) or a transocular (open lid) approach may be used
- One should never refrain from screening other related system and also for other associations, if documented in literature.

Systematic Evaluation (Fig. 17.2.1)

- A standard examination starts at the equator, first focusing the optic nerve and then sweeping anteriorly to reach the lens
- One should never forget to see the consensuous light reflex from other eye, the pupil becoming small and the iris become thicker
- Except for the optic nerve and the muscle all intraorbital structure are echogenic while the lens are mostly hypoechoic
- Under normal circumstances only the posterior lens capsule is seen as a curvilinear line behind the iris
- Aqueous fluid is a gelatinous structure with few floaters
- Choroid is hypoechoic while retina and sclera are echogenic structures

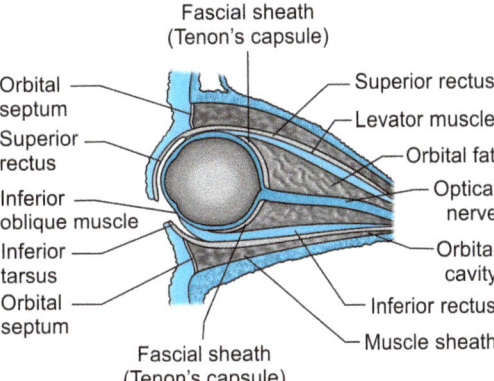

Fig. 17.2.1: Vertical section of the eye and orbit showing muscles and nerves.

- Retina itself is not normally seen, it is the interface of retina to vitreous which causes an echogenic line to appear
- Ciliary body is examined from the opposite side of the globe
- Optic nerve is usually an echopoor band with minimal internal echogenicity. Correlation with opposite nerve and clinical features are important to make the correct diagnosis
- Baum's bumps are artifacts due to the fractionation and increased propagation of ultrasound through lens. These are seen at the borders of lens in posterior segment.

Ultrasound Biomicroscopy (UBM)

This is the technique of sonological imaging of any tissue at microscopic resolution using B-mode ultrasonography. A 40-100 MHz transducer is used for this purpose (3 mm imaging pad diameter). The axial resolution is increased 5-10 times and measurements of fine structures can be made. Using the conventional 10 MHz probe, the superficial 5 mm layer is not seen, which can be clearly visualized thereof.

- All the layers of cornea can be seen
- Anterior chamber size and angle can be assessed by measuring angle opening distance and trabecular iris angle

- Iris can be measured on the trabecular–ciliary process distance line, its relation to anterior lens capsule can be seen nicely
- Superficial space-occupying lesions as iris nevi, melanoma, cysts and ciliary body tumors can be well-visualized
- Glaucoma can be better evaluated using UBM. The angle closure glaucoma, infantile glaucoma and plateau iris syndrome are all satisfactory evaluated by this technique
- Synechiae are equally well-depicted
- The main disadvantage is, however, the limited depth that can be assessed. One can see only uptill anterior lens capsule and anterior zonules.

Orbital Color Doppler

It is an extension of B-scan orbital sonography and should routinely be performed to add information on vascularity and flow. Doppler examination can suitably be done by using the same 7.5 MHz transducer, as for sonography.

Indications

- *Orbital trauma:*
  - Optic nerve avulsion
  - Intraocular hemorrhage
- *Inflammations:*
  - Iridocyclitis
  - Panuveitis
  - Endophthalmitis
- *Vascular disease:*
  - Central retinal artery occlusion
  - Central retinal vein occlusion
  - Ciliary artery occlusion
  - Diabetic retinopathy
  - Expulsive choroidal hemorrhage
- *Tumors—AVM:*
  - Retinal capillary hemangioma
  - Choroidal melanoma
  - Choroidal hemangioma
  - Metastasis
- *Orbital pathology—trauma:*
  - Cellulitis/abscess
  - Graves' disease
  - Tumors as metastasis, AVM, pseudotumor, lymph nodes
- *Caroticocavernous fistula:*
  - Central retinal artery (CRA) enters the optic nerve 10-12 mm posterior to sclera while ophthalmic artery is seen deep in the eyeball.
  - Peak systolic velocities (PSV):
    - Central retinal artery—9.5 cm/sec
    - Central retinal vein—4.2 cm/sec
    - Ophthalmic artery—37.7 cm/sec
    - Posterior ciliary artery—11.3 cm/sec
    - Superior ophthalmic vein—7.6 cm/sec
    - Vertical veins—5.8 cm/sec.
  - In central retinal artery block the flow in it decreases
  - In central retinal vein block while the PSV in CRA is decreased the diastolic flow is either absent or significantly reduced
  - In caroticocavernous fistula (CCF), a dilated superior ophthalmic vein with increased arterialized flow is seen in the vein. Doppler is also a useful technique for postembolization follow-up.

17.3 SONOPATHOLOGY

Lesions of eyeball and orbit have been classified according to their echogenicity (reflectivity and attenuation), as follow:
- *Extremely low reflectivity (anechoic):*
  - Silicone implants
  - Hematoma
  - Cysts (are also compressible)
  - Mucocele (is incompressible)
  - Peripheral nerve sheath (PNS) malignancy (has bone chips in it)
  - Varix (expands on Valsalva)

- *Low reflectivity (mild hypoechogenicity):*
  - Cellulities, abscess
  - Glioma
  - Lymphoma, sarcomas, pseudotumor
  - Neurilemmoma malignant/benign fibrous histiocytoma, pericytoma
  - Caroticocavernous fistula
  - Hemangioma (capillary)
- *Medium reflectivity (moderate hypoechogenicity/isoechoic):*
  - Dermoid
  - Meningioma.
- *High reflectivity (echogenic):*
  - Lymphangioma
  - Hemangioma (cavernous)
  - Pleomorphic adenoma
  - Foreign bodies
  - Metastasis.

17.4 SONOLOGICAL FEATURES OF ORBITAL DISEASES

Orbital Trauma

This is a field of orbital imaging where a sonologist plays a predominant role in diagnosis as most of the time ophthalmological examination is difficult due to hazy media. A clinical and plain film examination should always be one prior to USG examination.

Indications
- Detection and localization of a radiolucent foreign body
- Localization of radiopaque foreign body
- Assessment of other associated injury
- Determination of nature (magnetic or nonmagnetic)
- Extraction of foreign body by gliding
- Follow-up of management.

Ocular trauma can be divided as:
- *Nonpenetrating:*
  - Extraocular foreign body
  - Concussion/contusion
  - Abrasion.
- *Penetrating:*
  - Penetrating wound
  - Penetrating with retention of intraocular foreign body.
- *Sympathetic ophthalmitis:*
  - Small extraocular foreign body should be looked for its presence in sulcus subtarsalis, fornix or surface of cornea and completed by applying thick gel or using a water bath
  - Abrasion to eyelid, conjunctiva and cornea may be noted as areas of inhomogeneity and anechoic areas suggestive of edema. A heteroechoic hematoma may also be seen
  - Tissue inhomogeneity in contour and echogenicity because of disruption and protein coagulation may be seen in cases of chemical injury by acid, alkaline or gases
  - Adhesions formed are also examined by changing the gaze
  - Noxious gases (as mustard gas, ethyl iodoacetate, bromobenzyl cyanide and chloroacetophenone) usually cause only blepharospasm and watering.
  - *Other features:*
    - Hyphema: Early and uniformly distributed blood in anterior chamber can be easily detected
    - Angle widening and recession: Due to severe injury to anterior chamber
    - Lens dislocation/injury: A partial/complete zonular tear may lead to subluxed/dislocated lens which is usually seen as an echogenic ovoid structure floating in posterior segment. The anterior chamber is deep and iridodonesis (freely fluttering iris) can be appreciated. If (rarely) the lens has gone in anterior chamber, then there might be an anterior uveitis or glaucoma associated. Lens may even come in

episcleral space, if sclera has also ruptured

Contracture develops due to injury to lens fibers and capsule which usually tears at posterior pole letting in the liquefied vitreous. This vitreous seeps along the sutures and forms a feathery rosette-like slowly progressing or static opacity known as rosette cataract or posterior subcapsular cataract

- *Vitreous hemorrhage*
- *Retinal detachment:* Subretinal fluid is a common accompanying feature
- *Scleral injury:* This is not adequately imaged by B-scan sonography. An indirect indication as subretinal fluid, suprachoroidal hematoma, lens and vitreous prolapse, angle recession, retinal detachment may be seen. Sclera is usually injured at the canal of Schlemm, which is a relatively fixed
- *Choroidal detachment*
- *Optic nerve avulsion:* Normal movement of optic nerve is lost while changing the gaze

    Sometimes this may not be evaluated adequately by B-scan
- Injury to muscle bone vessels, etc. are better evaluated by other modalities
- *Prephthitic eyeball:* The eyeball is small, soft and disorganized. The coats appear wrinkled and thickened. The ciliary body is elevated while hypoechoic edema is seen in Tenon's capsule
- *Phthisis bulbi:* The eyeball is totally disorganized and calcification is present
- *Foreign body:*
Inert—glass, plastic, porcelain
Inorganic—iron, copper, brass
Organic—wood
While the former two lead to mechanical or chemical effects only, the latter leads to infective changes
Glass, wood, plastic due to low mass and velocity are usually anteriorly located
Foreign bodies more than 2 mm is size are capable of causing significant disruption
Foreign bodies are echogenic particles with distal acoustic shadowing or duplication artifacts. If laying on retina a mass of soft tissue suggesting inflammatory response is seen.
A low gain setting may be used to indentify foreign bodies by suppressing other structures, especially if it is surrounded by inflammatory response
A magnetic foreign body can be studied by magnet test (using a pulsed magnet). Every time a pulse is generated, there is flickering movement in magnetic foreign body
Echogenic air in eyelid suggests fracture ethmoid
Rounded foreign bodies show a trail of spikes due to many surfaces
False-negative results may be seen, if the surface area of foreign body is very small or the body is within 2 mm of sclera
- *Sympathetic ophthalmitis:* It is a bilateral diffuse granulomatous panophthalmitis, occurring within 3–12 weeks (mean = 2 week) after a perforating injury, especially if ciliary body is injured. The injured eye is known as the exciting eye while the other eye having this reaction is known as the sympathizing eye

The earliest sonological evidence is floaters in aqueous and vitreous. Later on plastic exudates at pupil, synechia, etc. may form. Meticulous search and proper gain settings may detect even a small orbital foreign body. Surrounding inflammatory reaction is an important indirect indicator
- Orbital hemorrhage may be seen as a hyperechoic resolving mass lesion or may take the form of a diffuse inflammatory disease.

Common Congenital Condition

- *Persistent hyperplastic primary vitreous (PHPV)*
  - A developmental anomaly where the embryonic vitreous does not get converted to normal adult vitreous and hyaloid vascular system persists
  - The eyeball and lens are small with a thick opaque echogenic membrane in posterior segment
  - Retrolental membrane may also be seen
  - Sometimes a thick membrane traversing from lens to disk may be seen which might lead to tractional retinal detachment. Hyaloid artery may be seen in these bands
  - Usually unilateral
  - It may be anterior (commoner) or posterior type.
- *Congenital cataract:* Lens becomes swollen and echogenic
- *Orbital cyst*
- *Cryptophthalmos:* Eyeball is only a cystic structure with no differentiation of various structure. Lens is absent while the eyelids are also not developed
- *Anophthalmia (agenesis):* A small cystic structure representing rudimentary eyeball in orbital fat with a small fissure on the face suggestive of rudimentary lids may be seen.

Common Ocular Tumors

- *Retinoblastoma:* It is most common primary malignant intraocular tumor of childhood and second to melanoma in adult. It arise from primitive cells in retina and may grow anteriorly (endophytic) or posteriorly (exophytic). The tumor has good prognosis and has no sex predilection. About 6% are autosomal dominant, sporadic cases are also seen. This tumor is usually unilateral and unifocal but may be multifocal and 1/3rd cases may be bilateral. Sonologically, well-defined irregular mass lesion arising from retina. A total retinal detachment may be seen in exophytic lesions. Abundant calcification is quite commonly seen. Optic nerve involvement diagnosed on by CT or MRI.
  - Differential diagnosis is from PHPV, Coat's disease, toxocara infection, retinopathy of premature.
  - Coat's disease—most severe form of retinal telangiectasia. Intra- or subretinal exudates, retinal detachment, uveitis and subretinal cholesterol crystals may be seen. Mean age is older than that for retinoblastoma. It is more hypoechoic than retinoblastoma and almost always unilateral.
  - Retinopathy of premature—a bilateral condition having retrolental fibroplasia following history of oxygen therapy and prematurity. Early on the eye may be larger but later may collapse and become small.
  - Toxocara infection—tractional RD with granulomatous chronic endophthalmitis and vitreous membrane are seen.
  - Orbital cysticercosis is also a common lesion in India and may mimic early retinoblastoma.

- *Uveal melanoma:* Usually, presents in 5th and 6th decade of life. About 85% arise from choroids while the rest arise posterior to equator and are unilateral. Sonographically, the tumor is lentiform, well-defined hypoechoic homogeneous and with very less incidence of cystic area or calcification. A waist or mushroom head may form, if the lesion breaks through the Bruch's membrane. "Choroidal excavation" is an important sign. Blood flow by Doppler may further confirm the diagnosis (only if lesion >3 mm).

  Associated subretinal or vitreous hemorrhage may be seen. The tumor may lead to retinal detachment, posterior vitreous detachment and vitreal degeneration. One should also try to look for scleral breech and extension in orbital fat as a hypoechoic lesion. Color Doppler is very useful in following the effect of radiotherapy on the tumor.

  Differential diagnosis is from Fuchs spots which are echogenic lesions developing in response to choroidal tear and subretinal bleed. Disciform lesions, which are macular or paramacular degenerative patches of fibrosis with subretinal fluid, also have to be differentiated. All such lesions regress on their own, unlike uveal melanoma.

- *Choroidal metastasis* are commoner than primary lesion. These are located posteriorly and may be diffuse in nature. Common primary sites are breast, bronchus, testis, kidney and gastrointestinal tract (GIT).
  - Opposite eye should always examined. These are broad-based lesion. May be associated with exudative retinal detachment.
- *Choroidal osteoma (choristoma):*
  - In young females
  - Bilateral > unilateral
  - Peripapillary area
  - Well-defined, dense echogenic lesion with acoustic shadow
  - Differential diagnosis to optic disk drusen (by clinical features).
- *Choroidal hemangioma:*
  - Associated to cutaneous angioma and Sturge-Weber syndrome
  - Located posteriorly temporal to disk
  - Multiple blood-filled spaces show blood flow
  - Overall a broad-base echogenic lesion
  - Calcification commonly seen.

Disease of Lens

- *Ectopia lentis:* Bilateral upward dislocation of lens in Marfan's syndrome (associated with retinal detachment). Downward dislocation is seen in homocystinuria. During imaging, the dislocated lens throws lot of artifacts.
- *Cataract:*
  - Developmental/hereditary
  - Nutritional
  - Inflammatory
  - Degenerative (senile)
  - Endocrine
  - Traumatic
  - Congenital.

According to distribution site of opacity, it may be classified as nuclear, subcapsular, and cortical.

Features

- Increased echogenicity of lens
- "Nicely" seen lens capsule
- Thick posterior acoustic shadow
- Two thin acoustic shadow at margins
- Thick posterior capsule
- Rough posterior capsule with low level echoes
- Internal echoes in lens
- Anterior capsule seen

- *Distorted and/or dislocation lens:*
  - A dislocated lens has to be differentiated from malignant melanoma, dislocated lens moves with changing of gain
  - By decreasing the gain, we can judge which part of lens is more affected, and hence judge the cause.

Disease of Vitreous

Aging

- Liquefaction with formation of dark areas known as lacunae
- Prominence of fibers posteriorly
- Shrinkage of gel due to contraction of particles within the gel
- Posterior vitreous detachment.

Vitreous Detachment

- Most commonly posterior vitreous detachment
- Associated vitreous hemorrhage, floaters and opacities noted
- Presents as a thin mobile sheet
- Some opacities may be adherent to the sheet
- Usually not attached to nerve head
- In absence of, opacities may missed.

Vitreous Opacities

These opacities may be:
- *Intravitreal:*
  - Developmental
  - Degenerative
  - Inflammatory
  - Hemorrhagic
  - Neoplastic
- *Retrovitreal:*
  - Degenerative
  - Hemorrhagic
  - Inflammatory

Various opacities that may be seen are:
- *Floaters:*
  - Highly echogenic
  - Pinpoint
  - Posteriorly located
  - Due to condensation of filaments
- *Asteroid hyalosis:*
  - Tiny crystal like
  - Few to many in number
  - Calcium soaps containing sulfur and phosphorus in an amorphous matrix
  - Most common in a zone between lens and nerve head (as it is more common in primary vitreous)
  - Are dense and mobile, therefore show smooth wavy movement
  - A spare zone is seen between these opacities and retina
  - Seen even on low gain setting, a very important point of diagnosis
  - Associated with diabetes
  - Seen more in old females
  - Vision may even be normal
  - It is unrelated to eye disease and may even be seen in normal patients
  - Usually unilateral.
- *Subhyaloid hemorrhage:* Red blood cells between posterior vitreous and retina (i.e. in subhyaloid space)
- *Endophthalmitis:*
  - Highly mobile pinpoint opacities
  - Diffusely, scattered inflammatory cells
  - An H-shaped echo is typical. A central thick opacity with two vertical dotted bands are seen
  - Differential diagnosis to choroidal detachment (where the vertical bands are curved)
  - Differential diagnosis to amyloidosis where strand-like opacities are noted.
- *Membranes and adhesion:*
  - Old pathologies such as vitreous hemorrhage may organized to form membrane

- Such membranes are thin peripherally located and thick posteriorly
- No specific location and attachment are there
- Motility is also variable depending upon thickness
- Adhesion connects posterior vitreous to retinal and can cause retinal detachment, retinal tear, etc.
- Adhesions may form due to inflammation, phototherapy techniques, neovascularization.

- *Vitreous hemorrhage:*
  - Early hemorrhage in clear vitreous appears as free-floating pinpoint opacities
  - These are located more at the bleeding points and more posteriorly
  - Late hemorrhage and clots are thick and coarse. Organization leads to restriction of movement
  - Finger-like projection may appear from point of bleeding
  - May be associated to subhyaloid hemorrhage but likes longer time to organize, especially if vitreous is in gel state
  - Cause of vessel tear may be a localized or generalized disease
  - Vitreous hemorrhage is echopoor and disappear on reducing gain therefore making its differentiation from mass, adhesion, membrane easy
  - Vitreous hemorrhage (VH) may also simulate retinopathy; again reducing gain shows that the former looses contact to posterior surface while latter does not. Movement with change in gaze, is not a very reliable criteria for this purpose.

Classification

- Vitreous hemorrhage without retinal detachment and fibrin
- VH without retinal detachment (RD) but with fibrin, structural changes as dislocated lens may be seen
- VH with RD but no evidence of any organization as a cyclitic membrane. The main role of USG in VH is to:
  - Decide operability (contraindicated in type 3)
  - Planning the type of operation
  - Planning the site of puncture.

17.5 DISEASE OF RETINA

Ultrasonography is an important tool for differential diagnosis of retinal detachment.

- Retinal detachment appears as a thin membrane attached at ora serrata and optic nerve head ballooning forwards to variable degree
- Later on there is contraction of membrane which leads to its thickening and reduction in motion forming the morning glory appearance (V-shaped)
- Cysts and tractional bands may develop in very late stages. There are more common at site of holes in the rhegmatogenous RD (i.e. RD with tear in retina)
- In nonrhegmatogenous RD (RD with no tear), a solid mass like lesion (that is to be differentiated from melanoma), may be formed
- B-scan should be done in case of RD even, if ophthalmoscopic diagnosis has been made with reasonable surety, in order to detect the following points which may be still missed, and by all these we want to confirm or refute the presence of a mass as the cause of RD
  - To rule out retinal breaks
  - To rule out smooth ballooning and shifting fluid is noted
  - To rule out increased intraocular tension
  - To rule out a large iris nevi present (which may be associated with melanoma)

- After any operation for RD, USG should be done to assess the success and complications as choroidal effusion
- A cyclitic membrane, that is seen in chronic infections and comes in differential diagnosis appears as a T-shaped or triangular structure
- Partial RD is not attached in its center to nerve head
- Common causes of RD are high myopia, trauma, an associated subretinal fluid is seen in Coat's disease, Harada's disease, malignant hypertension, melanoma, subretinal hemorrhage in Coat's and von Hippel-Lindau disease. This fluid is exudative in tractional RD and is seen in diabetes and sickle cell anemia
- In cases where a subretinal fluid is suspected scanning in sitting position is must as the fluid settles and bows the lower leaf more anteriorly
- In certain ocular inflammatory diseases, vaso-occlusive disease and degenerative disease crumpled membrane may form
- In central serous retinopathy, RD may occur at macula
- Disciform macular degeneration shows heterogeneously hypoechoic, rounded or flat elevation at macula. These occur due to a subretinal scar formed secondary to bleeding. It may be a senile condition. This condition is bilateral, associated with drusen, constant in size and rarely associated with RD
    - Differential diagnosis is to melanoma, which may change in size and show vascularity, choroidal excavation by Bruch's membrane. Macular degeneration is an irregular focal elevation with underlying hypoechoic area
    - Macular edema is another differential diagnosis
    - Acquired retinoschisis is a commonly seen condition especially in hypermetrops. It is a splitting of sensory retina in two layers. This may be a precursor to RD. This splitting usually starts at periphery inferotemporal to macula and increased circumferentially. The condition is usually located anterior to equator (plexiform) or rarely posterior to it (reticular). It usually presents as a thin echogenic membrane, unlike RD which is seen as a thick definite membrane.

Disease of Choroid

Choroidal Detachment (CD) and its Differential Diagnosis

It is caused basically due to globe hypotony:
- Postoperative
- Trauma
- Tumor
- Lens dislocation/swollen lens
- Papillary block
- In association to rhegmatogenous RD.

Features

- Flat anterior chamber, signs of RD, VH, etc.
- Hazy media and choroidal effusion
- CD is seen as an echogenic line attached at ora serrata, vertical vein and disk margins. This is in differentiation to RD, which is attached at disk center
- Step signs are typical of CD which presents as an echogenic elevation at all points of attachment
- Kissing choroids is a condition when due to bowing opposite membranes touch each other.

Disease of Sclerocornea

Staphyloma and ectasia are the main conditions requiring evaluation by USG.
- Formed due to decreased intraocular tension and/or focal weakness in sclerocornea, and presents as a focal. This bulge,

if associated with uveal bulge is known as staphyloma or else simply an ectasia
- Corneal staphyloma is thus a misnomer
- Ectasia is seen in congenital glaucoma (total) or in high myopia (posterior)
- Staphyloma is usually located at points of entry/exit of nerves and vessels
- A band in posterior chamber may exert pull leading to pseudostaphyloma in diabetic retinopathy, vitreous hemorrhage, etc.

Disease of Optic Nerve Head

- Papilla and its disease are best evaluated from lateral approach
- Papilledema, papillitis, pseudopapilledema, drusen and melanocytoma present with an increased echogenicity
- In papilledema, fluid may be seen in subretinal space and along optic nerve sleeve
- Drusen is a congenital or acquired condition which is usually asymptomatic but may be symptomatic if there is associated intraocular bleed. Acquired drusens may increase in number with increasing age
  This has to be differentiated from foreign body and dislocated lens. Both of these conditions are more echogenic and are seen even at low gain setting
- Optic atrophy can only seen by narrow beam transducers which do not cause beam width artifacts
- Inflammatory conditions like neuritis show:
  - Echogenic nerve sheath
  - Hypoechoic zone between nerve and its sheath known as "doubling of wall"
- Such signs associated with rectus muscle thickening indicated Graves' disease. If Tenon's capsule inflammation is associated then pseudotumor may be the cause
- Such findings are also seen in orbital congestive conditions like caroticocavernous fistula, ophthalmic artery aneurysm, etc.
- In neuritis, the thickness of nerve is increased as opposed papilledema due to increased intracranial tension, where doubling of wall is very prominent.

17.6 ORBITAL PATHOLOGIES

Sonographic Classification of Orbital Lesions

- Except muscles, nerves and vitreous all normal orbital structures are hyperechoic
- Pathologies are usually hypoechoic apart few which are hyperechoic but not as much as the normal orbital structures. Also the pathologies are heterogeneous.

A. Extremely Low Reflectivity Lesions

- Cysts
- Mucocele (noncompressible)
- Hematoma
- Varix (alters shape with Valsalva)
- Paranasal sinus malignancy (has bony chips in it).

B. Low Reflectivity Lesions

- Cellulitis, abscess, pseudotumor
- Lymphoma
- Glioma
- Capillary hemangioma
- Caroticocavernous fistula.

C. Medium Reflectivity Lesions

- Dermoid
- Meningioma.

D. High Reflectivity Lesions

- Metastases
- Foreign body
- Cavernous hemangioma
- Lymphangioma
- Pleomorphic adenoma
  - Pathologies may also be classified according to their edge definition.

E. Well-Circumscribed Masses/Lesions

- Cavernous hemangiomas
- Hemangiopericytomas
- Dermoids **(Fig. 17.6.1)**
- Meningioma
- Foreign body **(Fig. 17.6.2)**
- Nerve sheath tumors.

F. Infiltrative Lesions

- Pseudotumor
- Lymphoma
- Metastases

- Capillary hemangioma
- Lymphangioma
- Wegener's granulomatosis.

G. Serpiginous Lesions

- Arteriovenous malformation **(Figs. 17.6.3A and B)**
- Varix
- Plexiform neurofibroma.

H. Differential Diagnosis of Orbital Muscle Enlargement

- Graves' disease
  - Look for thyroid
  - Look for thyroid function tests
- Myositis/pseudotumor **(Figs. 17.6.4A and B)**
  - Look for signs of inflammation
- Lymphoma **(Fig. 17.6.5)**
- Leukemia
- Metastasis
- Rhabdomyosarcoma/myoma
- Hemangioma
- Lymphangioma
- Caroticocavernous fistula
- Dural arteriovenous malformations (AVM)
- Injury/hematoma
- Acromegaly
- Infective cysticercosis **(Fig. 17.6.6)**.

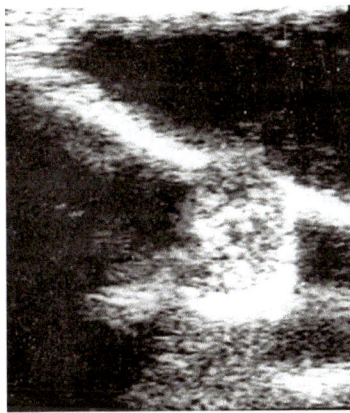

Fig. 17.6.1: Epidermoid cyst—a large space-occupying lesion (SOL) with predominant cystic areas with internal debris is seen anterosuperiorly to the eyeball. The lesion is seen to extend intracranially and causing bone destruction. The intracranial part is predominantly solid with foci of calcification in it. The eyeball is not involved. Fine-needle aspiration cytology (FNAC) confirmed the case.

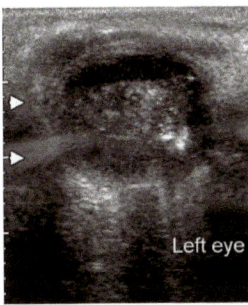 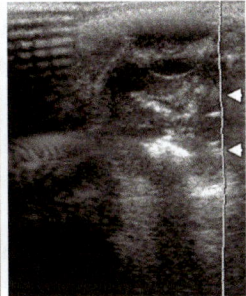

Fig. 17.6.2: US scans show vitreous hemorrhage and foreign body secondary to trauma (arrowheads).

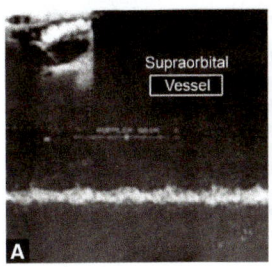 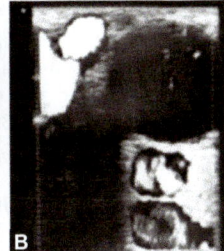

Figs. 17.6.3A and B: There is evidence of dilatation of superior ophthalmic vein and dilated vessels in the superorbital region and within extraconal compartment. The dilated vessels on duplex showed a mixed arteriovenous turbulent signal.

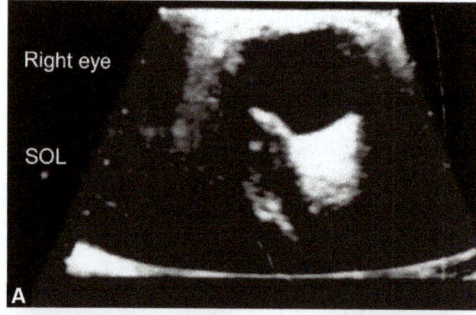

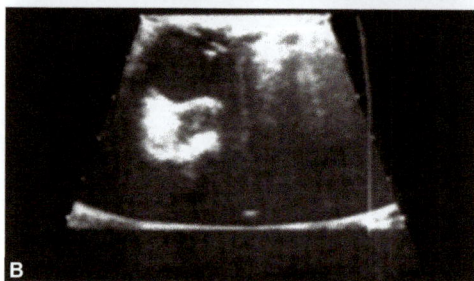

Figs. 17.6.4A and B: Pseudotumor—(A) Longitudinal; (B) Transverse scan shows well-defined, spindle-shaped hypoechoic solid mass with foci of calcification in the lateral rectus muscle. (SOL: space-occupying lesions)

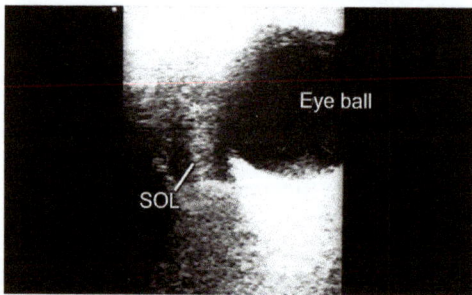

Fig. 17.6.5: Follow-up case of Hodgkin's lymphoma showing a well-defined round hypoechoic SOL adjacent to the eyeball FNAC—confirmed lymphomatous origin. (SOL: space-occupying lesion)

I. Differential Diagnosis of Unilateral Proptosis

Lesions of eyeball
- *Retinoblastoma* **(Figs. 17.6.7A and B):**
  - Echogenic
  - Calcification present, coarse

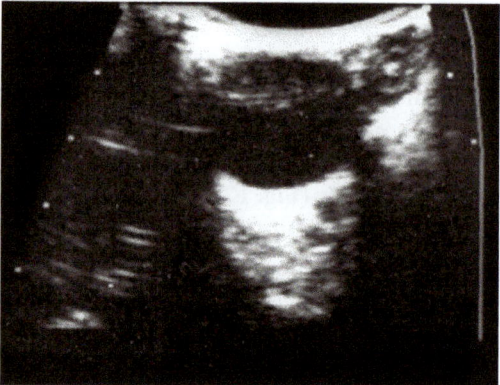

Fig. 17.6.6: Orbital cysticercosis—a well-defined round cystic space-occupying lesion (SOL) with focus of calcification seen in muscle adjacent to eyeball.

  - Associated with retinal detachment **(Figs. 17.6.8 and 17.6.9)**.
- *Melanoma:*
  - Iso to hypoechoic
  - Adults
  - May breech the Tenon's capsule **(Figs. 17.6.10 to 17.6.13)**
- Metastasis
- Hematoma **(Fig. 17.6.14)**
- Episcleritis
- Scleritis
- Uveitis
- Lens (calcification) **(Fig. 17.6.15)**.

Lesions of optic nerve
- *Glioma:*
  - Thickened optic nerve, focally
  - Protruding optic disk
- Meningioma: Thickened nerve shadow but smoothly **(Fig. 17.6.16)**.

Lesions of Extraocular Muscles

- Myositis
- *Graves' disease:*
  - Increased intraorbital echogenic fat
  - May be associated with muscle thickening
  - No fat stranding

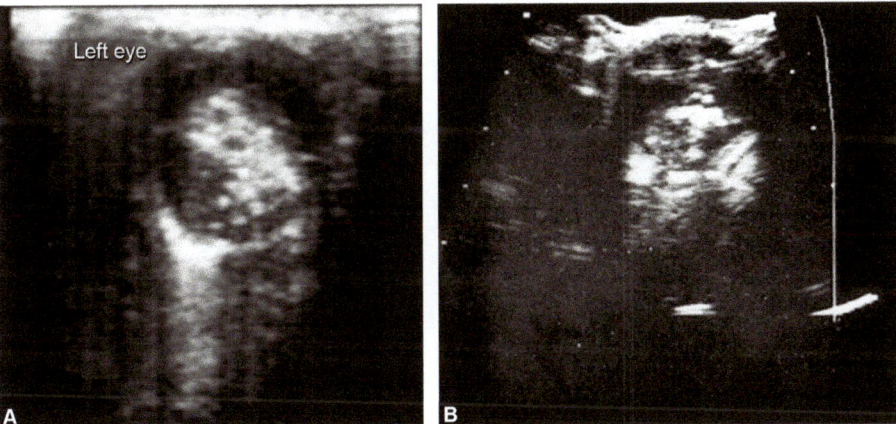

Figs. 17.6.7A and B: (A) Retinoblastoma—6-month-old male child showing a heterogeneous echotexture mass in the left eye with multiple dense echogenic and anechoic areas; (B) Retinoblastoma—transverse scan of left eye in a 3-year-old female child showing a solid intraocular mass attached posteriorly with areas of calcification in it.

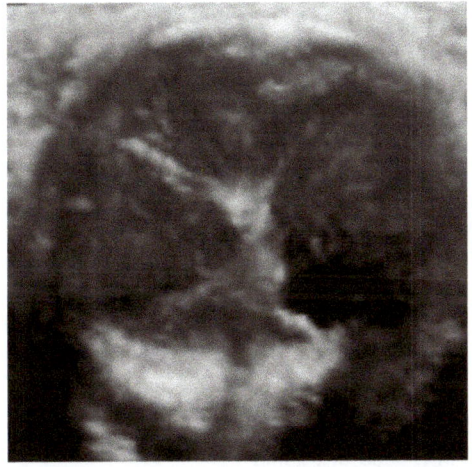

Fig. 17.6.8: Three-dimensional (3D) US scan shows retinal detachment.

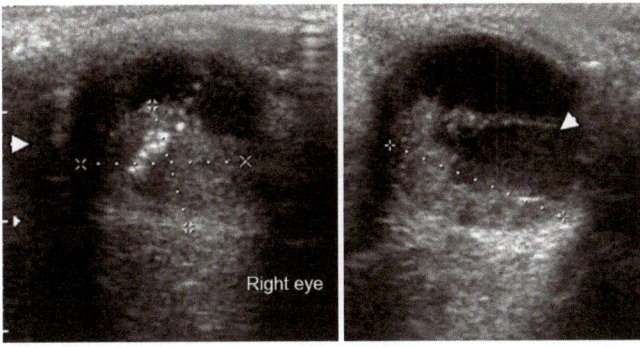

Fig. 17.6.9: US scan shows retinoblastoma with retinal detachment (arrowheads).

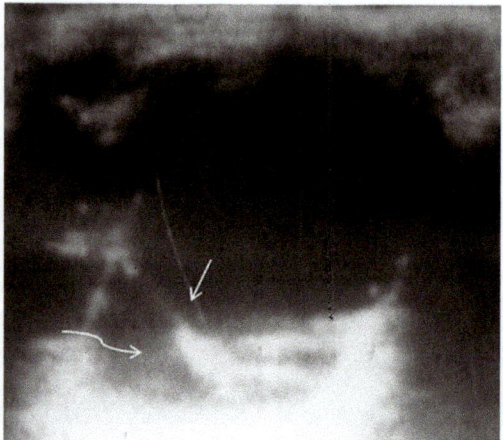

Fig. 17.6.10: USG eye globe showing subretinal fluid (curved arrow) with retinal detachment (straight arrow).

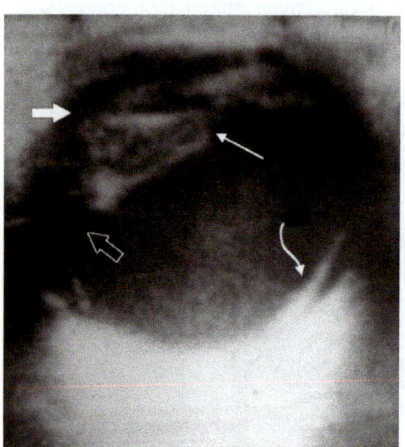

Fig. 17.6.11: USG eye globe showing echogenic lesion in anterior (thick black arrow) and posterior chamber (thick white arrow) in a case of trauma suggesting hemorrhage (straight arrow) with retinal detachment (curved arrow).

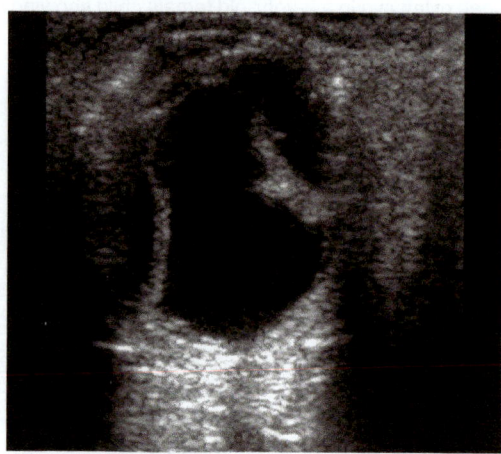

Fig. 17.6.12: US scan shows choroid detachment.

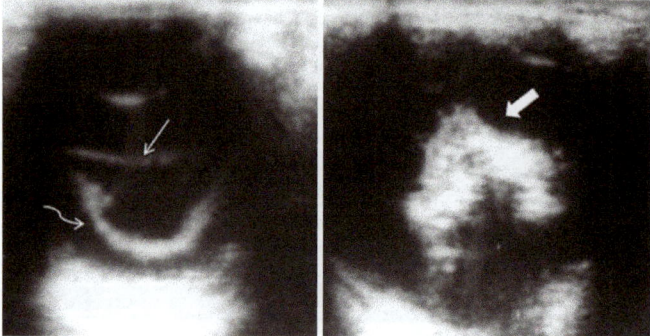

Fig. 17.6.13: USG eye globe showing choroidal melanoma (thick white arrow) with choroidal (straight arrow) and retinal detachment (curved arrow).

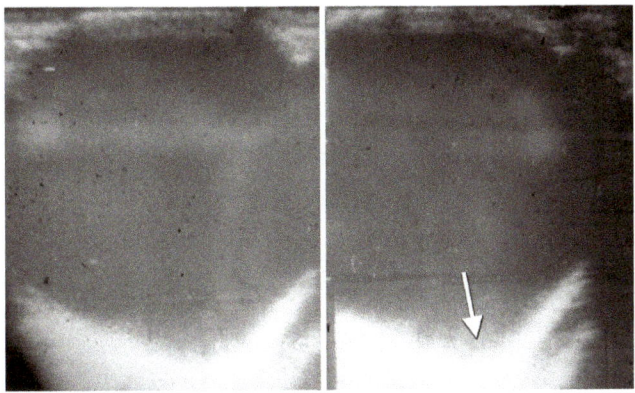

Fig. 17.6.14: USG eye globe showing posterior staphyloma (arrow).

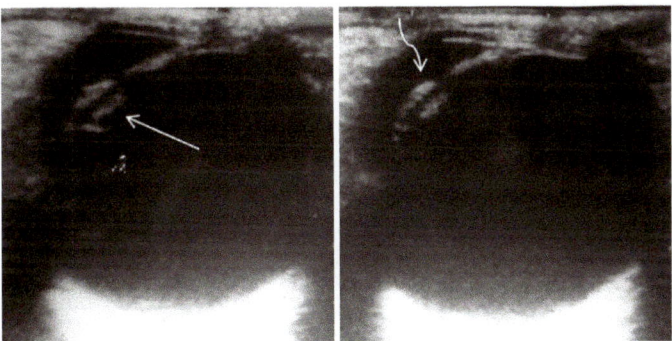

Fig. 17.6.15: USG eye globe showing increased echogenicity (straight arrow) of lens in a case of cataract (curved arrow).

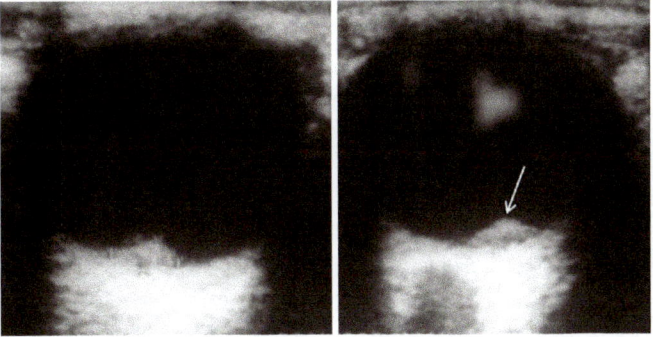

Fig. 17.6.16: USG eye globe showing echogenic lesion in area of disk-suggesting drusen (arrow).

- Rhadomyoma/sarcoma
- Hemangioma
- Trauma
- Lymphoma
- Leukemia.

Lesions of Lacrimal Glands

- *Dacryoadenitis:*
  - Bulky lacrimal glands
  - Edema in surrounding tissues

- Lymphoma
- Mucoepidermoid tumor
- Adenoid cystic tumor
- Pleomorphic adenoma
- Sarcoidosis
- Benign cysts.

Other Intraconal Space-occupying Lesions

- Vitreous lesions **(Figs. 17.6.17 and 17.6.18)**
- Fibroma

- Hemangioma
- Lymphangioma
- Lipoma/sarcoma
- Lymphoma
- Varix
- Neurofibroma
- Abscess
- Hydatid/cysticercosis **(Fig. 17.6.19)**
- Granuloma.

Extraconal Lesions

- Fibrous dysplasia
- Nonossifying fibroma
- *Subperiosteal abscess:*
    - Extraconal fluid (heterogeneous collection)
    - Broad-based towards bone
- Mucocele
- Carcinoma maxilla/sinonasal malignancies
- Hematoma
- Orbital cellulitis
- Aneurysmal bone cysts
- Epidermoid/dermoid.

Differential Diagnosis of Bilateral Proptosis

- *Graves' disease:*
    - Intraorbital fat
    - Abnormal thyroid function tests

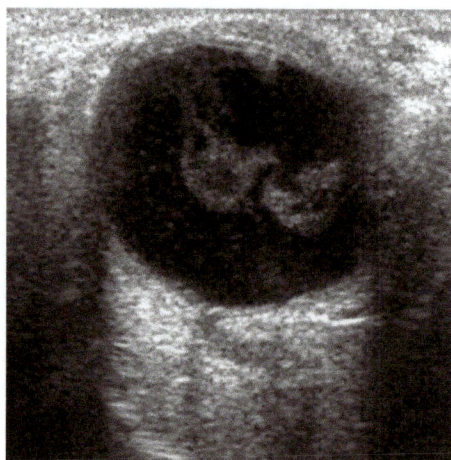

Fig. 17.6.17: US scan shows vitreous exudates.

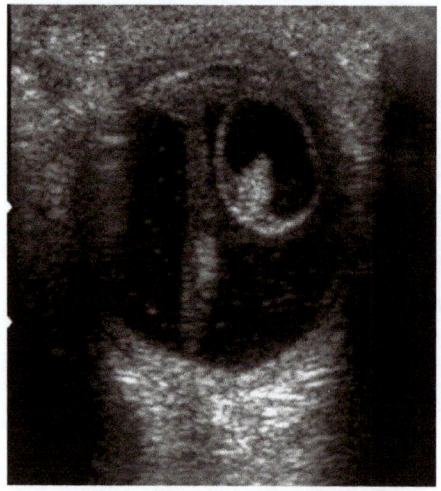

Fig. 17.6.18: US scan shows vitreous cyst and persistent hyaloid artery.

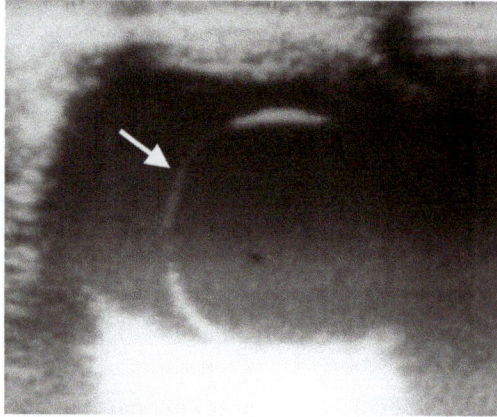

Fig. 17.6.19: USG eye globe showing intraocular (arrow) neurocysticercosis.

- Metastasis
- Lymphoma/sarcoma:
  - Diffuse infiltrative hypoechoic lesion involving both intra- and extraconal structures
- Leukemia
- Histiocytosis
- Late phase of cavernous sinus thrombosis
- *Developmental lesions of skull:*
  - Oxycephaly
  - Apert's syndrome
  - Cruzon's syndrome.

Differential Diagnosis of Pulsatile Proptosis

- *Caroticocavernous fistula:*
  - Serpiginous tortuous hypoechoic vascular structures showing flow towards orbit are seen
  - Waveforms are one of arterialized veins
- Arteriovascular malformations
- Aneurysms
- *Varix:* Avascular channel that inflates on Valsalva is seen
- Cephalocele
- Neurofibromatosis with sphenoid wing dysplasia
- Base of skull fracture.

Differential Diagnosis of Intraorbital Calcification

Calcification within globe:
- Cataract
- Trauma
- Infection
- Retinoblastoma.

Calcification outside globe:
- Phleboliths
- Dermoid
- Meningioma
- Neurofibroma
- Lacrimal gland carcinoma.

CHAPTER 18

Neonatal and Infant Brain

18.1 CYSTIC LESIONS

- Porencephalic cyst
- Hydranencephaly
- Cystic encephalomalacia.

Ventriculomegaly

- Hydrocephalus
- Atrophy
- Colpocephaly.

Congenital/Developmental Malformations

- Holoprosencephaly **(Fig. 18.1.1)**
- Schizencephaly
- Dandy-Walker malformation
- Arachnoid cyst
- Midline interhemispheric cyst
- Mega cisterna magna
- Choroid plexus cyst
- Subependymal cyst.

Infections

- Abscess **(Fig. 18.1.2)**
- Subdural effusion
- Empyema **(Fig. 18.1.3)**.

Vascular

- Vein of Galen malformation
- Varix of vein of Galen
- AV malformation.

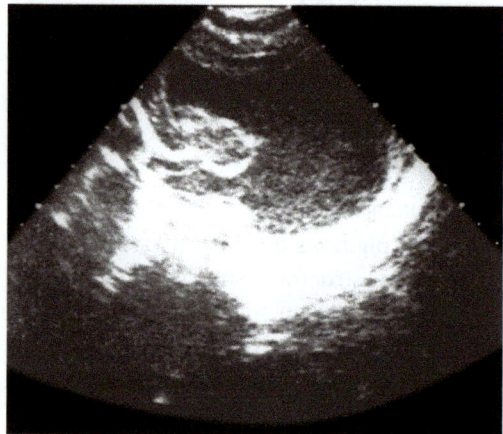

Fig. 18.1.1: Semilobar holoprosencephaly.

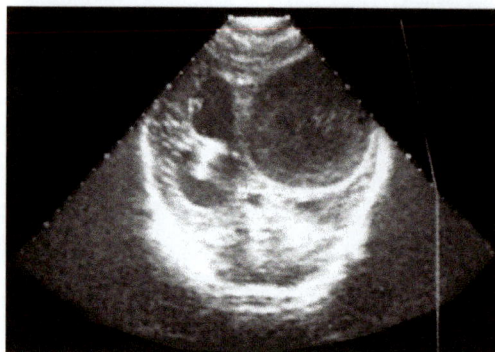

Fig. 18.1.2: Anechoic lesion in left parietal region compressing lateral and third ventricles—brain abscess.

Trauma

- Leptomeningeal cyst
- Chronic hematoma.

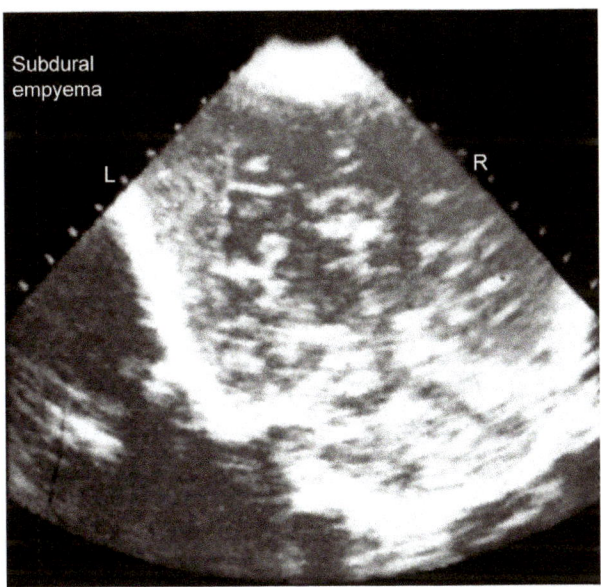

Fig. 18.1.3: Brightly echogenic meninges seen overlying the left frontal lobe with extra-axial collection containing echoes overlying it—subdural empyema.

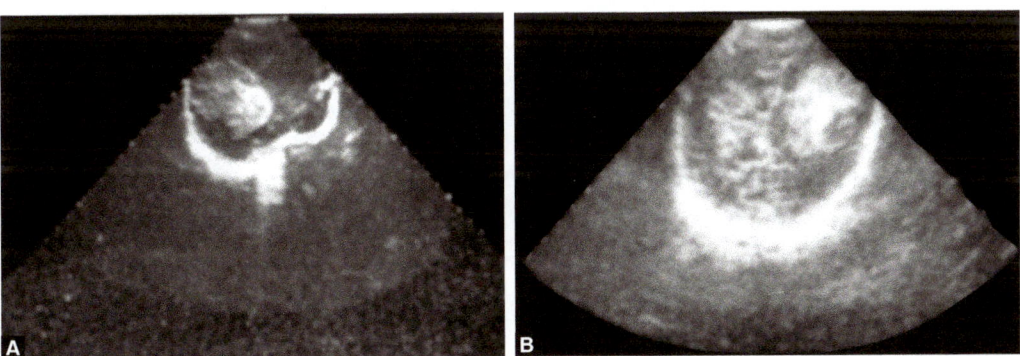

Figs. 18.2.1A and B: (A) Intracranial hemorrhage in right parietal area—longitudinal and sagittal scan; (B) Intracranial hemorrhage in left cerebral hemisphere parietal area.

18.2 SOLID LESIONS

- Intracranial hemorrhage (**Figs. 18.2.1A and B**)
- Asphyxia
- Infection (cerebritis and edema)
- Tumors.

18.3 PROMINENT CHOROID PLEXUS

- Intraventricular hemorrhage (**Figs. 18.3.1 and 18.3.2**)
- Infection
- Choroid plexus papilloma.

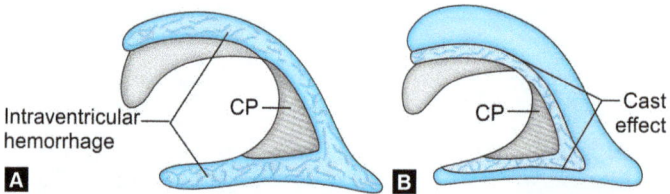

Figs. 18.3.1A and B: Intraventricular hemorrhage. (A) Lateral sagittal view. An intraventricular hemorrhage fills the entire lateral ventricle. The choroid plexus (CP) is difficult to distinguish from the hemorrhage; (B) With time, the hemorrhage takes on a cast effect and adopts the shape of the ventricle as the blood resolves. The choroid plexus is still difficult to distinguish from the clot.

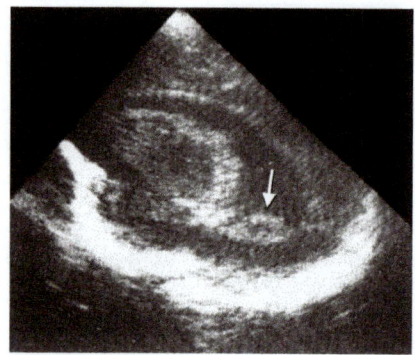

Fig. 18.3.2: Intraventricular hemorrhage (IVH).

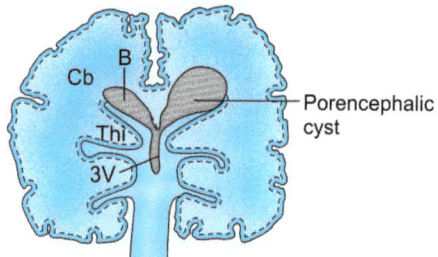

Fig. 18.4.1: The clot resolves completely, leaving a porencephalic cyst with lateral ventricular dilatation. (B: hemorrhage; Cb: cerebral cortex; Thi: thalamus; 3V: 3rd ventricle)

18.4 DESTRUCTIVE LESIONS OF BRAIN

Porencephalic Cyst (Fig. 18.4.1)

- It is an area of normally developed brain that has been damaged and heals with a lining of gliotic white matter
- It is seen as a cystic area which connects to ventricular system but does not extend to surface cortex
- Typically occurs after birth as a sequelae to hemorrhage, infection and trauma.

Hydranencephaly (Figs. 18.4.2 and 18.4.3)

- Result of occlusion of bilateral internal carotid arteries in fetal life
- Regarded as severest form of porencephaly
- USG shows calvarium filled with cerebrospinal fluid (CSF) with total destruction of cerebral cortex and falx cerebri is preserved

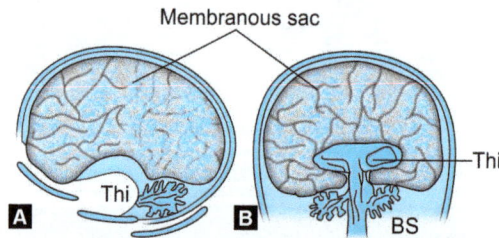

Figs. 18.4.2A and B: A hydranencephaly. Lateral sagittal (A) and midcoronal (B) views. There is no evidence of cortical tissue. A membranous fluid-filled sac replaces the brain. Only the brainstem (BS) and midbrain are present. (Thi: thalamus)

- Structures supplied by posterior circulation are spared, e.g. thalamus, cerebellum, brainstem and posterior choroid plexus
- Doppler USG shows absence of blood flow in carotid arteries
- Differential diagnosis (D/D)—Alobar holoprosencephaly and hydrocephalus.

Neonatal and Infant Brain

Cystic Encephalomalacia

- It is an area of focal or widespread brain damage with astrocytic proliferation and glial septations **(Figs. 18.4.4A and B)**
- May result from infection, anoxia and thrombus in neonatal brain
- Differential diagnosis—porencephalic cyst.

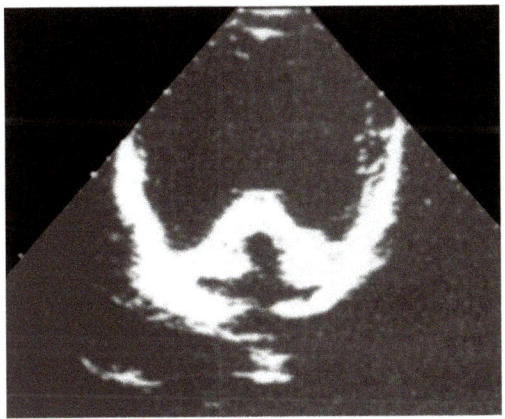

Fig. 18.4.3: Hydranencephaly.

Porencephalic cyst	Cystic encephalomalacia
Always connect with the system ventricular	Typically do not connect to ventricular system
Do not extend to surface cortex	May extend to surface cortex

18.5 VENTRICULOMEGALY

Hydrocephalus

- Enlargement of ventricles with decreased sulcal and cisternal space is identified as hydrocephalus.

Imaging findings are:
- Enlargement of 3rd ventricle especially anterior and posterior recesses
- Proportionate dilatation of the temporal horns with the lateral ventricle
- Narrowing of mammilopontine distance
- Narrowing of ventricular angle
- Widening of frontal horn radius
- Periventricular interstitial edema
- Effacement of cortical sulci.

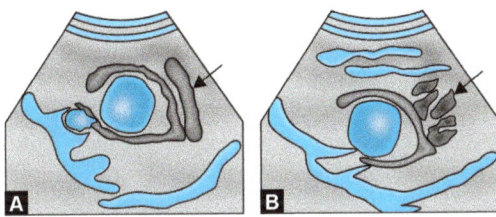

Figs. 18.4.4A and B: Periventricular leukomalacia. (A) An echogenic area surrounds the trigone of the lateral ventricle in its early stages (arrow); (B) Tiny cysts develop soon afterward to replace this echogenic area (arrow).

Differentiating Features

- Alobar holoprosencephaly
- Falx cerebri is absent in this but present in hydranencephaly
- *Hydrocephalus:* A thin rim of cortex is usually seen by sonography which is absent in hydranencephaly.

Causes of Hydrocephalus

Intraventricular obstruction	Extraventricular obstruction	Over production
Posthemorrhagic	Posthemorrhagic	Choroid plexus papilloma
Postfossa subdural hematoma Chiari II malformation **(Figs. 18.5.1A and B)**	Postinfectious	Achondroplasia – Absence or hypoplasia of arachnoid granulation
Aqueductal stenosis Postinfectious Vein of Galen malformation		
Tumor or cyst		Venous obstruction

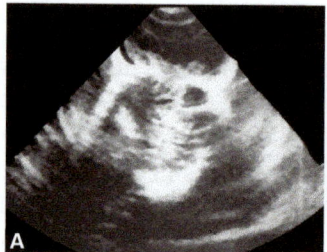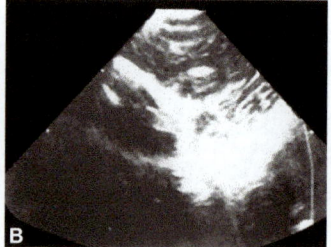

Figs. 18.5.1A and B: Arnold-Chiari malformation II is showing tonsillar herniation with downward shift of fourth ventricle.

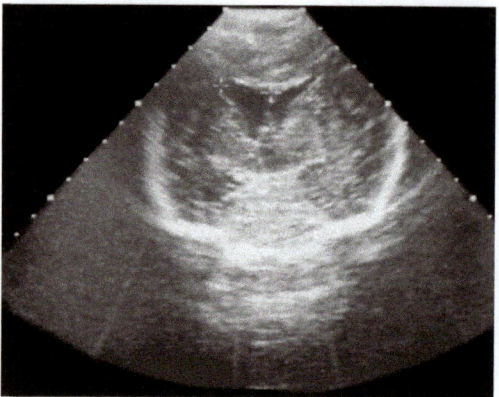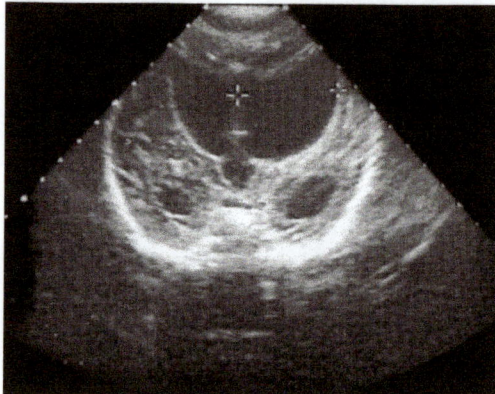

Fig. 18.5.2: Frontal horn of right lateral ventricles appears dilated. Left is normal suggestive of asymmetrical hydrocephalus due to obstruction at foramen of Monro.

Fig. 18.5.3: Congenital aqueductal stenosis—bilateral lateral ventricles appear dilated with funnel-shaped third ventricle.

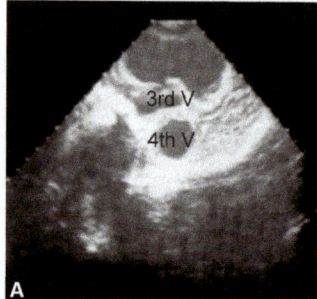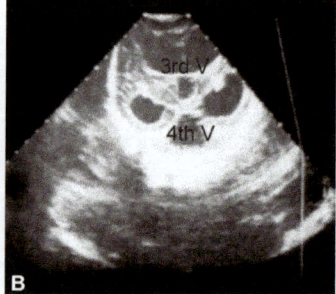

Figs. 18.5.4A and B: Communicating hydrocephalus. (3rd V: 3rd ventricle; 4th V: 4th ventricle)

Sonography is Useful for

- *Diagnosis of hydrocephalus (Figs. 18.5.2 to 18.5.6):*
  - Can be diagnosed in utero by 15 weeks of gestation
  - In utero, size of atrium >10 mm indicates ventriculomegaly
  - Progressive rounding and bulging of superolateral angles of frontal horns
  - Dilatation of occipital horns.

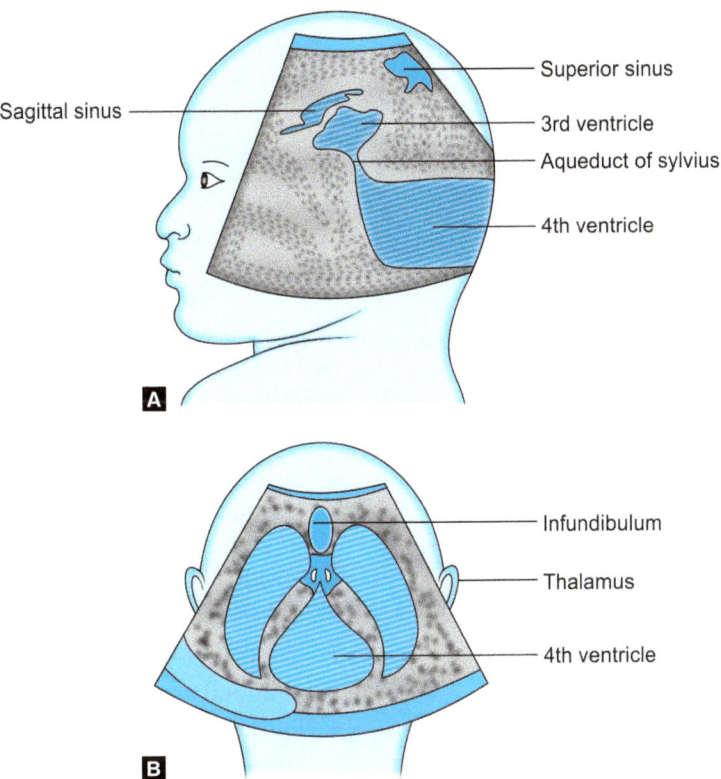

Figs. 18.5.5A and B: Dandy-Walker syndrome. (A) Midline sagittal view. There is cystic dilatation of the fourth ventricle; the third ventricle and aqueduct of Sylvius are dilated to some degree. Note the abnormal cerebellar shape; (B) Posterior coronal view: Massive IVth ventricular and lateral ventricular enlargement.

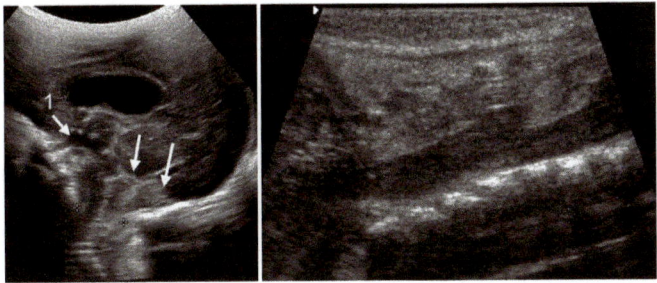

Fig. 18.5.6: US scans show Chiari malformation (arrows).

- *Level of obstruction:*
  - Site of obstruction in hydrocephalus is the point of transition from dilated to nondilated CSF containing spaces, e.g.
    - Dilatation of lateral and IIIrd ventricles indicates aqueductal obstruction
    - Dilatation of all ventricles indicates an extraventricular cause.
- *Causes of hydrocephalus:*
  - Presence of hemorrhage, ventriculitis is evident by intraparenchymal changes and intraventricular echoes and septations with irregular ependymal outline

- Other well-defined conditions associated with obstructive hydrocephalus, e.g. Dandy-Walker syndrome and Chiari II malformation are apparent on US.

Ventriculomegaly Secondary to Atrophy

- There is prominence of ventricles as well as CSF spaces
- Small or diminishing head circumference favors atrophy
- Anterior and posterior recesses of 3rd ventricle are not enlarged in atrophy whereas they are enlarged in case of hydrocephalus
- Temporal horns dilate less than the bodies of lateral ventricles in case of atrophy due to relatively small size of temporal lobes.

Colpocephaly

- Atria and occipital horns of lateral ventricles are disproportionately enlarged
- It is associated with Chiari II malformation and corpus callosum agenesis.

18.6 CONGENITAL AND DEVELOPMENTAL MALFORMATIONS

Holoprosencephaly (Fig. 18.6.1)

Can be alobar, semilobar or lobar types.

Sonographic Findings in Alobar Holoprosencephaly

- Single midline crescent-shaped ventricle
- Thin layer of cerebral cortex
- No falx
- No interhemispheric fissure
- No corpus callosum
- Fused thalami and basal ganglia
- Fused echogenic choroid plexus
- Absent third ventricle
- Large dorsal cyst

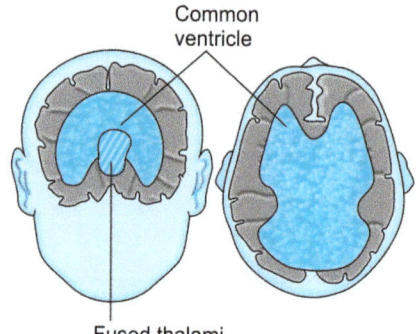

Fig. 18.6.1: Holoprosencephaly. Anterior coronal and axial views. A single misshaped ventricle is present.

- Severe facial anomalies—colpocephaly, cyclopia, ethmocephaly.

Sonographic Findings in Semilobar Holoprosencephaly

- Single ventricle but separate occipital and temporal horns
- Partially developed falx and interhemispheric fissure in the occipital cortex posteriorly
- Partially separated thalami
- Rudimentary 3rd ventricle
- Facial anomalies are less severe—hypotelorism, cleft lip.

Sonographic Findings in Lobar Holoprosencephaly

- Nearly complete separation of hemispheres with development of falx and interhemispheric fissure but part of frontal lobes may be fused anteriorly
- Genu and rostrum of corpus callosum is absent
- Mild or absent facial anomalies.

Schizencephaly

- Caused by a destructive process in utero leading to gray matter lined clefts that extend through the entire hemisphere from

ependymal lining of lateral ventricles to cortical surface
- Bilateral (BL) or unilateral (UL) clefts
- It can be open lip type or closed lip type. Closed lip type is identified by a nipple-like protrusion on the ventricular surface.

Arachnoid Cyst

- It is seen as an cystic extra-axial lesion producing mass effect with displacement of underlying brain parenchyma
- Does not communicate with ventricular system.

Mega Cisterna Magna

- In utero mega cisterna magna is diagnosed when its AP dimension measures 5 ± 3 mm
- It arches around cerebellum posteriorly and is usually widest in the midline where invagination of space occurs between the two cerebellar hemispheres
- Not associated with hydrocephalus or abnormal brain parenchyma.

Choroid Plexus Cyst

- Cystic well-defined mass within the choroid plexus measuring 4–7 mm in diameter
- Usually U/L, occurring more frequently on the left and situated in the dorsal aspect of choroid plexus
- Rarely can cause obstructive hydrocephalus.

Subependymal Cyst

- Discrete cysts in the lining of ventricles
- Commonly result from germinal matrix hemorrhage in premature infants, also due to infection with rubella, cytomegalovirus (CMV) and Zellweger syndrome.

Dorsal Interhemispheric Cyst (Fig. 18.6.2)

- Well-defined anechoic cystic structure in dorsal interhemispheric fissure
- Associated with corpus callosum agenesis, (Fig. 18.6.3) Dandy-Walker malformation and holoprosencephaly.

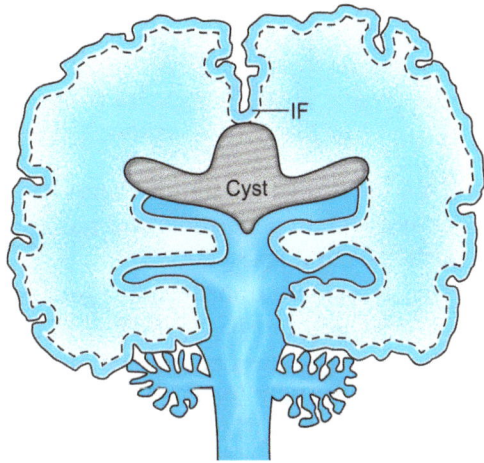

Fig. 18.6.2: Agenesis of the corpus callosum with cyst. In this variant, the lateral and third ventricles are joined by a cyst that extends superiorly from the third ventricle. (IF: infundibulum)

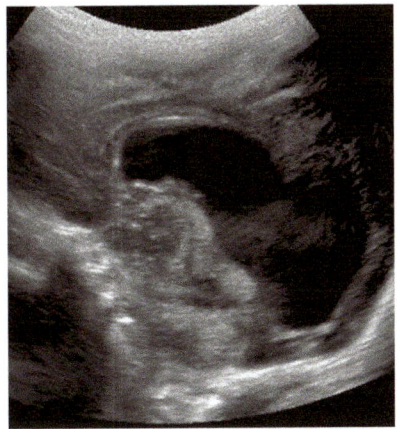

Fig. 18.6.3: US scan shows partial corpus callosum agenesis with hydrocephalus.

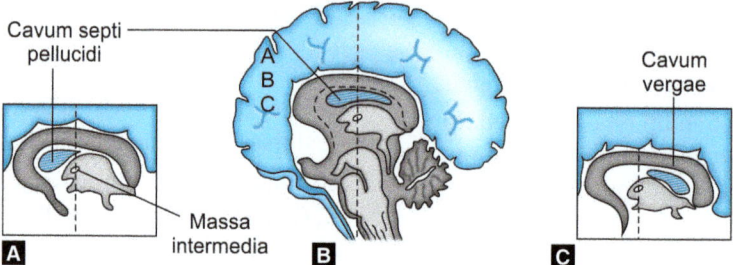

Figs. 18.6.4A to C: Cavum septi pellucidi. If the scanning angle is incorrect, this normal variant may be mistaken for a dilated ventricle. It may appear in one of three different patterns: (A) Cavum septi pellucidi; (B) Cavum septi pellucidi and cavum vergae; (C) Cavum vergae.

Cavum Septum Pellucidum and Cavum Vergae (Figs. 18.6.4A to C)

- Anterior to the foramen of Monro is the cavum septum pellucidum and posterior is the cavum vergae
- They are present normally early in gestation but they close from back to front starting at 6 months gestation and are completely closed normally by 3–6 months after birth.

18.7 INFECTIVE CYSTIC LESIONS

Brain Abscess

Well-defined hypoechoic lesion with internal echoes and distal enhancement showing mass effect.

Subdural Effusion (Fig. 18.7.1)

- There is leakage of protein and fluid in subdural space due to inflammation of subdural veins
- Seen as crescentic extra-axial hypoechoic fluid collection in subdural space
- Usually resolve spontaneously
- Subdural effusion has to be differentiated from prominent subarachnoid spaces seen in atrophy and benign intracranial collection of infancy.

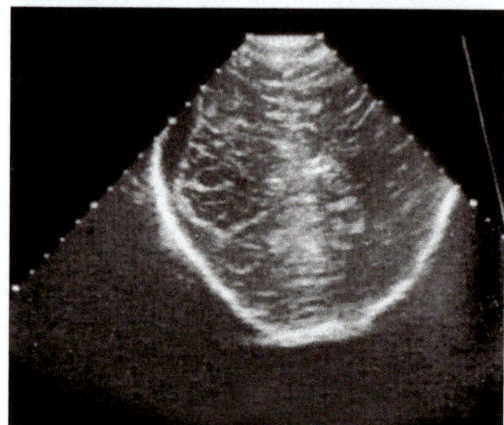

Fig. 18.7.1: Subdural effusion—small amount of fluid is seen in the right subdural space.

	Subdural effusion	Prominent subarachnoid spaces (Atrophy, benign extra-axial collection of infancy)
	Extra-axial fluid does not extend between the cortical sulci	Extra-axial fluid extends into the sulci
	Cortical veins are displaced away from the inner table of the calvarium	Cortical veins course through the fluid and lie adjacent to the inner table of calvarium
	Mass effect may be present	No mass effect
	May be asymmetrical	Usually symmetrical, if benign extracranial collection of infancy

Benign Extra-axial Collection of Infancy

- Also known as benign enlargement of subarachnoid space in infancy and occurs due to delay in maturation of subarachnoid space
- Present between 2 and 6 months of age
- Microcephaly with no clinical signs of raised intracranial pressure
- Cerebrospinal fluid spaces are disproportionately larger with only mild prominence of ventricles. Subarachnoid spaces are more prominent in fronto-parietal regions and are seen as widened cortical sulci, fissures and anterior interhemispheric fissure.

Empyema

Seen as crescentic or lentiform extra-axial fluid collection with internal echoes usually in region of cerebral convexities and interhemispheric fissure on sonography with mass effect on the adjacent brain parenchyma.

18.8 VASCULAR LESIONS

Vein of Galen Malformation (Figs. 18.8.1A and B)

- Aneurysmal dilatation of vein of Galen is the most common pathology of vascular causes
- Newborn usually presents with congestive heart failure (CHF)
- USG shows a sonolucent mass posterior to 3rd ventricle causing obstructive hydrocephalus
- Color Doppler demonstrates turbulent bidirectional flow within the enlarged vein of Galen.

Varix of Vein of Galen

- Presents in young infants as cardiac failure
- US reveals a midline cystic structure above quadrigeminal plate
- Enlarged straight sinus.

Arteriovenous Malformation

- This congenital condition is rarely seen in infancy
- Clinical presentation is with seizures and neurological deficit
- Commonly supratentorial in location
- Mostly solitary but may be multifocal in Wyburn-Mason and Rendu-Osler-Weber syndrome
- Seen as multiple dilated tortuous vascular channels with arterial and venous signature on pulsed and color Doppler. Adjacent brain may show focal atrophy. Associated hemorrhage has variable appearance on US depending upon its stage. Formation of

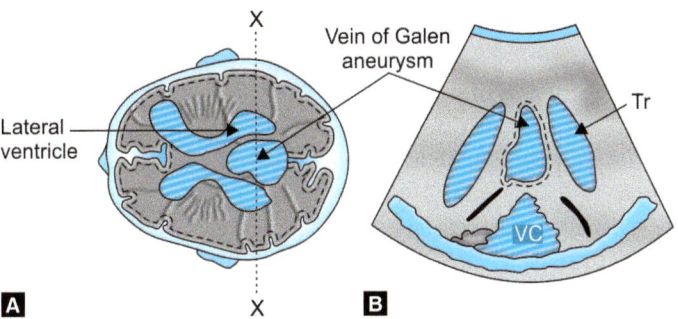

Figs. 18.8.1A and B: Aneurysm of the vein of Galen. Axial (A) and posterior coronal (B) views. An aneurysm of the view of Galen is usually associated with lateral ventricular dilatation. The posterior coronal view was performed along line X-X. (Tr: thalamus; VC: ventricle)

flow-related aneurysms appear as focally dilated vascular channels in the feeding vessels or intranidal vessels.

18.9 TRAUMATIC CYSTIC LESIONS

Leptomeningeal Cyst (Growing Fracture/Post-traumatic Cyst)

- Occurs as late complication of skull fracture with dural tear
- It is seen as an extra-axial, well-defined, cystic structure with adjacent focal brain atrophy. It herniates through the bone defect into the subgaleal tissues.

Chronic Hematoma (Extra-axial)

- It appears as a cystic, well-defined collection (crescentic-subdural, lenticular—epidural) in late stages of the hematoma due to clot lysis
- Extra-axial collection must be near 1 cm thick to be detected on sonography due to the near field artifact of 1 cm with most transducers.

18.10 INTRACRANIAL HEMORRHAGE

Cerebral hemorrhage is a common central nervous system (CNS) pathology in premature neonates due to presence of germinal matrix which involutes by 34 to 36 weeks of gestation.

Germinal Matrix Hemorrhage (Fig. 18.10.1)

- Germinal matrix is a region of very thin-walled veins and actively proliferating cells located in the subependymal layer of lateral ventricle
- Infants at greatest risk are those at gestational ages < 30 weeks, of birth weight <1500 g.

Causes

Prematurity with:
- Hypoxia
- Hypertension

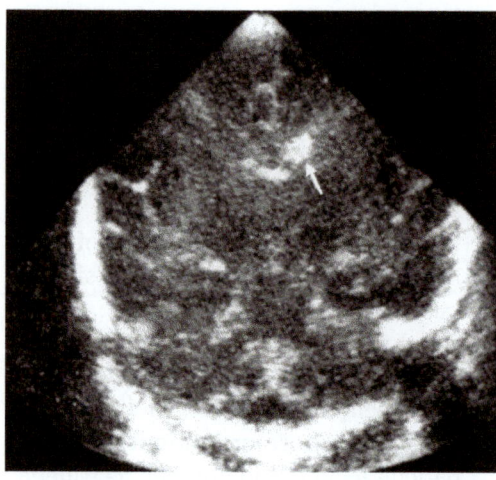

Fig. 18.10.1: Germinal matrix hemorrhage originating in germinal eminence (arrow).

- Hypercapnia
- Hypernatremia
- Pneumothorax
- Rapid volume increase.

Germinal matrix hemorrhage may extend to:
- Subependymal
- Intraventricular.

Intraparenchymal regions and is accordingly graded as follows:

 Grade I : Subependymal hemorrhage
 Grade II : Intraventricular extension without hydrocephalus
 Grade III : Intraventricular hemorrhage with hydrocephalus
 Grade IV : Intraparenchymal hemorrhage with or without hydrocephalus

- *Imaging:*
  - Echogenic focus in the region of caudate nucleus or caudothalamic groove.

Subependymal Hemorrhage

- *Imaging:*
  - Echogenic clot in subependymal space, which may cause focal enlargement of choroid in caudothalamic groove
  - As clot ages, it becomes less echogenic with center becoming hypoechoic.

Sequelae of Subependymal Hemorrhage

- May resolve completely
- Subependymal cyst
- Parenchymal/intraventricular extension leading to porencephaly/hydrocephalus respectively.

Intraventricular Hemorrhage without Hydrocephalus

- Hyperechoic material that fills a portion of ventricular system
- Clot forms a cast of ventricle may obscure the ventricle due to complete filling of the lumen
- Thick echogenic choroid plexus
- Later echolucent center
- Low level echoes floating in a ventricle
- Cerebrospinal fluid blood fluid levels.

Imaging after Development of Hydrocephalus

- As ventricles dilate, clot and choroid plexus become better defined
- Echogenic clot adherent to the ventricular wall
- Clot movement may be seen with change in head position if clot is free
- Chemical ventriculitis due to presence of blood in CSF is seen as thickening of subependymal lining of ventricle.

Intraparenchymal Hemorrhage (Fig. 18.10.2)

- Most common sites are frontal and parietal lobes
- It is usually due to periventricular hemorrhagic venous infarction:
  - Large subependymal hemorrhage
  - Compresses subependymal veins
  - Hemorrhagic venous infarcts

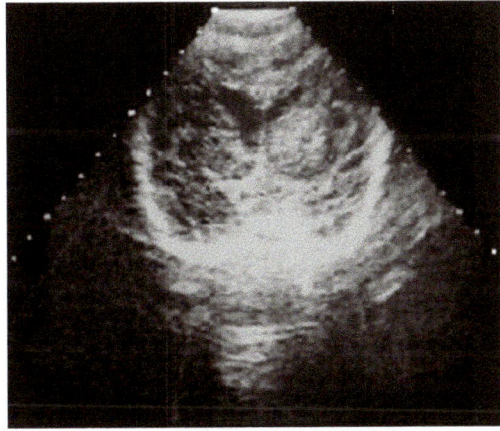

Fig. 18.10.2: Intracerebral bleed—a well-defined echogenic lesion seen in the caudate region causing mass effect on frontal horn.

  - Intraparenchymal damage
  - Later-porencephaly
- *Imaging:*
  - Homogeneously echogenic mass extending into brain parenchyma usually associated with intraventricular hemorrhage
  - As clot retracts, rim becomes echogenic with sonolucent center
  - After 2–3 months of injury encephalomalacia or porencephalic cyst is formed.

18.11 ASPHYXIA

Birth asphyxia or perinatal hypoxia leads to:
- Hemorrhage (intraparenchymal or subarachnoid).
  Imaging features of subarachnoid hemorrhage (SAH)
  - Enlarged sylvian and interhemispheric fissure
  - Thickened sulci
  - Increased echogenicity within the sulci.
- *Periventricular leukomalacia (<34 weeks gestation)* **(Fig. 18.11.1):**
  - It occurs in the watershed zone of periventricular area. These are bilateral symmetrical lesions mainly around trigone but also extending to frontal lobes
  - On US, periventricular areas of increased echogenicity is the first visible change

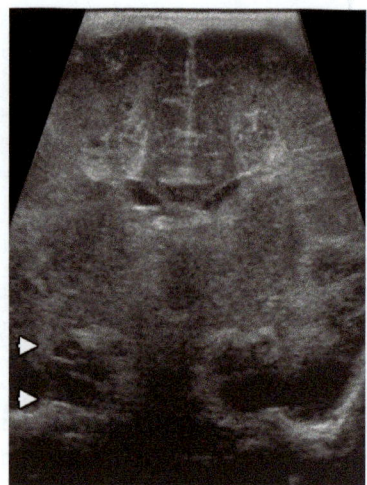

Fig. 18.11.1: US scan show periventricular leukomalacia (arrowheads).

  - On follow-up, echogenicity may subside or may be replaced by cavitations
  - After several weeks, cyst collapse and disappear with reduction of periventricular white matter, deep cortical sulci and ventricular dilatation.
- *Ischemia (>34 weeks gestation)*
  Imaging features of infarction:
  - Arterial territorial distribution of injury
  - Echogenic parenchyma with mass effect from edema
  - Decreased sulcal definition
  - Lack of arterial pulsation at real-time examination
  - Lack of a vascular waveform and flow on pulsed Doppler and color Doppler respectively
  - Increased pulsation in the periphery of the infarcted with early collateral arterial vasculature.

Focal	Diffuse
Subcortical leukomalacia	Diffuse encephalomalacia
On USG, focal hypoechoic area is seen	Diffusely bright brain on USG
	There may be echogenic thalami in severe cases

18.12 SOLID INFECTIVE LESIONS

Cerebritis is the Focal or Diffuse Swelling with Mass Effect

- Focal cerebritis is seen as an echogenic area with mass effect in the cortex
- It leads to abscess formation in later stages.

Cerebral Edema

Imaging Features

- Diffusely echogenic brain parenchyma
- Poorly defined sulci
- *Slit-like ventricles*
  The cause can be enumerated as:
  - Hypoxic-ischemic and other encephalopathy
  - Meningoencephalitis
  - Trauma.

18.13 TUMORS

- *Common neoplasms in this age group are:*
  - Astrocytoma (optic chiasm and hypothalamus)
  - Choroid plexus papilloma
  - Primitive neuroectodermal tumors (PNET)
  - Ependymoma.
- Most CNS neoplasms are rare in infants
- If present, mostly supratentorial
- On US, they appear as highly reflective lesion with a mixed echopattern
- Mass effect and hydrocephalus are usually present.

18.14 CONGENITAL INTRACRANIAL INFECTION OF INFANT AND CHILDREN

Toxoplasmosis, others, rubella, cytomegalovirus, herpes (TORCH) organisms are most common cause of congenital CNS infections (**Fig. 18.14.1**).

Neonatal and Infant Brain

Sl. No.	Cytomegalovirus (CMV)	Toxoplasmosis
Incidence	Most common	Second most common
Sites affected	• Periventricular germinal matrix • Cerebellum • Brainstem • Spinal cord	• Basal ganglia • Periventricular white matter • Cortex
Clinical features	• Hepatosplenomegaly • Jaundice • Chorioretinitis • Seizures • Optic atrophy • Hearing loss • Mental retardation	• Seizures • Microcephaly
Calcifications	Periventricular	Scattered in basal ganglia and cortex
Ventricles	Enlarged due to atrophy	Hydrocephalus due to aqueductal stenosis
Migration anomalies	Present	Absent
Cerebral atrophy	Present	Not a feature

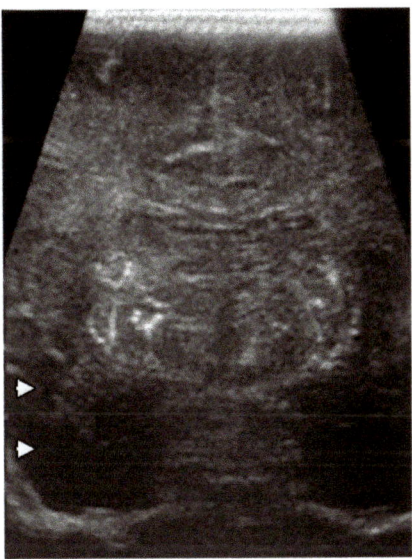

Fig. 18.14.1: US scan shows congenital CMV infection (arrowheads).

Rubella

- Incidence decreasing due to immunization
- *Clinical features:*
    - Cataract, glaucoma, chorioretinitis
    - Microphthalmia
    - Cardiac malformations
    - Microcephaly
    - Deafness
- *Ultrasonography:*
    - Echogenic calcifications in basal ganglia and cortex with microcephaly
    - Subependymal cysts in basal ganglia.

Herpes Simplex

- Neonatal herpes is HSV II

	HSV II (Genital herpes)	HSV I
Age	Usually affects neonates	Usually affects adults
Site of involvement	Diffuse brain involvement	Predilection for limbic system (Temporal lobe cingulate gyrus)

- *Imaging in HSV II:*
    - Cystic encephalomalacia of periventricular white matter
    - Hemorrhagic infarctions
    - Scattered parenchymal calcification
    - Relative sparing of lower neuronal axis of thalamus, basal ganglia, cerebellum, brainstem.
    - *In utero infection leads to:*
        - Microcephaly
        - Intracranial calcification
        - Retinal dysplasia.

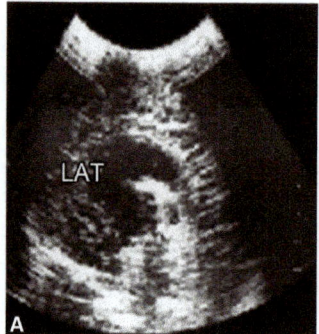 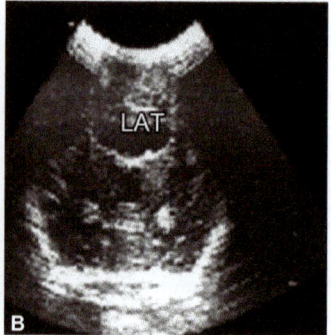

Figs. 18.15.1A and B: Postmeningitis hydrocephalus lateral and third ventricles appear dilated, 4th ventricle is normal. (LAT: lateral ventricle)

18.15 MENINGITIS (FIGS. 18.15.1 AND 18.15.2)

Infecting agents are:
- *Neonates:* Group B *Streptococcus, Escherichia coli, Listeria*
- *Infants: Haemophilus influenzae*
  - Imaging.

Ultrasonography—In Acute Stage

- Increased echogenicities in basal cisterns inter-hemispheric tissue and cortical sulci
- Lateral and 3rd ventricles are symmetrically compressed and subarachnoid spaces are effaced (due to diffuse brain edema)
- Focal echogenic areas representing edema may be seen
- USG may be normal in uncomplicated cases.

Complications
- Hydrocephalus
- Ventriculitis.

Ultrasonography Shows
- Hydrocephalus
- Echogenic debris within ventricle
- Echogenic shaggy ependymal lining
- Fibrous septae in ventricles that can cause trapped ventricle
- Subdural effusion
- Empyema
- Cerebritis and abscess

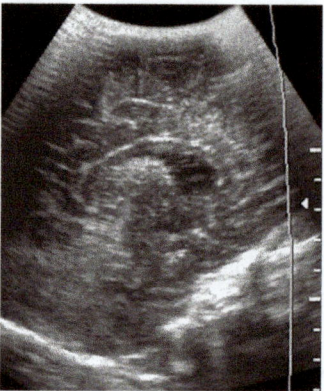

Fig. 18.15.2: US scan shows dilated lateral ventricle with ventriculitis.

- Cerebrovascular complications, e.g. cerebral infarction, venous infarct, dural sinus thrombosis, mycotic aneurysm.

18.16 ENLARGED CHOROID PLEXUS

- Adherent clot (intraventricular hemorrhage)—serial scanning may reveal complete resolution of the clot with or without development of hydrocephalus
- Infection (ventriculitis and choroid plexitis)
- *Choroid plexus tumor (CPP):*
  - Most common site for CPP is lateral ventricle
  - Papilloma is well-defined lobulated masses causing enlargement of ventricular system.

CHAPTER 19

Neonatal and Infant Spine

Indications for ultrasound of the neonatal spinal canal:
- Midline or paramedian masses
- Midline skin discolorations
- Skin tags
- Hair tufts
- Hemangiomas
- Small midline dimples and paramedian deep dimples
- Caudal regression syndrome
- Cord retethering, diastematomyelia, hydromyelia, and syringomyelia
- Detection of sequelae such as hematoma following birth injury, infection or hemorrhage secondary to prior instrumentation and post-traumatic leakage of cerebrospinal fluid (CSF)
- Visualization of blood products within the spinal canal in patients with intracranial hemorrhage. Guidance for lumbar puncture
- Postoperative assessment for cord retethering.

Complete visualization of spinal cord is possible in infant (due to presence of incompletely ossified vertebral arches) or in a child with a congenital or surgical bony defect. Various pathological conditions can be evaluated as:
- Spinal dysraphism
- Postoperatives spine
- Spinal trauma
- Vascular*
- Tumors.

19.1 SPINAL DYSRAPHISM

Overt Spinal Dysraphism

Nonskin Covered Back Mass (Spina Bifida Aperta)
- Myelomeningocele
- Myelocele.

Skin Covered Back Mass (Spina Bifida Cystica)
- Lipomyelomeningocele (**Fig. 19.1.1**)
- Myelocystocele
- Posterior meningocele.

Occult Spinal Dysraphism
- Diastematomyelia
- Dorsal dermal sinus
- Spinal lipoma
- Tight filumterminale
- Anterior sacral meningocele
- Lateral thoracic meningocele
- Hydromyelia (**Fig. 19.1.2**)
- Split notochord syndrome
- Caudal regression syndrome.

---

*NB: Vascular anomalies do not usually present during infancy. However, if present, US reveal the anomaly and color Doppler helps in the hemodynamic assessment of the lesion.

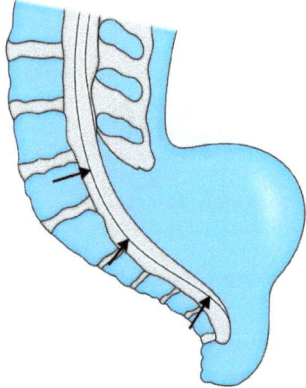

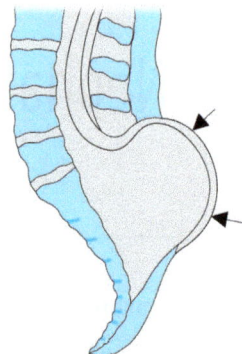

Fig. 19.1.1: A lumbosacral spine (sagittal) lipomyelomeningocele.
Note: The large defects in the neural arches of the lumbosacral vertebrae with a skin-covered herniated sac that is composed of fat contiguous with the subcutaneous fat that is growing into the dorsal aspect of the low-lying tethered spinal cord (arrows).

Fig. 19.2.1: Sagittal view of myelomeningocele at the level of the lumbosacral region with large defect in the neural arches of the lumbosacral vertebrae that has a herniated sac of exposed neural tissue (arrows) posteriorly and CSF anteriorly.

Ultrasound (US) clearly distinguishes meningocele from myelomeningocele by demonstrating the presence of neural tissue in the protruding sac.

Myelocele

It has almost the same appearance as myelomeningocele (**Fig. 19.2.1**) but the herniated sac is flush with the plane of the back.

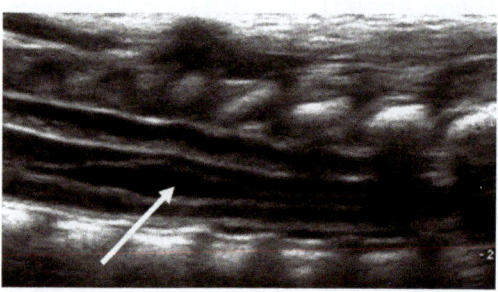

Fig. 19.1.2: US scan shows hydromyelia (arrow).

19.3 SPINA BIFIDA CYSTICA

Lipomyelomeningocele

Present as skin-covered lumpy back masses. US reveals the subarachnoid space and cord bulging through the spina bifida into the subcutaneous tissues. The spinal canal is widened at the level of the defect. Common locations are lumbosacral, lumbar, and lumbothoracic regions.

19.2 SPINA BIFIDA APERTA

- Most common congenital anomaly of central nervous system
- Occurrence 2 per 1000 live births
- About 98% have hydrocephalus.

Associated anomalies of brain are present—Chiari, type II malformation, hydromyelia, arachnoid cyst, diastematomyelia.

In myelomeningocele, the exposed part of the neural tissue (placode) is pushed above the surface of the back by the distended ventral subarachnoid space through the defect in the posterior arches of the spine soft tissues and dura.

Myelocystocele (Fig. 19.3.1)

- Most common location is lumbosacral region.
- Associations—cloacalexstrophy, partial sacral agenesis, hydromyelia.

Neonatal and Infant Spine

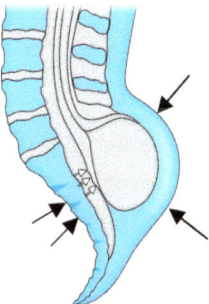

Fig. 19.3.1: Sagittal diagram of myelocystocele at the lumbosacral region in which a large dysraphic defect within the bone and a skin-covered back mass (the herniated sac) that contains the low-lying caudally splayed (small black arrows), spinal cord with a cyst (small white arrows) terminally are present. The subcutaneous fat (large black arrows) of the back is separated from the cyst by a tissue plane.

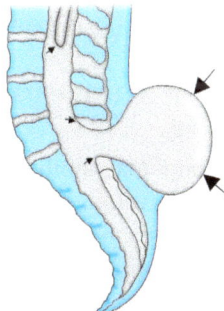

Fig. 19.3.2: Sagittal view of posterior meningocele herniation of a CSF sac (large black arrows) through a spina bifida at 1.5 (small black arrows). The conus is in the normal location.

US reveals the herniated sac consists of the dilated central canal of the distal end of the low-lying and tethered spinal cord, CSF, and meninges.

The subcutaneous fat is clearly separated from the sac by a tissue plane.

Simple Posterior Meningocele (Figs. 19.3.2 and 19.3.3)

This is a skin-covered back mass consisting of herniated sac of meninges (dura and arachnoid) with CSF protruding through

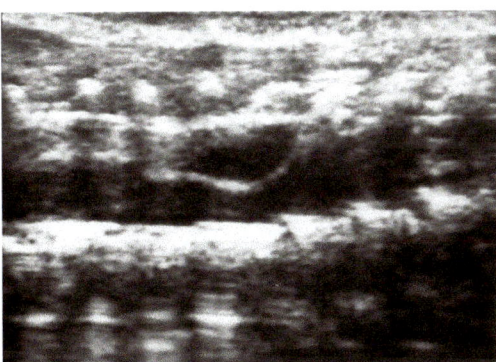

Fig. 19.3.3: US scan shows arachnoid cyst.

a posterior bony defect in the spine. Most commonly formed in lumbosacral region. The bony defect may involve the anterior aspect or lateral aspect resulting into anterior sacral and lateral thoracic meningoceles respectively and are classified under occult spinal dysraphism.

19.4 OCCULT SPINAL DYSRAPHISM

Diastematomyelia (Figs. 19.4.1 and 19.4.2)

- Complete or partial sagittal clefting of the spinal cord. The two hemicords typically reunite below the cleft
- More frequent in girls and common location is D9 to S1
- Associated findings—segmentation anomalies of vertebral bodies
- US findings include clefting of spinal cord, spur (bony, fibrous, cartilaginous), hydromyelia (50%), fatty filumterminale, intraduralipoma and conus is low lying below L2 level. These findings are demonstrated well on US
- About 50% asymptomatic—this form of diastematomyelia does not have a spur and no duplication of meninges is seen.

Dorsal Dermal Sinus

Epithelial tract that extends to a variable length from skin surface anteriorly and downwards

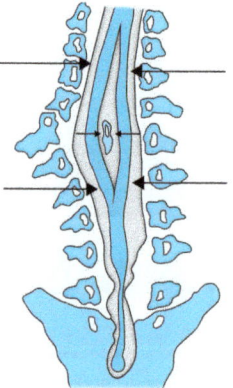
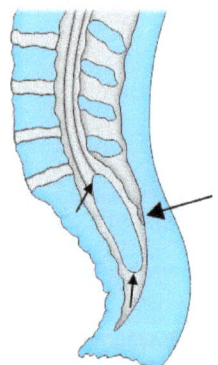

Fig. 19.4.1: Diagram (anteroposterior) of diastematomyelia with the area of clefting of the spinal cord (large black arrows), bony spur (small black arrow), and thickened filum.

Fig. 19.4.3: Intradural lipoma (large black arrow) tethering a low-lying spinal cord (small black arrows) which is separated from the subcutaneous fat of the back by an obvious tissue plane.

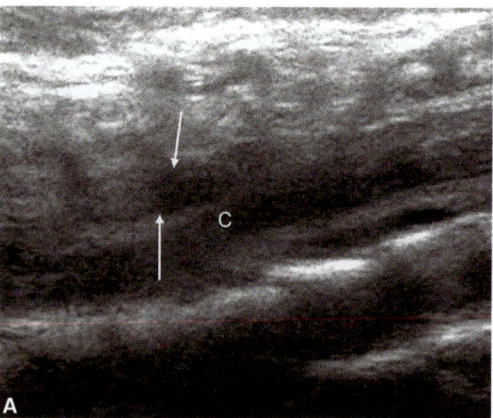
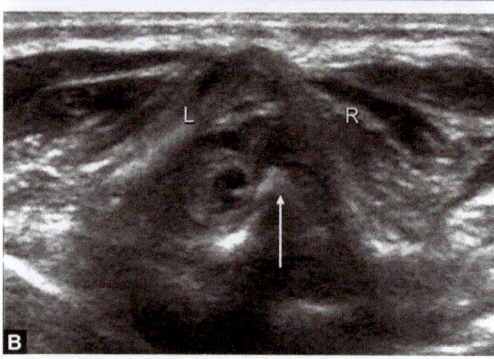

Figs. 19.4.2A and B: US scans show diastematomyelia (arrows show cord). (C: cord; L: left; R: right)

into the associated soft tissue of the back. On US, it is seen as a linear or curvilinear echogenic tract reaching the spinal canal.

Spinal Lipomas (Fig. 19.4.3)

- Lipomyelocele
- Leptomyelolipoma: Another form of spinal lipoma is lipomyelomeningocele which is an overt spinal dysraphism
- Lipomas are lumps of subcutaneous soft tissues (connective tissue and fat) covered by skin and found most commonly in the lumbosacral region
- They may be associated with dermal sinuses, hemangiomas, hairy nevi and hair tufts
- Extension of the lesion is variable into the spinal canal through the defect in the midline dura, bone, muscle, and fascia.

Lipomyelocele

- Cord is intracanalicular and meninges, which do not bulge into the soft tissues
- On US, the echogenic lipoma is attached to the cord tethering, the cord which is low and eccentric is in the position

- The lipoma may be limited to the filum or dura or extend into the central cord or along the cord.

Leptomyelolipoma

- A term used when the lipoma has a large area of direct interface with the spinal cord
- This is a form of occult spinal dysraphism.

Intradural Lipoma

Intraspinal lipoma lie adjacent to the dorsal aspect of spinal cord. A tissue plane separates it from the adjacent subcutaneous fat of the back. Associated findings are spina bifida and a tethered cord.

Tight Filum Terminale

- On US, it appear as a thickened filum terminal >2 mm in thickness
- Associated findings—spina bifida (50–70%) cases, low-lying tethered cord (50%).

Anterior Sacral Meningocele (Figs. 19.4.4 and 19.4.5)

- Defect anteriorly in sacrum with herniation of meninges and CSF into the presacral or pelvic area
- It may be associated with an anterior sacral teratoma.

Lateral Thoracic Meningocele

- Sac protruding laterally into posterior mediastinum through intervertebral foramen or a lateral defect
- Commonly seen in patients with neurofibromatosis type I.

Hydromyelia

- Dilatation of central canal
- It may be focal, localized, multiple or diffuse

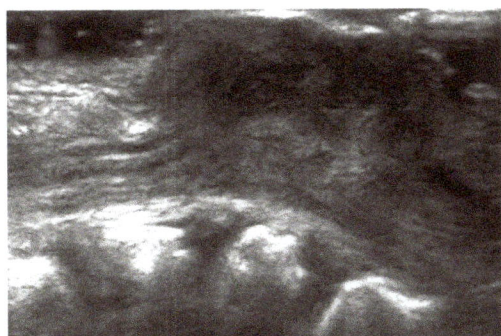

Fig. 19.4.4: US scan shows complex meningomyelocele.

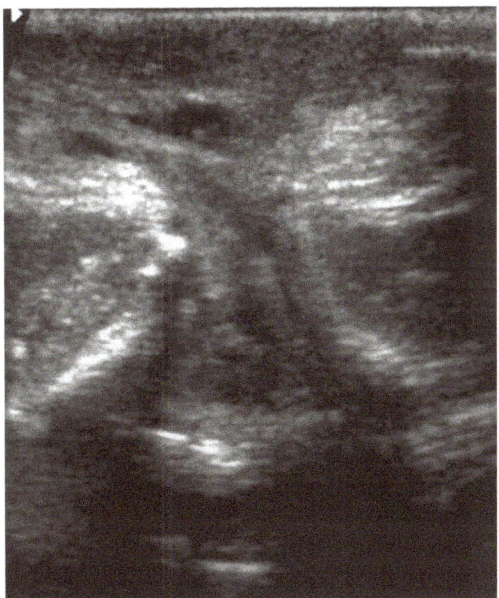

Fig. 19.4.5: US scan shows spina bifida with meningocele.

- It usually seen in association of other dysraphic states
- US reveals the dilated central canal as a separation of the normal echogenic line by an anechoic space.

Split Notochord (Fig. 19.4.6)

- Abnormal splitting or deviation of notochord covered by persistent partial or complete connection between any part

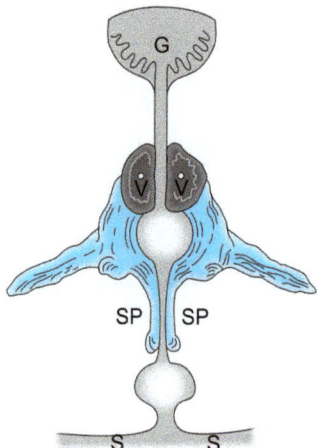

Fig. 19.4.6: Axial view of the split notochord syndrome: A tract extending from the gut (G) produces a sagittal cleft in the vertebral body (V) and spinous process (SP) to the skin (S) surface of the back.

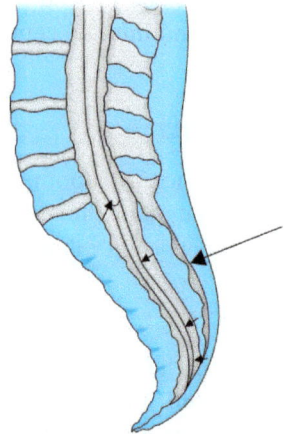

Fig. 19.5.1: Sagittal view of lumbosacral region. Conus (large black arrow) of the spinal cord which is low-lying and tethered by a thickened fatty filum terminale (small black arrows) is detailed.

of gut with spine, cord and/or skin of back. Connection may be a tract, diverticulum, cyst, fistula or sinus
- Presentation may be with a mass in chest, posterior mediastinum, spinal cord or abdomen
- Most common abnormality is mediastinal, dorsal enteric cyst presenting in childhood with respiratory symptoms (dyspnea, cyanosis), pulmonary infection, and posterior mediastinal mass.

Caudal Regression Syndrome

- Characterized by absence of portions of the lower bony spine and spinal cord
- Associated findings are renal aplasia/dysplasia, neurogenic bladder, malformed external genitalia, atresia, and sirengomelia, clubfoot
- On US, conus ends abnormally high in spinal canal. Segmentation anomalies of vertebra and spina bifida are also seen.

19.5 TETHERED CORD (FIG. 19.5.1)

- It is a pathologically fixed spinal cord in an abnormal caudal location
- Child may be asymptomatic at birth but develops progressive neurological deficit with growth of the child.

Causes of Tethered Cord

- Lipomeningocele
- Intraspinal lipoma
- Thickened filum terminale
- Dermal sinus.

Risk Factors for Tethered Cord

- Atypical sacral dimples
- Subcutaneous lipomas
- Skin defect
- Hair tufts
- Skin tag
- Hemangioma
- Pigmented nevi
- Occult spinal dysraphism
- Dermal sinus
- Anorectal malformation
- Lipomeningocele
- Leptomyelolipoma
- Lipomyeloschisis.

Findings on US

- Level of conus below L3
- Position of conus—eccentric especially dorsal
- Decreased cord oscillations (except in 1st 2 months).

19.6 SPINAL TRAUMA

Etiology

- Birth trauma
- Severely shaken infant
- *Mechanism—longitudinal stretching of cord (hyper-extension of head) and rotational forces (forceps application):*
  - Parts affected
  - Brainstem—(severely shaken infant)
  - Upper cervical cord—(cephalic delivery)
  - Lower cervical cord and upper thoracic segments (breech delivery).

Mode of Injury

- Cord laceration
- Transection
- Vascular injury at watershed areas.

US Features

Acute Stage

- Cord discontinuity
- Cord swelling
- Abnormal reflectivity in swollen cord with nonvisualization of central canal
- Extra-axial hemorrhage within spinal cord, cisterna magna, soft tissues.

Chronic Stage

Cord atrophy—heterogeneous appearance and cysts.

19.7 TUMORS

- Spinal childhood tumors are rare especially during infancy
- Presentation—often nonspecific and non-neurological, motor weakness, spinal deformity, cutaneous markers-dermoid, lipoma

US findings depends upon the location of tumor:

- Extradural—displacement of dura inwards away from margins of spinal canal
- Intramedullary—discrete, diffuse heterogeneous area in a uniformly echopoor cord
  - Cord expansion is present
- Extramedullary and intradural—the lesion compresses and displaces the cord and widens the subarachnoid space.

Extradural Tumors

US findings—expansion, disruption of vertebral body, dumbbell tumor with extension of paravertebral lesion into the canal that may be expanded due to tumor. Tumor appears to be of mixed echogenicity with areas of calcification.

Sacrococcygeal Tumors

- Rare congenital tumors (80% are benign, occurring more commonly in females)
- Association—anorectal malformation, anomalies of genitourinary tract, sacral vertebral anomaly
- Commonly occur as purely dorsal lesion or have a presacral mass as well.

US Reveals

- Heterogeneous mass with calcification and spinal cord expansion
- Displacement or encasement the spinal roots
- Sacral erosion.

CHAPTER 20

Gynecology and Obstetrics

20.1 FREE FLUID IN CUL-DE-SAC

- Normal ovulation
- Follicular rupture **(Fig. 20.1.1)**
- Ruptured ectopic pregnancy or hemorrhagic cyst
- Generalized ascites
- Pelvic inflammatory diseases
- Following culdocentesis
- Pelvic abscess or hematoma.

The posterior cul-de-sac is the most posterior and inferior-most reflection of the peritoneal cavity.

Normal Findings

In asymptomatic woman and can be seen during all phases of menstrual cycle.

Possible sources are:
- Blood or fluid caused by follicular rupture
- Blood caused by retrograde menstruation
- Increased capillary permeability of the ovarian surface caused by the influence of estrogen.

Pathological Fluid Collection

Ruptured Ectopic Pregnancy (Figs. 20.1.2 and 20.1.3)

- Sonographic signs
- Live embryo in the adnexae
- Empty uterus
- Pseudogestational sac of ectopic pregnancy
- Particulate ascites
- Adnexal mass—rounded and complex
- Ectopic tubal ring
- Color Doppler imaging shows characteristic fire ring appearance.

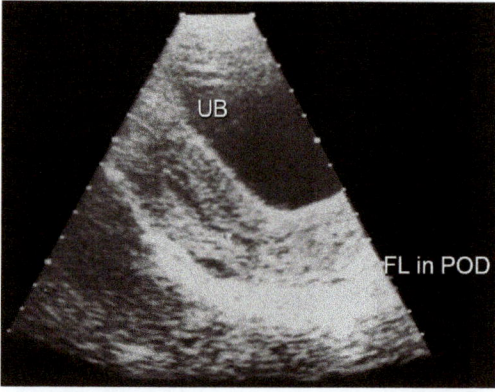

Fig. 20.1.1: Minimal fluid is seen in the pouch of Douglas (PoD) following follicular rupture. (UB: urinary bladder; FL: fluid)

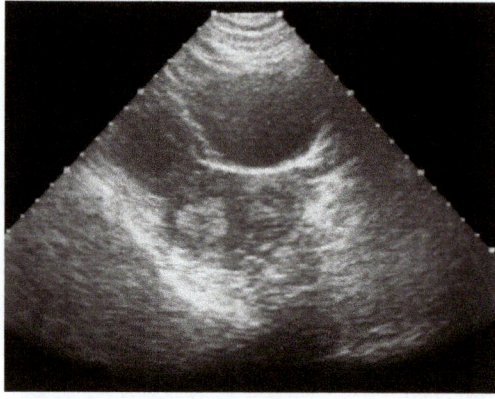

Fig. 20.1.2: Hyperplastic endometrium in uterus with cystic lesion in left ovary—ectopic pregnancy cannot be ruled out in such case.

Gynecology and Obstetrics

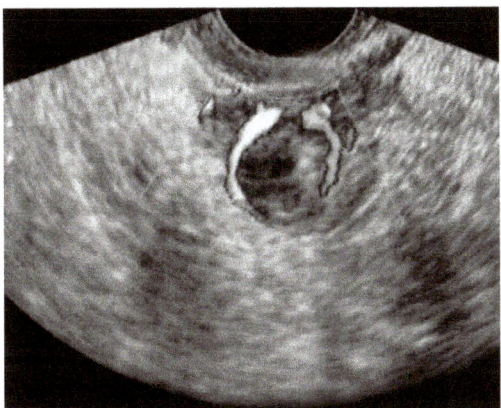

Fig. 20.1.3: Ectopic pregnancy—on color Doppler "ring of fire" appearance is seen.

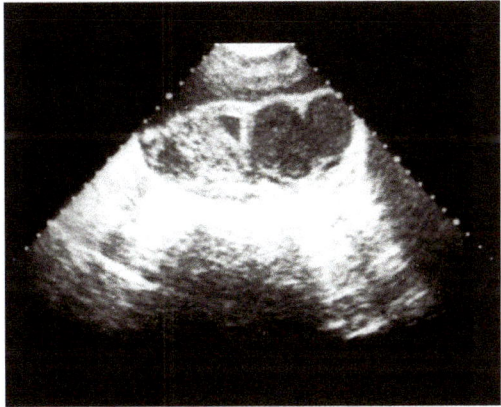

Fig. 20.1.5: Oblique scan showing, markedly dilated and thickened left fallopian tube filled with fluid with internal echoes. The endometrial cavity also contains fluid.

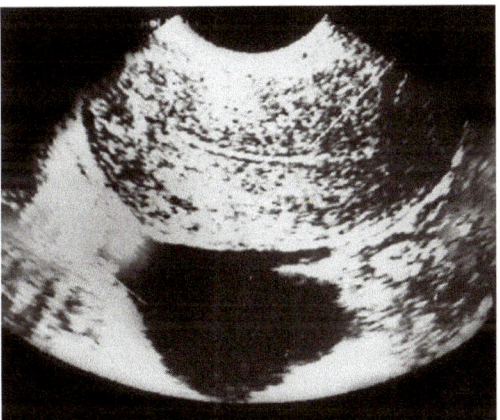

Fig. 20.1.4: Longitudinal scan shows markedly dilated fluid-filled right fallopian tube.

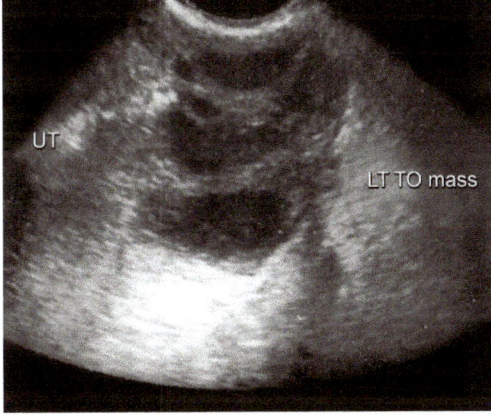

Fig. 20.1.6: Multiseptated complex heterogeneous tubo-ovarian mass is seen in transverse section.

Pelvic Inflammatory Disease

- Shows particulate fluid in the cul-de-sac
- Other findings of PID
- Endometritis—endometrial thickening or fluid, air if present, is diagnostic of endometritis
- Periovarian inflammation—enlarged ovaries with multiple cysts and indistinct margins. Pyosalpinx or hydrosalpinx—fluid-filled fallopian tubes **(Figs. 20.1.4 and 20.1.5)** with or without internal echoes
- Tubo-ovarian complex
- Tubo-ovarian abscess—complex multiloculated mass **(Figs. 20.1.6 and 20.1.7)** with variable septations, irregular margins, and scattered internal echoes and debris-fluid level
- Pelvic abscess or hematoma—can occur in cul-de-sac and sonographic appearance is similar to these conditions elsewhere in the body.

Generalized Ascites

The posterior cul-de-sac is a potential space and because of its location it is frequently the initial site for intraperitoneal fluid collection.

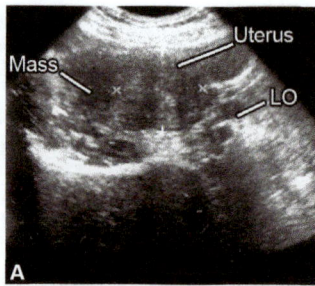 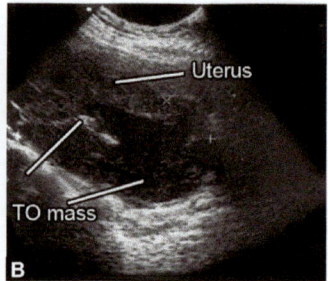

Figs. 20.1.7A and B: Tubercular tubo-ovarian (TO) mass—longitudinal and transverse scan of pelvis showing normal left ovary (LO) and a complex adnexal mass on right side with heterogeneous echotexture. The mass blends with posterior uterine wall. Also evidence of calcification is seen in mass.

20.2 CYSTIC PELVIC MASSES

- Obstructed uterus
- Cystic adnexal masses
- Extra-adnexal cystic masses.

Obstructed Uterus

Obstructed genital tract results in collection of blood and/or reactions in the uterus and/or vagina. Before menstruation hydrometrocolpos while after menstruation hematometrocolpos **(Figs. 20.2.1A and B)** result from various causes, such as imperforate hymen, vaginal atresia/stenosis or blocked rudimentary uterine horn. Endometrial or cervical tumors, postradiation fibrosis may also result in hemato/hydrometra.

Before puberty, US reveals anechoic collection within the genital tract, while hemorrhage and infection result in echoes, echogenic material or fluid–fluid level within the collection.

Cystic Adnexal Masses

Include both non-neoplastic and neoplastic lesions.

Non-neoplastic Lesions

- Functional cysts—include follicular, corpus luteal, hemorrhagic **(Fig. 20.2.2)**
- Endometriosis and theca lutein cysts
- Paraovarian (paratubal) cysts
- Tubal lesions as hydro/pyosalpinx.

Functional cysts are the most common cause of ovarian enlargement in young women. Most functional cysts usually resolve within one or two menstrual cycle and follow-up is usually not required for small simple cysts.

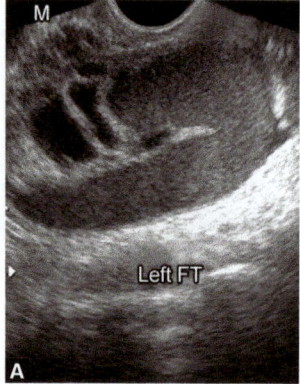 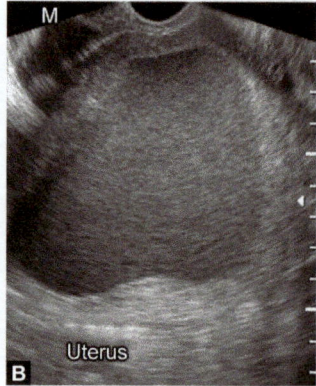

Figs. 20.2.1A and B: US scans show hematometra and hematocolpos. (M: mass; Left FT: left fallopian tube)

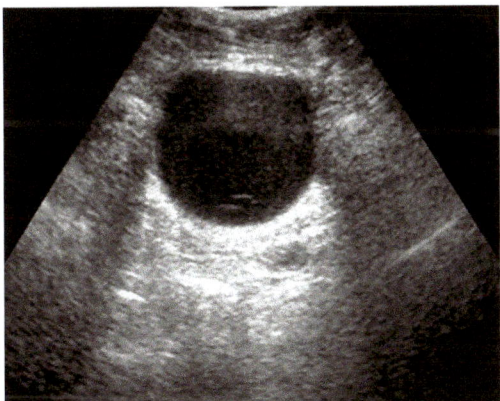

Fig. 20.2.2: US scan shows ovarian cyst.

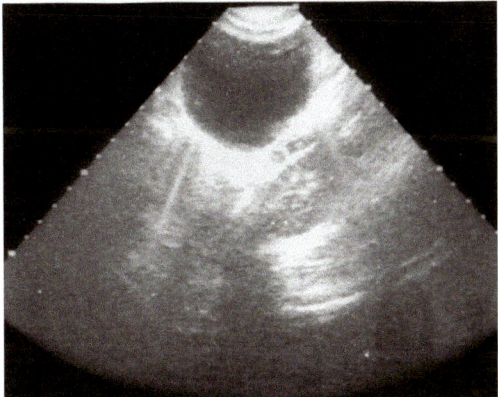

Fig. 20.2.3: Mesenteric cyst—a large cystic anechoic space-occupying lesion (SOL) with thin wall seen displacing the bowel loops.

However, follow-up is usually required in larger or hemorrhagic cysts at a different phase of menstrual cycle usually in six weeks.

Neoplastic lesions like serous and mucinous variety of ovarian cystadenoma can present as simple cystic mass in adnexal region. One or two thin septa may be present in it. Mucinous variety also shows low level echoes in the cysts.

Extra-adnexal Cystic Mass

- Peritoneal inclusion cysts
- Mesenteric cyst
- Urinoma
- Lymphocele
- Hematoma
- Bladder diverticulum, dilated distal ureters
- Ectopic gestation
- Fluid distended bowel
- Loculated pelvic abscess.

Peritoneal inclusion cyst—on sonography, peritoneal inclusion cyst appears as multi-loculated cystic masses. The diagnostic finding is presence of an intact ovary amid septations and fluid. This indicates an extraovarian origin of the mass. The ovary may be located centrally or displaced peripherally.

Mesenteric or Omental Cysts

Mesenteric cyst **(Fig. 20.2.3)** usually found in root of mesentery, omental cyst usually seen adjacent to the bowel.

Sonographically, they appear as unilocular cystic mass that may be septated. Rarely, a fat–fluid level may be seen. Differentiation from other cystic lesion may be difficult.

Lymphocele—disruption of lymphatic vessels following surgery or trauma results in the development of lymphocele.

Most commonly seen in pelvis, in the abdominal peritoneal recesses or in the retroperitoneum.

Uncomplicated lymphocele appears as echo-poor collection mimicking loculated ascites or mesenteric cyst. Septation or floating debris seen when they are complicated by hemorrhage or infection.

Bladder Diverticulum

Most result from bladder outlet obstruction **(Fig. 20.2.4)**. Bladder mucosae herniate through weak areas in the wall.

On sonography, cystic lesion is seen to communicate with the UB. Internal echogenicity varies depending on the diverticulum contents.

Fluid-distended Bowel

Can mimic adnexal mass but continuation with bowel loop may help in identification. Presence of peristalsis also confirms bowel.

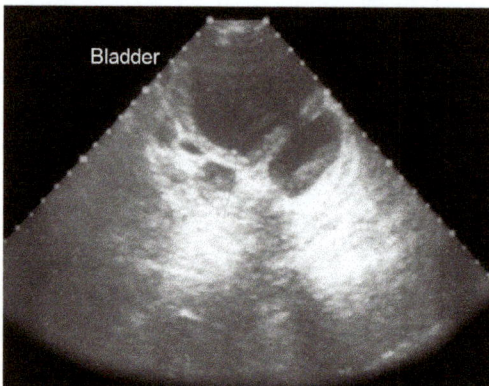

Fig. 20.2.4: Narrow neck diverticulum as seen from the posterior wall of urinary bladder with evidence of debris inside.

Loculated Pelvic Abscess

Appendiceal, diverticular and postoperative abscess. Appear as fluid collections having echoes, ± septa and well-defined irregular wall. Presence of air appears as highly reflective foci with reverberation artefacts and is specific of an abscess **(Fig. 20.2.5)**.

20.3 COMPLEX PELVIC MASS

- Uterine lesions—complex uterine collection, large necrotic tumors like fibroids, leiomyosarcoma
- *Ovarian lesions:*
  - Hemorrhagic cyst **(Fig. 20.3.1)**
  - Endometrioma **(Figs. 20.3.2A and B)**
  - Ectopic pregnancy

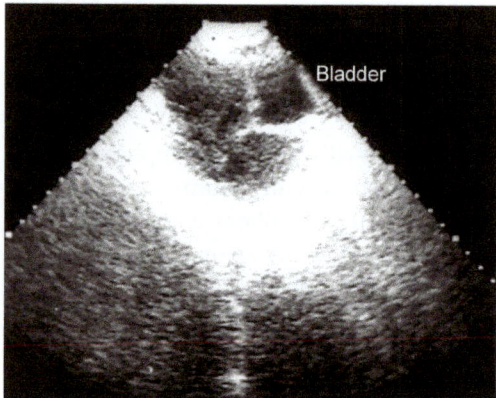

Fig. 20.2.5: Pelvic abscess—collection seen adjacent to bladder with debris inside it. It was a postoperative case of acute appendicitis.

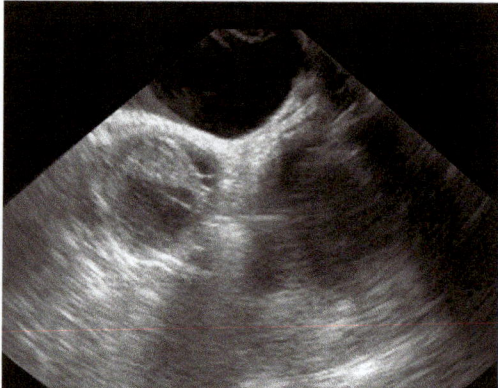

Fig. 20.3.1: US scan shows hemorrhagic unruptured follicular cyst.

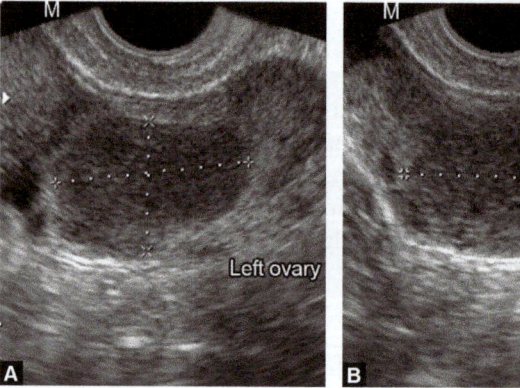

Figs. 20.3.2A and B: US scans show endometrioma. (M: mass)

- Tubo-ovarian abscess **(Fig. 20.3.3)**
- Tumors-like teratoma/dermoid **(Figs. 20.3.4A and B)**, malignant tumors like cystadenoma and necrotic germ cell tumors.

- Extra-adnexal lesions like complex collections (abscess), hematoma, **(Fig. 20.3.5)** loculated ascites, complex bowel masses **(Figs. 20.3.6A and B)**, necrotic soft tissue tumors, etc.

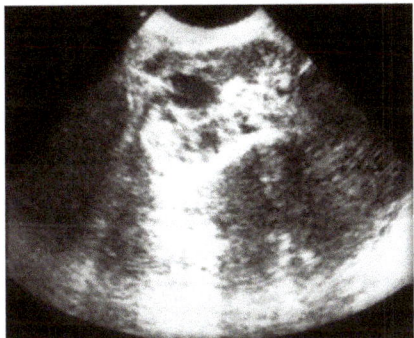

Fig. 20.3.3: Tubo-ovarian abscess.

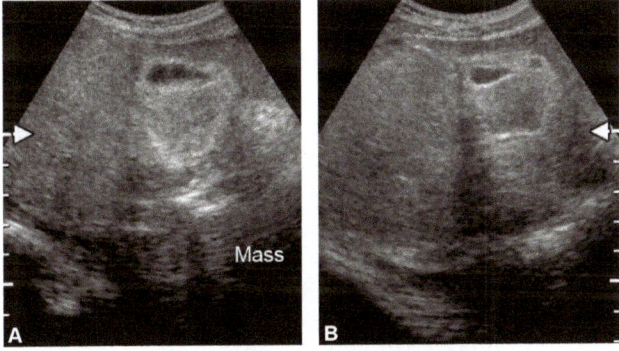

Figs. 20.3.4A and B: US scans show ovarian dermoid with fluid debris level.

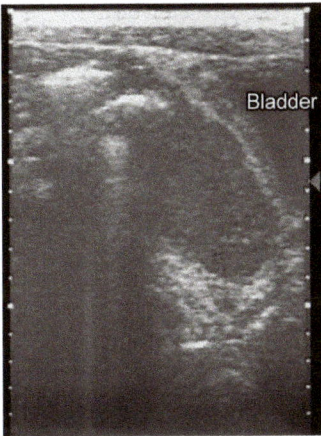

Fig. 20.3.5: Pelvic hematoma—in this case of blunt abdominal trauma. A collection is seen in the pelvis with internal echoes inside it.

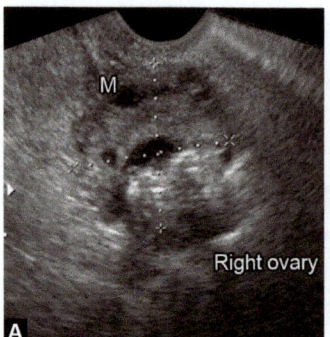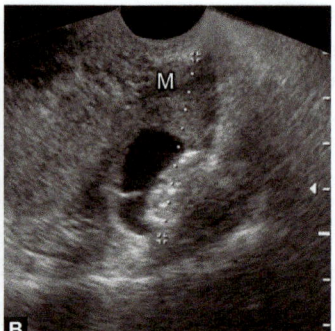

Figs. 20.3.6A and B: US scans show inflammatory mass in ovary. (M: mass)

20.4 SOLID PELVIC MASSES

Uterine (usually midline):
- Fibroids
- Adenomyosis
- Endometrial hyperplasia
- Endometrial carcinoma
- Cervical—fibroid, carcinoma
- *Off-midline:* Adnexal
- *Ovarian:*
  - Non-neoplastic-ovarian torsion, oophoritis, polycystic ovary
  - Neoplastic—benign (fibroma, thecoma, Brenner tumor) and malignant (surface epithelial tumors—cystadenocarcinoma, endometroid carcinoma; germ cell tumors; sex cord tumors).
- *Tubal:* Fallopian tube carcinoma
- *Broad ligament:*
  - Fibroid
  - Nonadnexal
  - Bowel masses
  - Soft tissue tumors
  - Bladder masses
  - Nodal masses.

20.5 ADNEXAL MASSES

Cystic Ovarian Mass
- Completely cystic.
  - Functional cyst—follicular cyst, corpus luteal cyst (uncomplicated)
  - Endometrioma
  - Hydrosalpinx
  - Cystadenoma **(Figs. 20.5.1A and B)**
  - Cystic teratoma
  - Paraovarian cyst **(Fig. 20.5.2)**
  - Serous/mucinous cystadenoma
  - Serous/mucinous cystadenocarcinoma.
- Multiple cysts—endometriomas
- Septated—cystadenomas, theca lutein cysts, massive edema of ovary.

Solid
- Ovarian tumors
- Ovarian torsion
- Oophoritis
- Polycystic ovaries
- Fallopian tube carcinoma.

Follicular cysts are discovered incidentally on sonographic examination. They appear as unilocular anechoic cyst with more than 2.5 cm in diameter.

Corpus luteal cyst is less common but larger and more symptomatic than follicular cyst. They are more prone to rupture and hemorrhage like corpus lutein cysts, hemorrhage cyst **(Fig. 20.5.3)** clinically present with acute pelvic pain. On US, they may appear as a cyst with internal echoes, complex cystic lesion with internal echoes and septae, fluid–fluid level within it or a hyperechoic lesion (in an acute, hemorrhagic cyst) mimicking a solid lesion.

Gynecology and Obstetrics

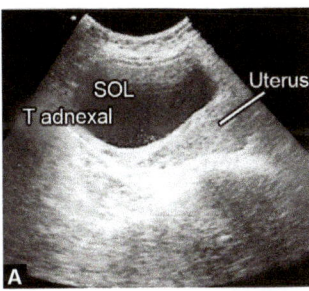
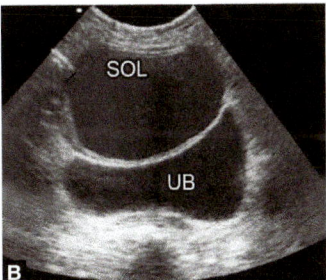

Figs. 20.5.1A and B: Transverse and oblique view—a well-defined anechoic cyst—serous cystadenoma. (UB: urinary bladder; SOL: space-occupying lesion)

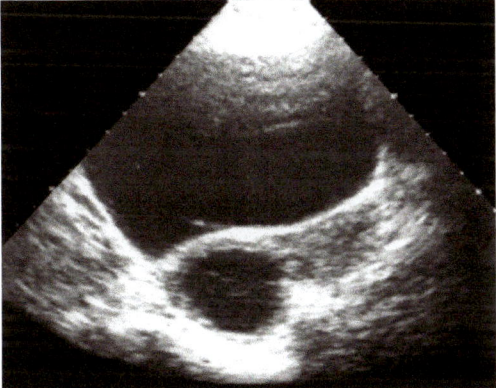

Fig. 20.5.2: Functional ovarian cyst with internal hemorrhage is seen as well-defined rounded lesion with internal echoes inside it.

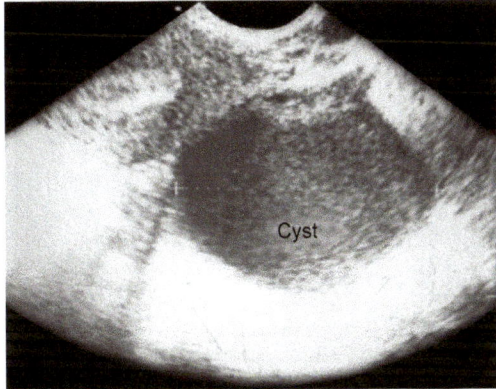

Fig. 20.5.3: Hemorrhagic cyst of ovary well-defined rounded hypoechoic cystic lesion with low-level echoes and forming a level seen on the left of scan.

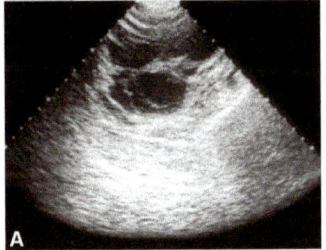
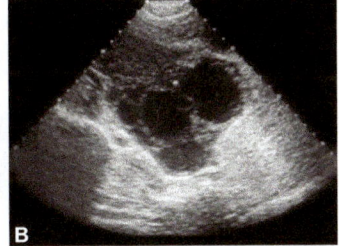

Figs. 20.5.4A and B: Theca lutein cyst seen on follow-up case of hydatidiform mole. Bilateral adnexal lesions are showing multiseptated appearance.

Theca Lutein Cyst (Figs. 20.5.4A and B)

These are associated with high levels of hCG (patients with trophoblastic disease, ovarian hyperstimulation syndrome) **(Figs. 20.5.5A and B)**. On US, bilateral, multilocular large cysts are seen.

Endometrioma **(Fig. 20.5.6)**—defined as presence of functional endometrial tissue outside the uterus. Localized form is referred to as endometrioma or chocolate cyst.

Diffuse form is usually asymptomatic and multiple and not evident on ultrasound.

In the localized form, ultrasound reveals a unilocular or multilocular (due to satellite

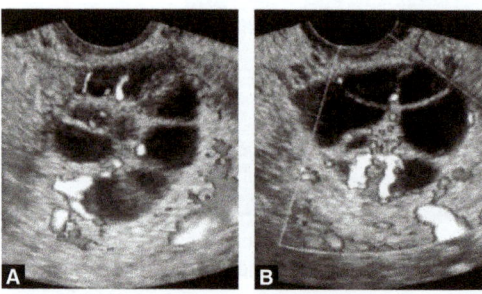

Figs. 20.5.5A and B: Intraovarian perfusion seen in a case of ovarian stimulation.

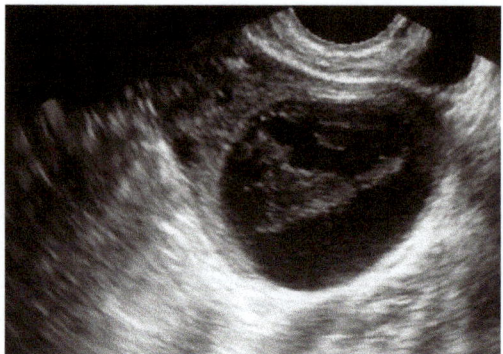

Fig. 20.5.7: Hemorrhagic ovarian cyst.

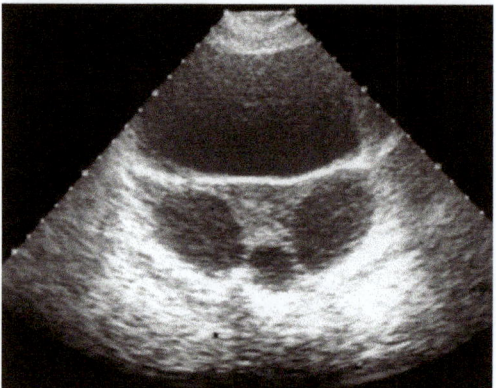

Fig. 20.5.6: Endometrioma.

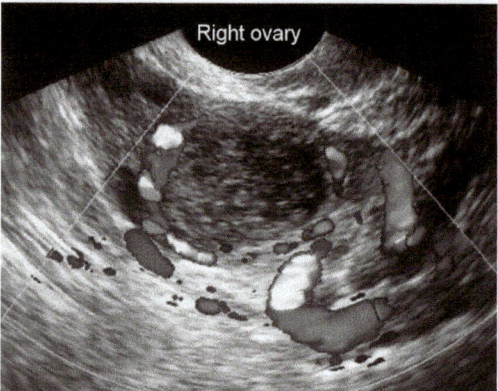

Fig. 20.5.8: Hemorrhagic cyst—showing no internal vascularity.

cysts) predominantly cystic mass containing diffuse homogeneous low-level internal echoes. A fluid–fluid level may be seen. Bright reflectors may be seen in the wall. Endometriomas are commonly confused with hemorrhage cyst or tubo-ovarian abscesses. Significant decrease in size is noticed in hemorrhagic cyst **(Figs. 20.5.7 and 20.5.8)** unlike in endometrioma **(Figs. 20.5.9 and 20.5.10)** Tubo-ovarian abscess is present with acute pelvic pain associated with fever.

Dermoid Cyst

- Seen in young patients
- Completely anechoic form can also be seen.

Paraovarian or Paratubal Cyst

- About 10% of all adnexal mass, mesothelial or paramesonephric in origin, most common in 3rd decade
- Unilocular cystic lesion in the broad ligament
- Frequently located superior to the uterine fundus
- Normal ipsilateral ovary.

Massive Edema of the Ovary

- Rare condition, resulting from partial or intermittent torsion of the ovary/causing venous or lymphatic but not arterial obstruction

Gynecology and Obstetrics

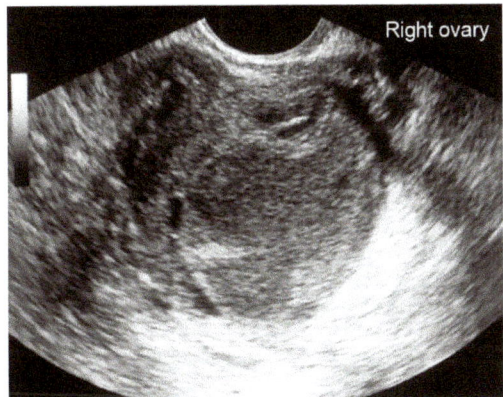

Fig. 20.5.9: Endometriotic cyst in ovary showing diffuse homogeneous low-level echoes.

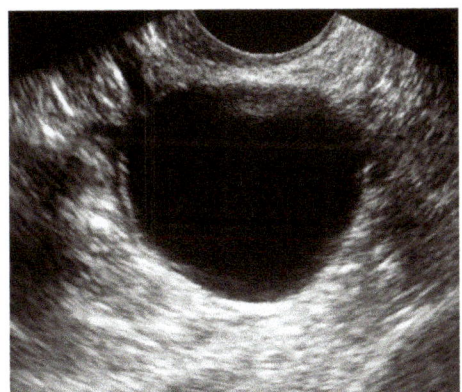

Fig. 20.5.11: Functional ovarian cyst having completely anechoic appearance.

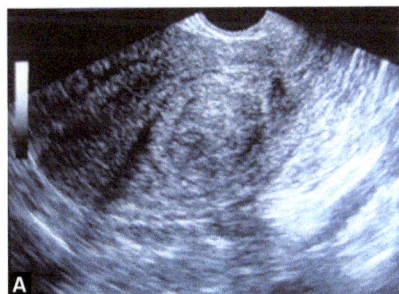
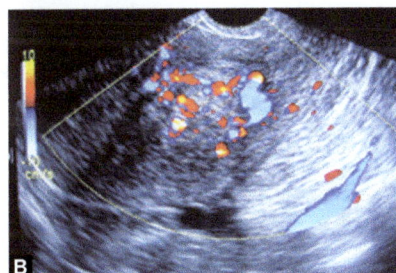

Figs. 20.5.10A and B: Focal adenomyosis—a heterogeneously hyperechoic SOL in submucosal region of uterus with increased intralesional vascularity and perilesional hypovascularity.

- This results in ovarian enlargement due to marked edema of ovarian stroma
- Sonography shows multicystic adnexal mass.

Hydrosalpinx

Fluid-filled dilated fallopian tube seen in adnexal as a well-defined walled tubular, ovoid with kinked configuration collection. Pyosalpinx demonstrates internal echoes as well.

Solid masses: Ovarian tumors discussed later.

Ovarian Torsion

- It is an acute abdominal condition of childhood or adolescence. May occur in association with ovarian cysts (**Figs. 20.5.11 to 20.5.14**) and tumors most common with teratomas
- Caused by partial or complete rotation of the ovarian pedicle on its axis.

Sonography shows:
- Unilaterally enlarged ovary
- Multiple cortical follicles in an enlarged ovary—considered as specific sign but not always present
- Color Doppler shows absent flow from the affected ovary.

Polycystic Ovarian Disease (PCOD) (Fig. 20.5.15)

- This complex endocrinologic disorder results in chronic anovulation
- Bilateral enlarged spheroidal ovaries containing multiple small follicles and

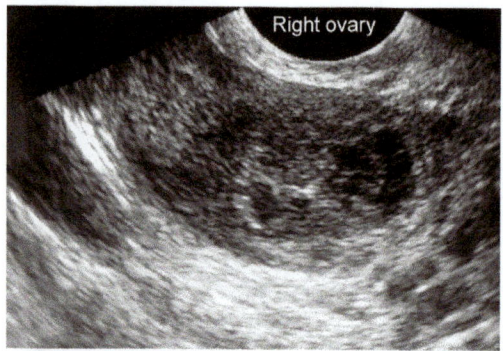

Fig. 20.5.12: Thick-walled cyst with heterogeneous appearance in ovary sign of corpus luteal cyst.

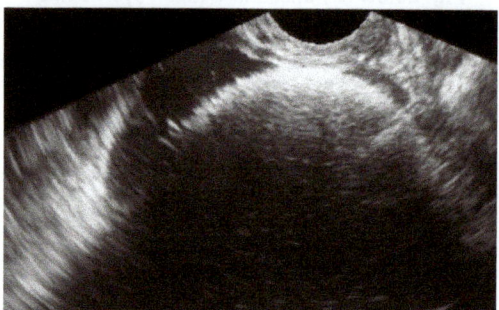

Fig. 20.5.13: Dermoid: Tip of iceberg sign—cystic mass with echogenic area with ill-defined posterior acoustic shadowing obscuring posterior wall.

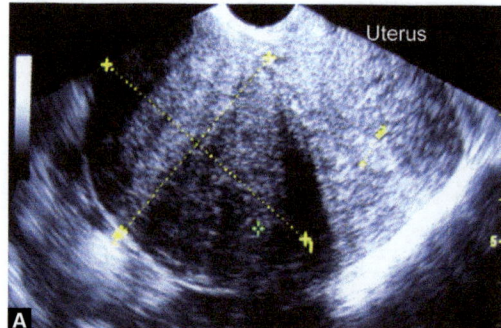

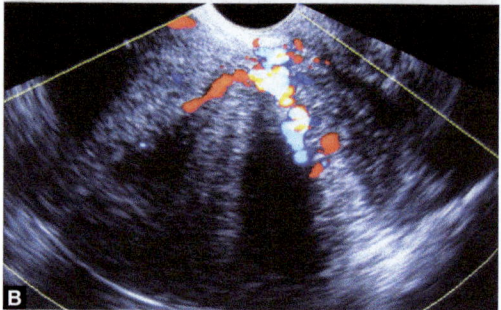

Figs. 20.5.14A and B: Large ovarian cyst (A) with increased peripheral vacularity (B).

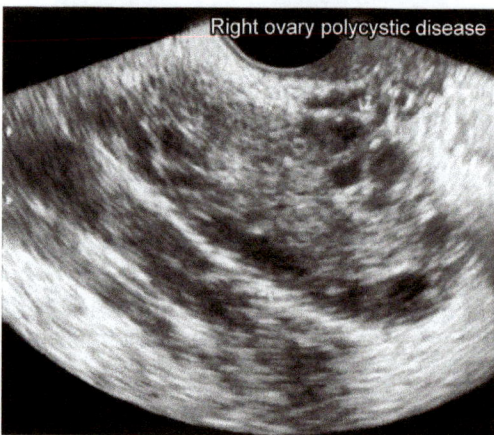

Fig. 20.5.15: Polycyctic ovarian disease: Gray scale image showing an enlarged right ovary (volume: 28.78 mL) with small peripheral follicles and increased stromal echogenicity.

stromal hypertrophy and increased echogenicity
- The follicles measure from 0.5 to 0.8 cm in size with more than five in each ovary
- Follicles persist on serial studies as a string of pearls
- An elevated LH/FSH ratio is characteristic.

Carcinoma of Fallopian Tube

- Least common (<1%) of all gynecological malignancy
- Most frequent in postmenopausal woman
- Usually involves the distal end of the tube
- Present as sausage-shaped solid or cystic mass with papillary projection.

20.6 OVARIAN TUMORS

Benign	Malignant
• Cystic	• Cystic
– Serous cystadenoma (Fig. 20.6.1)	– Serous cystadenocarcinoma (Fig. 20.6.2)
– Mucinous cystadenoma	– Mucinous cystadenocarcinoma endometrioid
– Teratoma/ dermoid cyst (Fig. 20.6.3)	
• Solid	• Solid
– Brenner	– Endometroid granulosa cell tumor. Dysgerminoma
– Thecomas	– Endodermal sinus tumor (yolk sac tumor)
– Fibromas	– Metastatic

BENIGN TUMORS

Cystadenoma

- Most common cystic ovarian tumor
- May be serous or mucinous
- Sonographically, appears as a large thin-walled unilocular cystic masses ± thin septations and papillary projections
- Multilocular lesion containing low-level echoes in its dependent part suggests the mucinous variety.

Cystic Teratoma

- Most common ovarian neoplasm seen in reproductive age group
- About 10–20% are bilateral.
  Sonographic appearance is variable ranging from completely cystic appearance to erroneously interpreted solid lesion.

On Ultrasound

- Unilocular anechoic/hypoechoic cyst with thick/thin walls
- Hyperechoic mural nodule may be present

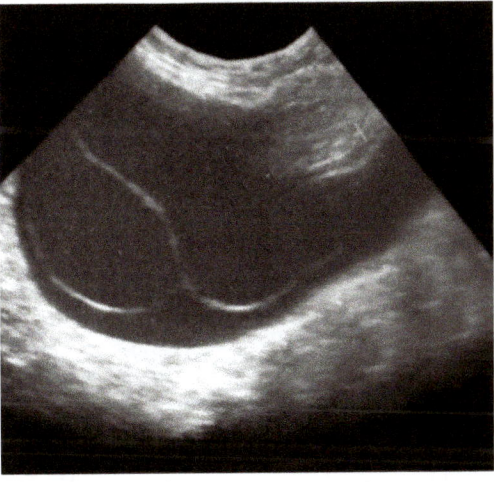

Fig. 20.6.1: Serous cystadenoma—large anechoic lesion with thin septae in right adnexal region.

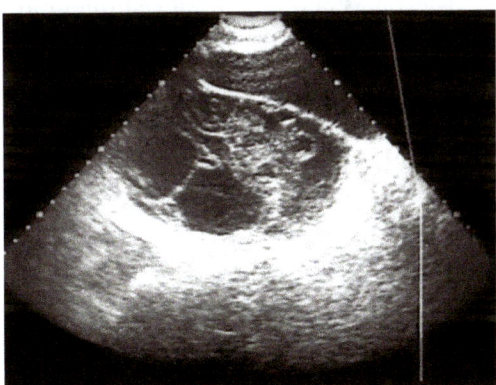

Fig. 20.6.2: Cystadenocarcinoma—large complex mass with cystic and solid areas and multiple septae in right adnexa.

- Focal/diffuse area of greatly increased echogenicity often with shadowing
- Demonstration of teeth, fat-fluid level, hair-fluid level is a specific sign
- Echogenic dermoid may be misinterpreted for bowel gas and missed completely.

Solid Benign Ovarian Tumor

- Brenner tumor, granulosa cell tumor, thecomas and fibromas are indistinguishable from each other and from pedunculated uterine fibroid

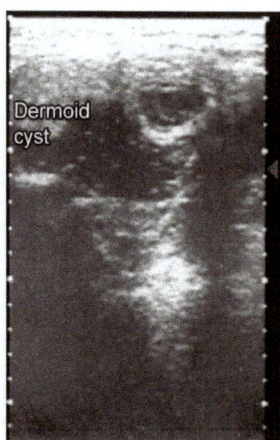

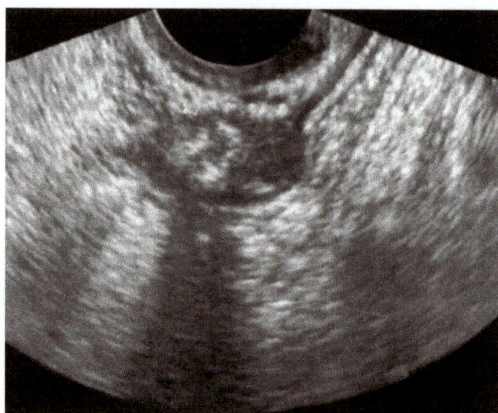

Fig. 20.6.3: Dermoid cyst—a complex mass lesion in right adnexa with solid and cystic areas. Multiple linear hyperechogenic interfaces floating in the mass.

Fig. 20.6.4: Gray scale image showing an ovarian dermoid.

- Thecomas and granulosa cell tumor are estrogenically active
- On US, they appear as well-defined, rounded, solid lesion causing attenuation of sound beam
- Left-sided pleural effusion and ascites associated with fibroma is called Meig's syndrome.

MALIGNANT OVARIAN NEOPLASM (FIGS. 20.6.4 TO 20.6.6)

Third most common gynecologic malignancy and has the highest mortality rate.

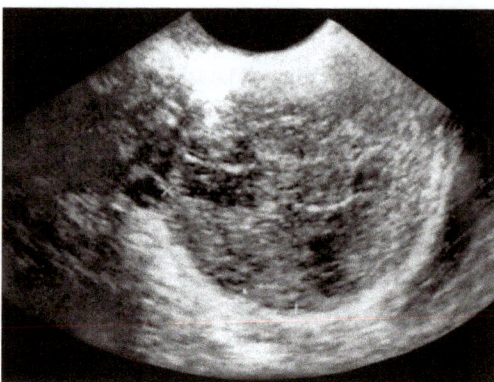

Fig. 20.6.5: Solid ovarian mass lesion suggestive of ovarian malignancy.

ULTRASOUND FEATURES OF MALIGNANT OVARIAN LESIONS

- Solid mass
- Mass more than 10 cm (except thin-walled unilocular cyst)
- Thick septa (>3 mm)
- Mural nodule
- Thick irregular solid mass
- Poorly defined margins
- Adherent bowel loops
- Ascites
    - Cystadenocarcinoma (serous and mucinous) **(Figs. 20.6.7 and 20.6.8)**

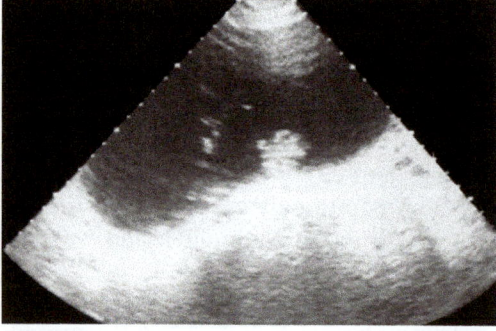

Fig. 20.6.6: Malignant ovarian mass—an irregular cystic lesion of right ovary with mural nodule and echogenic branching septae.

- Appear as multiloculated cystic masses having solid nodules and papillary excrescences
- About 8% are completely solid without cystic component
- *Endometroid tumors*
  - These tumors have better prognosis as they are detected early. About 30% of patients have associated endometrial carcinoma
  - *US reveals:* Cystic mass with papillary projections or predominantly solid mass with necrosis
- *Malignant germ cell tumors (dysgerminoma and endodermal sinus tumors):*
  - Younger age group is affected
  - α-fetoprotein is raised in endodermal sinus tumors

US reveals solid echogenic masses having small areas of necrosis
- *Metastatic tumor:*
  - Metastasis to ovaries arises most commonly from gastric, colonic and breast malignancies
  - Gastric and colonic metastases contain mucin-secreting 'signet ring' cells and are called Krukenberg tumors.

US shows bilateral solid lesion. A complex mass may be seen.

20.7 UTERINE MASSES

Benign

- Uterine fibroids (90%) rest are cervical **(Figs. 20.7.1 to 20.7.6)**

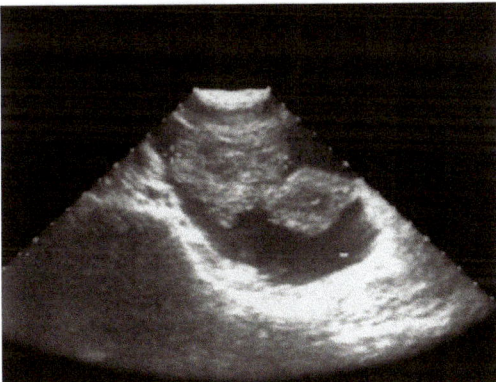

Fig. 20.6.7: Transverse scan of pelvis shows heterogeneous, predominantly echogenic ovarian mass surrounded by free fluid.

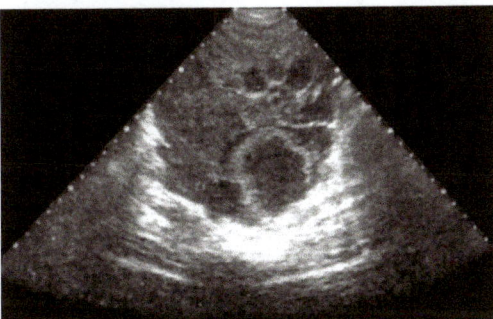

Fig. 20.6.8: Mucinous cystadenoma and cystadenocarcinoma of ovary.

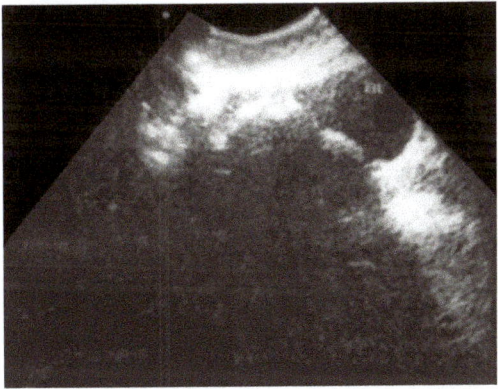

Fig. 20.7.1: Fibroid uterus.

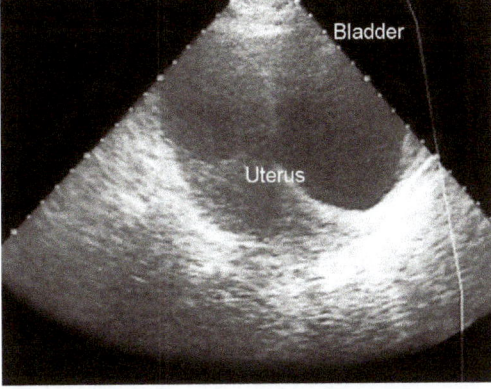

Fig. 20.7.2: Fibroid uterus—well-defined round hypoechoic solid lesion seen in the region of fundus.

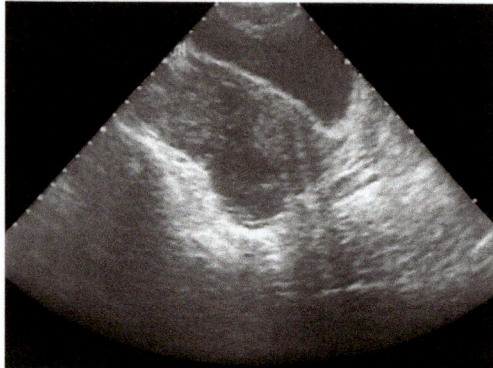

Fig. 20.7.3: Multiple uterine fibroids showing degeneration.

- Pyometra
- Hematohydrocolpos (**Fig. 20.7.7**)
- Transient uterine contraction (during pregnancy)
- Bicornuate uterus/Arcuate uterus/Septate uterus (**Figs. 20.7.8 and 20.7.9**)
- Adenomyosis (**Figs. 20.7.10 and 20.7.11**)
- Intrauterine pregnancy
- Lipoleiomyoma (**Figs. 20.7.12 and 20.7.13**).

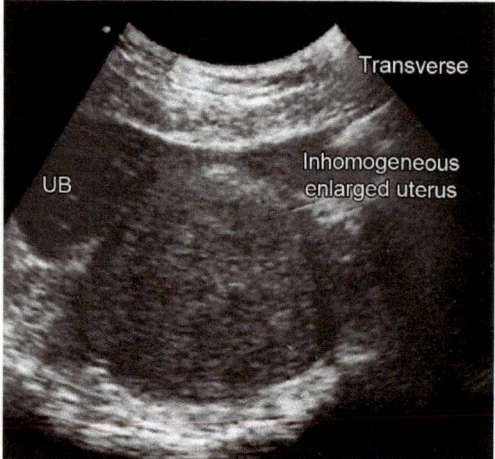

Fig. 20.7.4: Multiple fibroids—inhomogeneously enlarged uterus with posterior lobulated margin in longitudinal section with multiple poorly resolved hypoechoic areas. (UB: urinary bladder)

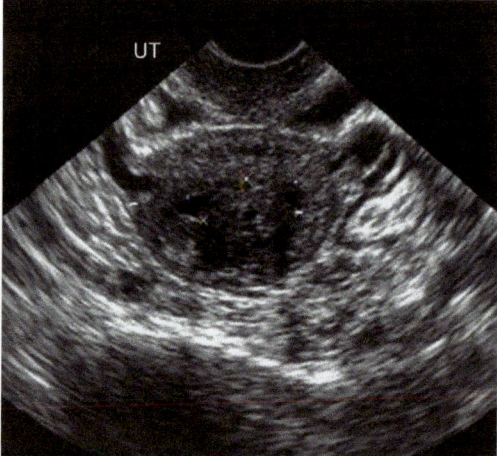

Fig. 20.7.6: US scan shows submucosal fibroid with fluid in endometrial cavity. (UT: uterus)

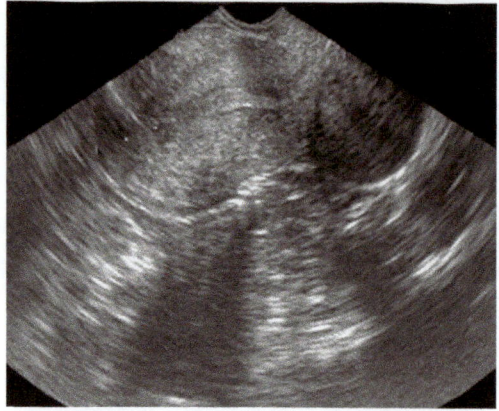

Fig. 20.7.5: US scan shows cervical fibroid.

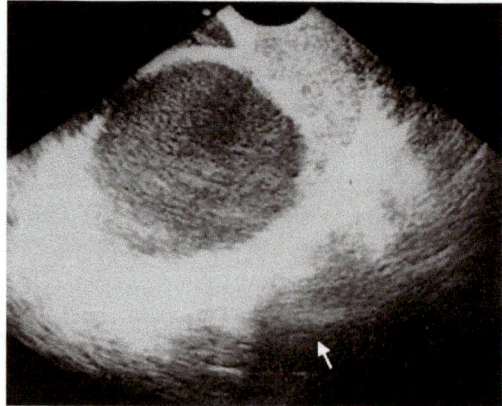

Fig. 20.7.7: Hematometrocolpos.

Gynecology and Obstetrics

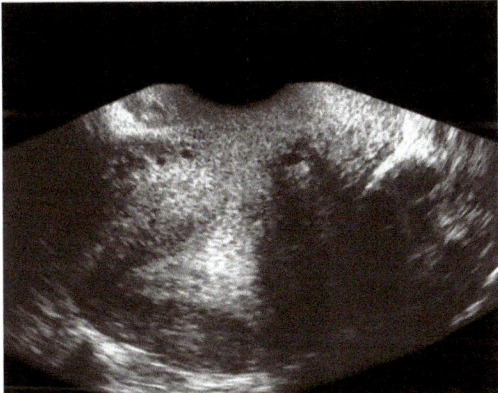

Fig. 20.7.8: USG image showing fundal indentation suggestive of arcuate uterus.

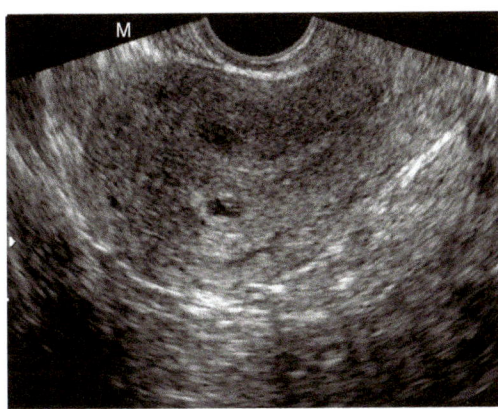

Fig. 20.7.11: US scan shows subendometrial myometrial cysts in adenomyosis of uterus. (M: mass)

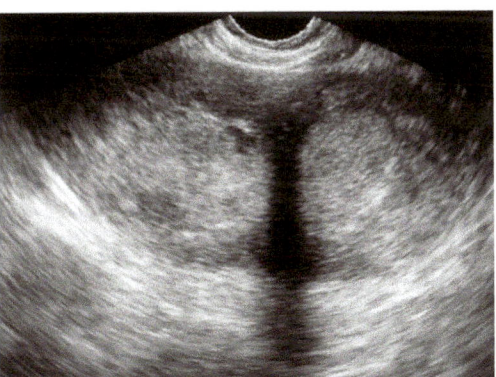

Fig. 20.7.9: Septate uterus: Two endometrial echocomplexes.

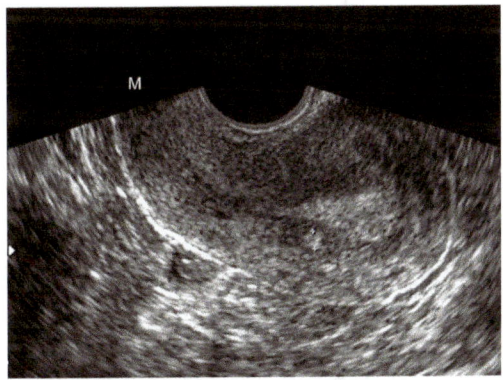

Fig. 20.7.12: US scan shows small lipoma of uterus. (M: mass)

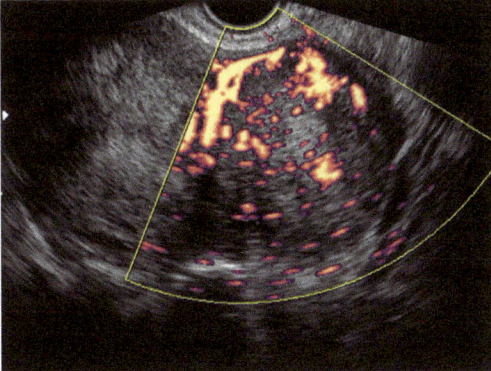

Fig. 20.7.10: US scan shows adenomyoma of uterus.

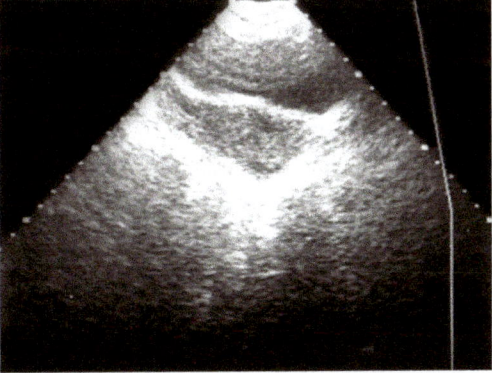

Fig. 20.7.13: Carcinoma cervix—longitudinal scan of the cervix shows an irregular growth. Base of the bladder is not involved.

Malignant

- Cervical carcinoma
- Endometrial carcinoma
- Leiomyosarcoma
- Invasive trophoblastic disease.

Leiomyoma

Most common neoplasm of uterus and most common cause of enlargement of non-pregnant uterus.

Clinical Features

- Usually asymptomatic
- However, pain and uterine bleeding are usual presenting features.

Types

- Subserosal
- Intramural (most common)
- Submucosal (most symptomatic).

Ultrasound

- Well-defined hypoechoic lesion with sound beam attenuation
- Uterine contour deformity, displaced/distorted endometrial echo.

As they are estrogen dependent:

- During pregnancy, 50% increase in size, decrease in echogenicity due to degeneration and necrosis
- Postmenopausal regression in size and calcification occur.

Focal Myometrial Contraction

This is a transient, focal contraction of the myometrium of pregnant uterus and commonly confused with an intramural fibroid.

On US, it appears similar in echotexture as the myometrium, no attenuation of sound beams is present. Disappears after some time.

Adenomyosis

Localized form of adenomyosis/adenomyomas (*see* Fig. 20.7.10) appears as inhomogeneous circumscribed areas in the myometrium having indistinct margins and containing anechoic spaces.

Lipoleiomyoma

Asymptomatic lesion: US shows a highly echogenic attenuating mass within the myometrium.

Cervical Carcinoma

A condition diagnosed clinically. US reveals a solid retrovesical mass which is hypoechoic or heterogeneous in echotexture. The lesion is indistinguishable from a cervical fibroid. Extension of lesion into endometrial canal causes cervical stenosis and pyometra formation.

Leiomyosarcoma

- Only 1% of leiomyomas undergo sarcomatous change
- Patients are usually asymptomatic or may present with uterine bleeding
- US shows a rapidly growing or degenerating leiomyoma with or without local invasion or distant metastasis.

Rudimentary Horn of Bicornuate Uterus

This congenital lesion may present as a mass lesion if it contains functional endometrium and then retention of menstrual blood can occur.

20.8 DIFFUSE UTERINE ENLARGEMENT

- Diffuse leiomyomatosis
- Adenomyosis
- Endometrial carcinoma.

20.9 THICKENED ENDOMETRIUM

- Early intrauterine pregnancy
- Incomplete abortion
- Ectopic pregnancy (*see* Fig. 20.9.6)
- Retained products
- Trophoblastic disease
- Endometrial hyperplasia.

Appearance of endometrium in a normal menstrual cycle (**Figs. 20.9.1A to E**).

- Endometrial polyp
- Endometrial cancer
- Endometritis
- Adhesions
- Foreign body (IUCD).

Date of cycle	Phase	Thickness (mm)	Appearance
1–4	Menstrual phase	1–4	Small amount of fluid may be seen endovaginally. Thin interrupted central echo
5–14	Proliferative phase	4–8	Central hyperechoic line with surrounding thin hypoechoic band
	Periovulatory phase	6–10	Trilayered appearance hypoechoic band becomes more prominent with thin echogenic lines on either side
15–28	Secretory phase	8–16	Thick, echogenic with thorough transmission

Sonographic appearance and thickness of endometrium varies with the phase of menstrual cycle.

Proliferative phase: Triple-line endometrium—4-8 mm thick.

Secretory phase: Hyperechoic—7-14 mm, acoustic enhancement.

Postmenstrual: Asymptomatic—up to 8 mm.

Symptomatic (P/V bleeding)—up to 4 mm.

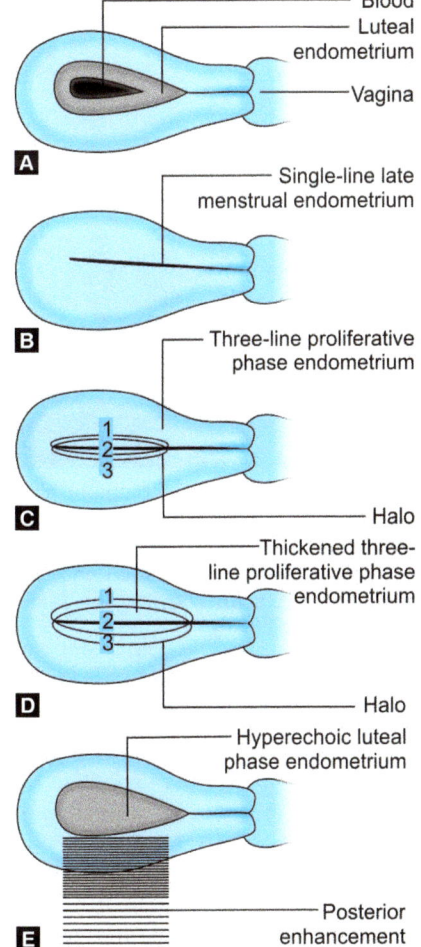

Figs. 20.9.1A to E: Uterine endometrium in different phases of menstruation.

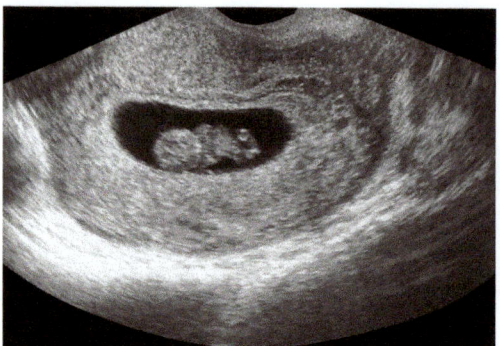

Fig. 20.9.2: USG image showing early intrauterine pregnancy.

Early Intrauterine Pregnancy (Fig. 20.9.2)

Earliest detection on US is at 4 weeks 3 days by transvaginal sonography (TVS), and 5 weeks by transabdominal sonography (TAS). The gestation sac is seen as a small collection surrounded by moderate level echoes of uniform thickness located eccentrically within the endometrium.
- Human chorionic gonadotropin level doubles every 2 days in early intrauterine pregnancy.

Incomplete Abortion: Retained Products (Figs. 20.9.3A and B)

An enlarged uterus with thickened endometrium with echogenic/heterogeneous material ± fluid in a proper clinical setting suggests the diagnosis **(Figs. 20.9.4 and 20.9.5)**.

Ectopic Pregnancy (Fig. 20.9.6)

- Clinical symptoms—missed period, P/V bleeding pain
- hCG—raised less than in normal pregnancy.

Ultrasound

- Thick echogenic endometrium ± fluid collection (pseudogestational sac)

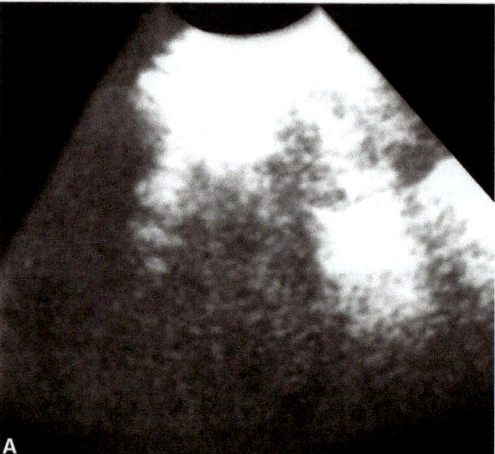
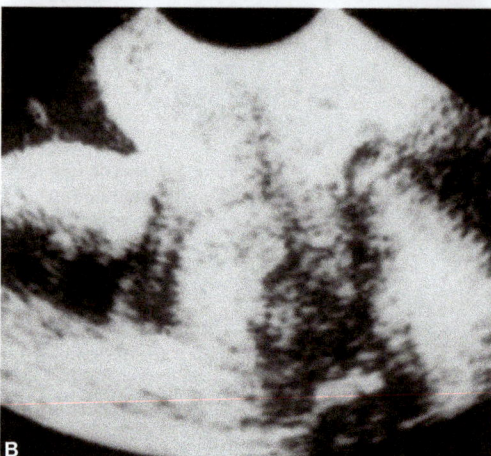

Figs. 20.9.3A and B: (A) Incomplete abortion: Thickened endometrium only, transabdominal scan showing uterus with thickened endometrium; (B) Incomplete abortion: Thickened endometrium only, transvaginal scan showing the thickened endometrium more clearly.

- Adnexal mass—cystic, complex ± live embryo, tubal ring on color Doppler imaging
  - Free fluid in POD.

Gestational Trophoblastic Disease

This is a proliferative disease of trophoblasts presenting as hydatidiform mole **(Figs. 20.9.7A and B)** (benign form) or as malignant forms—invasive mole or choriocarcinoma.

Most common form is hydatidiform mole.

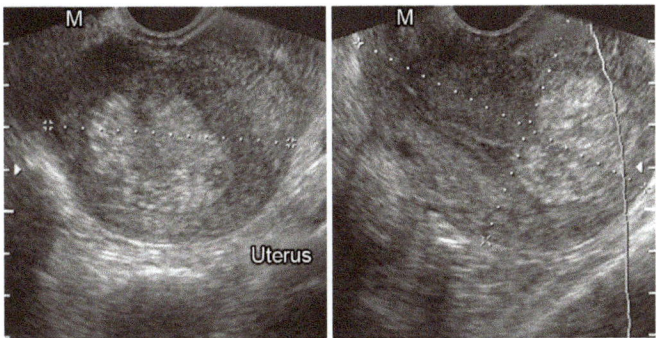

Fig. 20.9.4: US scans show retained placenta. (M: mass)

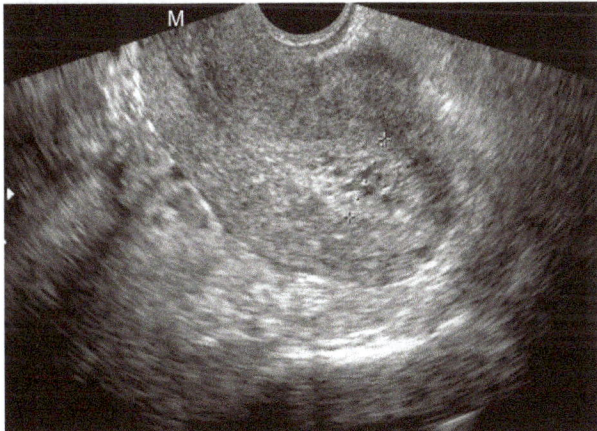

Fig. 20.9.5A: US scan shows cystic endometrial hyperplasia. (M: mass)

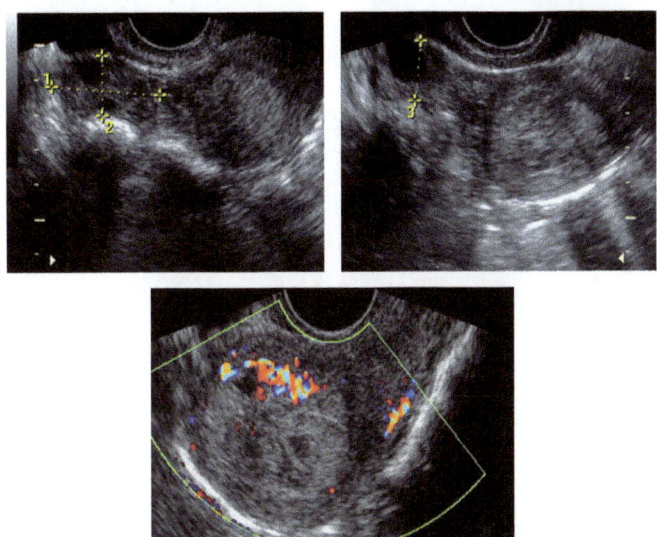

Fig. 20.9.5B: Hyperechoic lesion in the endometrial cavity with increased vascularity in post-D and C patient suggestive of retained products of conception.

Risk Factors

- Women at the end of their reproductive age group
- Previous similar history.

Ultrasound

- *Ist trimester mole:*
  - Simulates a blighted ovum
  - Threatened abortion
  - Small echogenic mass filling the uterine cavity.
- *IInd trimester mole:*
  - Large moderately echogenic mass filling the uterine cavity
  - Cystic fluid containing spaces within it.

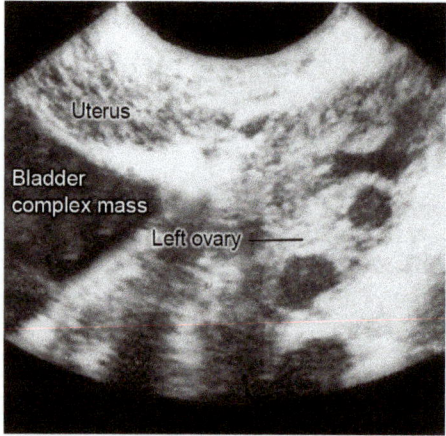

Fig. 20.9.6: Ectopic pregnancy: Adnexal mass—transvaginal scan reveals a complex mass in the (L) adnexa separate from the (L) ovary. Also seen as free fluid in the cul-de-sac.

- Doppler—low impedance, high flow with high systolic and diastolic velocities
- hCG is raised more than in a normal pregnancy
- Complications—hemorrhage seen as crescenteric anechoic regions surrounding the tumor.

Theca Lutein Cysts

Variations of molar pregnancy:
- *Coexistent mole and fetus:*
  - One normal fetus
  - Molar transformation of one binovular twin placenta
- *Partial mole (triploidy):*
  - Identifiable fetal tissue/fetus which is growth retarded or dystrophic
  - Formed placenta, which has numerous cystic spaces.
- *Invasive mole:*
  - Hydatidiform mole (villous pattern preserved) with local invasion
  - US—involvement of myometrium with or without extension into parametrium.
- Choriocarcinoma—50% cases are preceded by molar pregnancy
  - No identifiable villous pattern seen while necrosis and hemorrhage are present.

Ultrasound:
- Tumor extends into myometrium with or without parametrium
- Metastasis to lung, brain, liver, bone, GIT, skin.

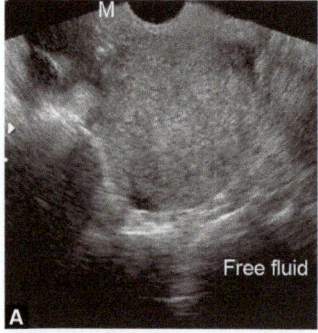 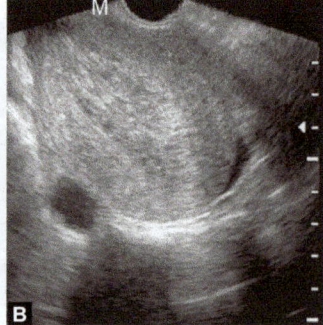

Figs. 20.9.7A and B: US scans show early hydatidiform mole. (M: mass)

- *Placental site trophoblastic tumor:*
  - Paucity of syncytiotrophoblasts and therefore low levels of β-hCG
  - Levels of human placental lactogen is increased
  - Lack of chorionic villi, lack of necrosis and hemorrhage
  US—No specific appearance.

Endometrial Hyperplasia (Fig. 20.9.8)

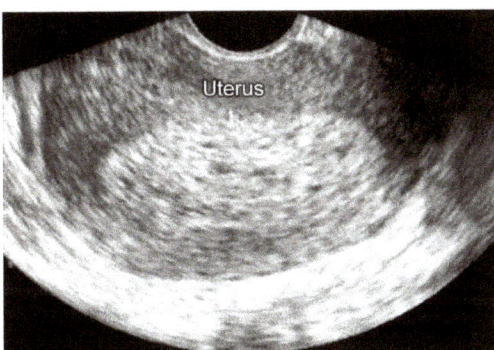

Fig. 20.9.8: Increased endometrial thickness in a case of endometrial hyperplasia.

- Proliferation of glands leading to increased gland/stroma ratio
- Diffuse involvement
- With or without cellular atypia, 25% of hyperplasia with atypia progresses to endometrial carcinoma
- Common cause of abnormal uterine bleeding developing from unopposed estrogen stimulation in post- or perimenopausal women.

Causes

- Estrogen hormone replacement therapy
- Persistent anovulatory
- Polycystic ovarian disease during reproductive age group
- Estrogen-producing tumors—granulosa cell tumors and thecoma
- Tamoxifen effect.

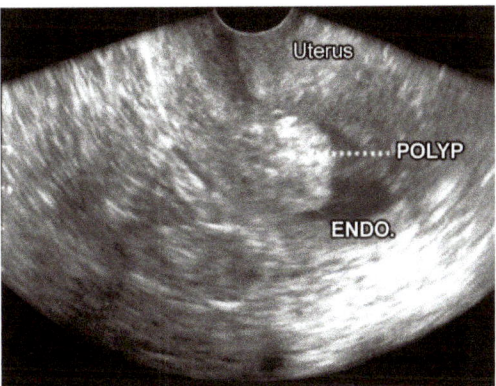

Fig. 20.9.9: Endometrial polyp seen as a localized echogenic lesion in the endometrium.

Ultrasound

- Reveals thickened echogenic endometrium having well-defined margins
- Small cysts may be seen in cystic hyperplasia.

Endometrial Polyp (Figs. 20.9.9 to 20.9.13)

- Important condition presenting in peri- or postmenopausal females as uterine bleeding

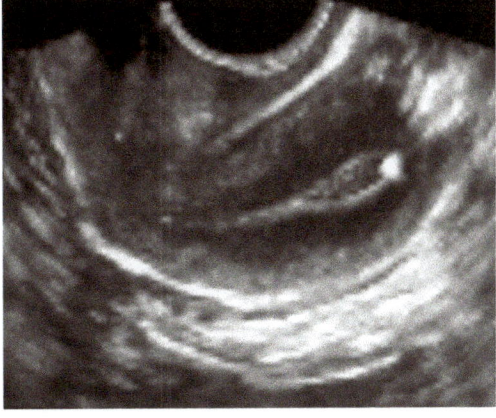

Fig. 20.9.10: 3D US scan shows calcified endometrial polyp.

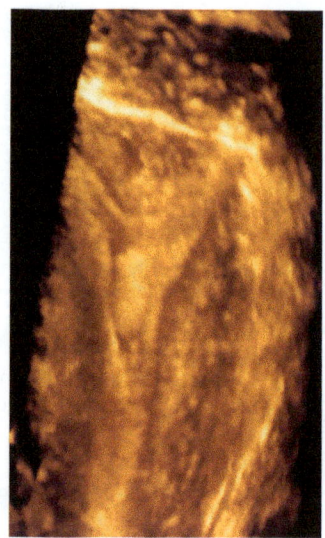

Fig. 20.9.11: 3D US coronal scan shows endometrial polyp.

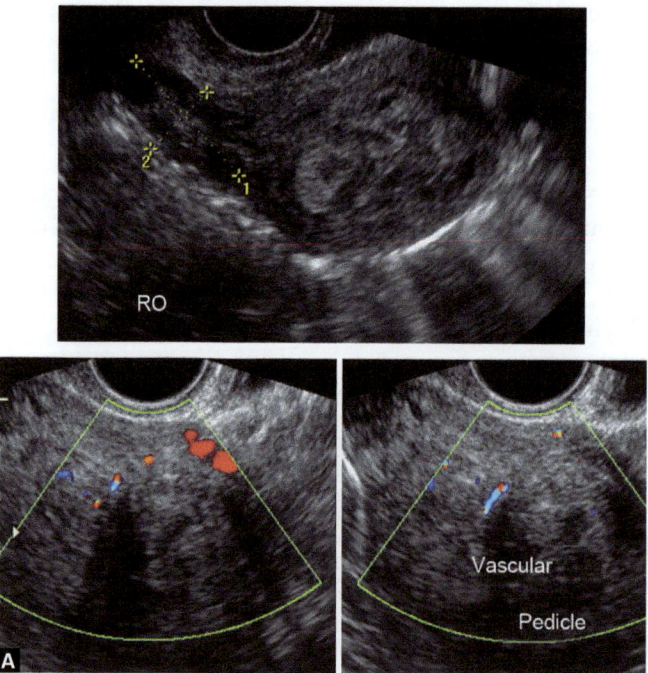

Fig. 20.9.12A: Hyperechoic lesion in the endometrial cavity with a feeding vessel s/o endometrial polyp. (RO: right ovary)

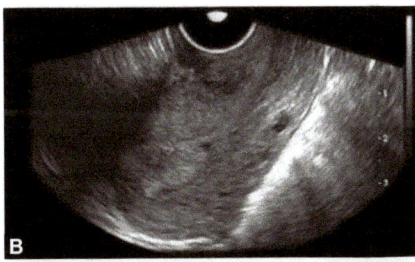
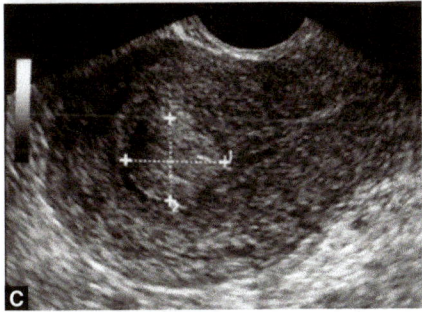

Figs. 20.9.12B and C: Endometrial polyp—echogenic polypoidal mass arising from endometrium protruding within uterine cavity.

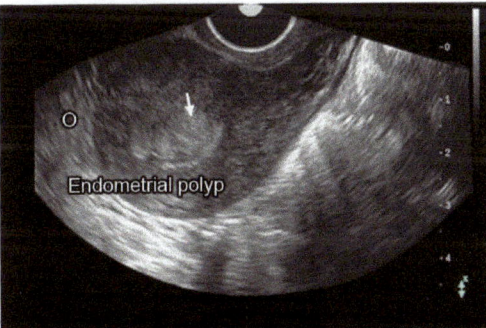
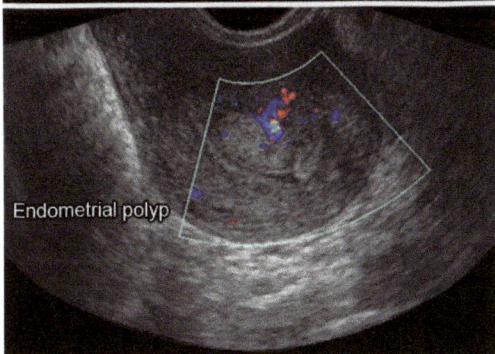

Fig. 20.9.13: Hyperechoic lesion in the endometrial cavity with a feeding vessel sign of endometrial polyp.

- In younger females—they present as intermenstrual bleeding or menometrorrhagia or infertility.

Ultrasound

- A nonspecific, echogenic, localized (central or eccentric) endometrial thickening with or without cysts
- Thickening may be diffuse
- On sonohysterography, it is seen as rounded, focal, echogenic mass within the endometrial cavity. Pedicle shows a feeding artery on color Doppler imaging.

It is easily differentiated from submucosal fibroids on sonohysterography which shows a rounded, hypoechoic sound attenuating lesion bulging into the endometrial cavity lined by normal thickness of endometrium.

Endometrial Carcinoma

- *The most common presentation is postmenopausal bleeding.*
    - It is the most common gynecological malignancy
    - Ultrasound is good for assessing endometrial thickness but not for staging
    - MRI is the modality of choice for staging endometrial carcinoma.

Ultrasound

- Thickened endometrium (>8 mm in asymptomatic or >4 mm in symptomatic postmenopausal females), mostly focal but can be diffuse
- Endometrium—echogenic/mixed echogenicity/hypoechoic
- Endometrial—myometrial interface—absence of subendometrial halo indicates deep invasion
- Cervical extension causes hemato- or pyometra

- It may appear as a heterogeneously enlarged uterus with lobulations.

Endometritis (Fig. 20.9.14)

Clinical presentation with features of pelvic inflammatory disease.

Ultrasound

Prominent echogenic endometrium with or without fluid with debris, debris-fluid level, presence of air is diagnostic.

Other features of PID like pyosalpinx (tubular shape cystic structure with folded configuration and echoes within it), complex tubo-ovarian masses, and fluid in POD.

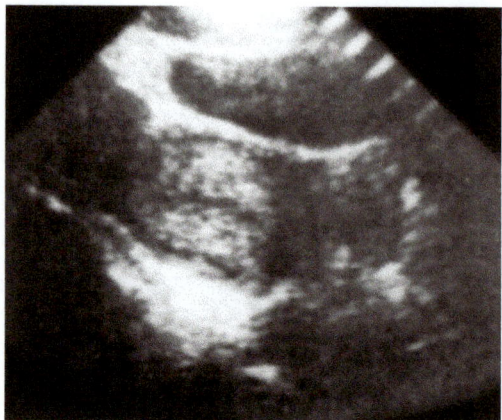

Fig. 20.9.14: Endometriosis.

Adhesions

- Clinical presentation is with history of infertility, scanty menstruation
- History of D/C is present
- US—irregular, echogenic, endometrium with areas of focal thickening
- Sonohysterography demonstrates the synechia **(Fig. 20.9.15)**
- Foreign body—IUCD **(Fig. 20.9.16)**.

Endometrial Fluid

- *Normal finding:*
  - Menstruation
  - Postmenopausally (small amount)
- Endometritis
- Early pregnancy
- Ectopic gestation
- *Obstructed uterus (Fig. 20.9.17):*
  - Congenital conditions like imperforate hymen, vaginal septum, vaginal atresia, rudimentary horn of bicornuate uterus
  - Cervical stenosis
  - Cervical carcinoma
  - Endometrial carcinoma
  - Post-irradiation fibrosis.

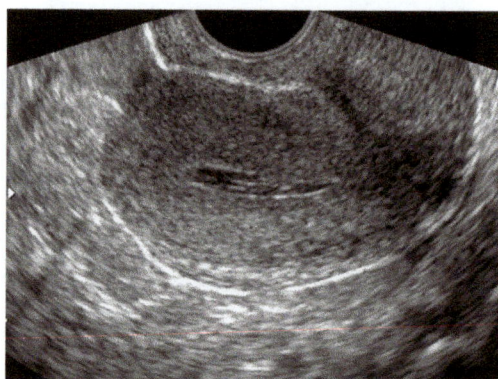

Fig. 20.9.15: US scan shows uterine synechia.

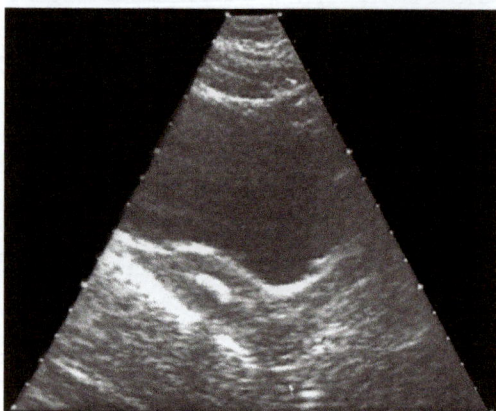

Fig. 20.9.16: Foreign body in uterus.

Gynecology and Obstetrics

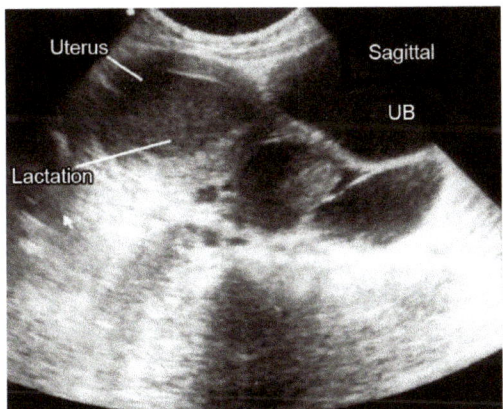

Fig. 20.9.17: Hematometra with hematosalpinx—uterine cavity is distended with fluid showing low-level echoes. Dilated fallopian tube is showing low-level echoes, septal and echogenic clot inside it. (UB: urinary bladder)

Foreign Body (IUCD)

It is seen as a thick linear echo with a distal shadowing.

Vaginal Lesions Detected on Ultrasound

- Hematocolpos
- Urethral diverticulae
- Gartner duct cyst.

20.10 DIFFERENTIAL DIAGNOSIS OF THICKENED PLACENTA

Causes

- Maternal diabetes
- Rhesus isoimmunization
- Fetal hydrops
- Triploidy
- Intrauterine infections
- Maternal severe anemia
- Fetal anemia
- Fetal hydrops
- Homozygous alpha thalassemia.

Salient Features

- Placenta is called thickened when it measures >4 cm in thickness at the cord insertion (Flowchart 20.10.1 and Fig. 20.10.1)
- Most of the above causes are better evaluated by microscopic and biochemical evaluation of maternal blood
- Karyotyping is an essential step in evaluation
- USG has a corroborative role in evaluating structural abnormalities in above conditions, e.g. fetal hydrops chromosomal abnormalities.

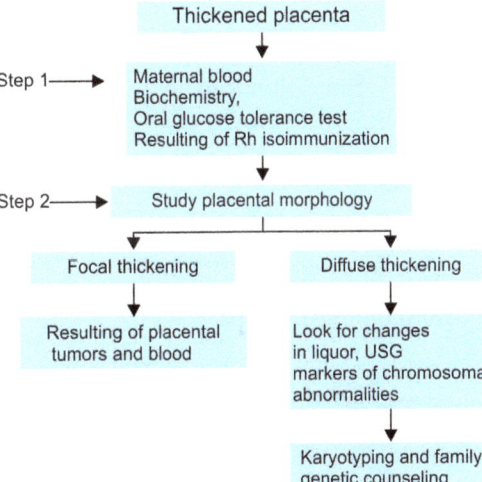

Flowchart 20.10.1: Thickened placenta.

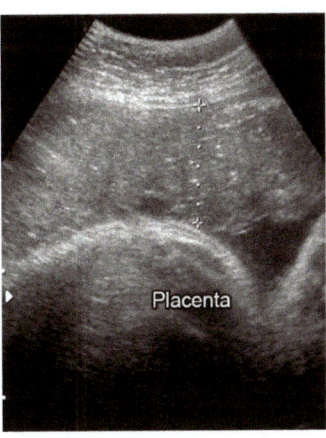

Fig. 20.10.1: US scan shows thickened placenta.

20.11 ULTRASOUND SIGNS OF CHROMOSOMAL ABNORMALITY

Generalized Signs

Which are important even if isolated (Flowchart 20.11.1):
- Borderline ventriculomegaly
- Posterior fossa abnormality
- Cystic hygroma
- Nuchal-fold thickness
- Nuchal translucency
- Atrioventricular septal defects
- Double outlet right ventricle
- Omphalocele
- Duodenal atresia
- Echogenic bowel
- Genitourinary abnormality
- Nonimmune hydrops.

Important Specific Signs

Trisomy 21

- Cystic hygroma
- Nonimmune hydrops
- Nuchal thickening
- Hydrothorax
- Gut atresias
- Protruding tongue
- Clinodactyly
- Increased distance between 1st and 2nd toes.

Trisomy 18

- Intrauterine growth restriction
- Single umbilical artery
- Cystic hygroma
- Microcephaly/dolichocephaly
- Megacisterna magna
- Omphalocele
- Renal dysplasias
- Rocker bottom feet.

Trisomy 13

- Cyclopia
- Anophthalmia
- Cleft lip/palate
- Low set deformed ear
- Holoprosencephaly

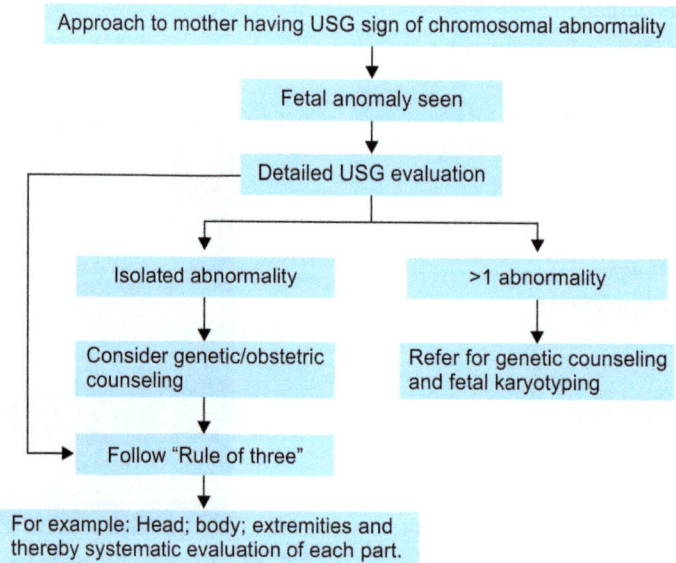

Flowchart 20.11.1: Approach in a case having chromosomal abnormal USG sign.

- Duplicated kidney
- Polydactyly
- Rocker bottom feet.

Triploidy

- Early onset IUGR
- Myelomeningocele
- Agenesis of corpus callosum
- Micrognathia
- Sloping forehead
- Postaxial polydactyly/syndactyly
- Molar placenta and other abnormalities (**Figs. 20.11.1 to 20.11.3**)
- Renal cortical cyst.

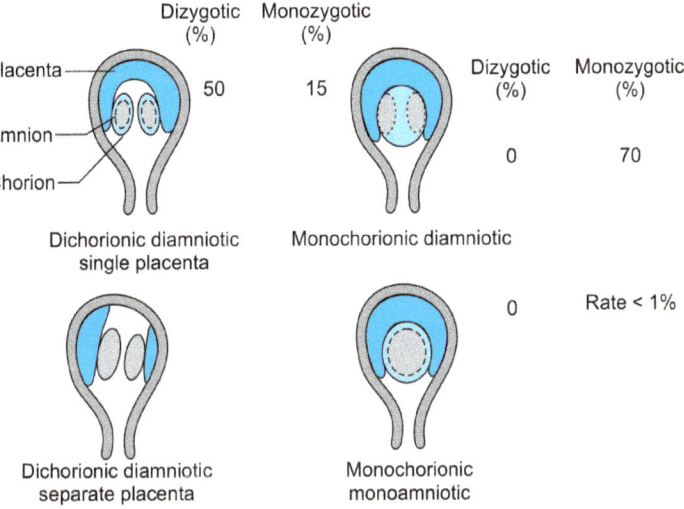

Fig. 20.11.1: Placenta and membranes in twin pregnancies.

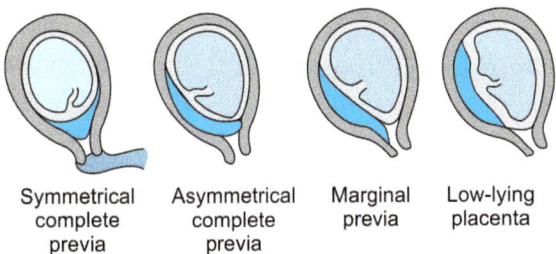

Fig. 20.11.2: Abnormalities of the placenta.

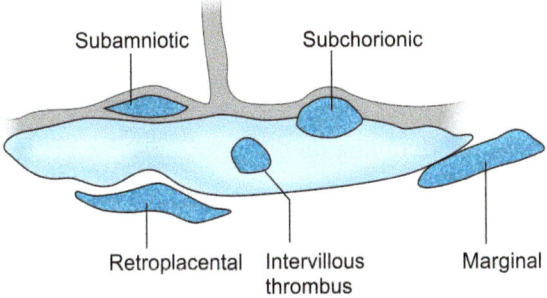

Fig. 20.11.3: Placental hemorrhage.

Turner's Syndrome

- Cystic hygroma
- Nonimmune hydrops
- Brachycephaly
- Small mandible
- Coarctation of aorta
- Horse-shoe kidney
- Cubitus valgus
- Short-stature.

20.12 ABSENT PREGNANCY TEST WITH ABSENT INTRAUTERINE PREGNANCY

Causes

- Ectopic pregnancy
- Very early I/U pregnancy
- Recent abortion
- Molar pregnancy/gestational trophoblastic neoplasia.

Salient Features

- *Ectopic pregnancy:*
  - Specific feature: Live embryo in the adnexa
  - *Nonspecific feature (Need β-hCG correlation):*
    - Empty uterus
    - Pseudogestational sac in uterus
    - Particulate ascites
    - Adnexal mass
    - Ectopic tubal ring.
  - *Nonsuppurative features:*
    - Live intrauterine pregnancy
    - Peritrophoblastic flow
    - Intradecidual sign/double decidual sac sign.
  - Slow rising β-hCG, i.e. doubling time <2 days.
- *Very early intrauterine pregnancy:*
  - Pregnancy test becomes positive at approximately 23 days. The earliest sonographic sign of pregnancy, i.e. intradecidual sign is detected at approximately 25 days. During this, window period of 2 days confusion may occur
  - It is always wise to screen after 72 hours in case of any confusion.
- *Recent abortion:* In case of positive pregnancy test with USG showing no intrauterine pregnancy serial monitoring of β-hCG should be done. In cases of abortion, a falling titer is seen in maternal serum
- *Gestational trophoblastic neoplasia:* Uterus is enlarged with cavity filled with multiple small vesicles and soft tissue nodules. Fetal parts and myometrial invasion may or may not be seen if hCG levels are quite high.

20.13 FETAL CAUSES OF ABNORMALITIES IN LIQUOR VOLUME

Causes

- *Oligohydramnios:*
  - Fetal demise/IUD
  - *Renal/bladder abnormalities:*
    - Posterior urethral valve
    - Prune-Belly syndrome
    - ARPCKD
    - BRA
  - IUGR
  - Postdated pregnancy.
- *Polyhydramnios:*
  - Cardiovascular decompensation
  - Diaphragmatic hernia
  - Anencephaly/other severe cranial anomaly, especially ONTD
  - Obstructive malformations of GIT, e.g. TOF duodenal stenosis/atresia
  - Bone dysplasias
  - Neuromuscular abnormalities
  - Chromosomal abnormality, e.g. trisomy 18.

Salient Features

- Amniotic fluid assessment (AFI)

	Single pocket	AFI
Oligohydramnios	<2 cm	<7
Reduced	2–3 cm	7–10
Normal	3–8 cm	10–17
More than average	>8–12 cm	17–25
Polyhydramnios	>12 cm	>25

- *Fetal demise:*
  - Fetal wastage after the time significant liquor production is seen leading to slow resorption of liquor
  - Urine production status at 9 weeks and renal function starts at 11 weeks. At 12 weeks, urine accumulates at the rate of 5 cc per day.
- *Signs of IUD are:*
  - *Spalding's sign:* Over-riding of skull bones
  - Gas in vessels
  - Sometimes associated hydrops
  - Extended limbs/lost tone
  - Absent cardiac activity
  - Gas in abdomen.
- *IUGR:*
  - Weight of neonate below 10 percentile of the expected fetal weight for that age
  - Usually detected after 32–34 weeks, i.e. the age of maximum fetal growth
  - May be due to uteroplacental insufficiency that leads to asymmetric IUGR
  - Asymmetric IUGR is early onset and leads to concordant reduction of all parameters
  - Criteria for IUGR:

	Sensitivity	Specificity
Advance placental grade	62%	64%
FL/AC (increased)	34–49%	78–83%
TIUV (decreased)	57–80%	72–76%
Small BPD	24–88%	62–94%
Slow increase in BPD	75%	84%
Low EFW	89%	88%
AFV decreased	24%	98%
HC/AC	82%	94%
Biophysical profile	<6 = Equivocal <4 = Fetal compromise	

  - Doppler indices
  - Uterine artery: S/D >2.3, difference of the two sides >1, RI >0.6
  - MCA: RI <0.7
  - Umbilical artery: RI – >0.7
- *Postdated pregnancy/Large for dates:*
  - When weight is >90th percentile for the expected fetal weight
  - Also when weight >4000 g
  - Sonographic criteria.

LGA	Sensitivity	Specificity
AD/BPD (increase)	46%	79%
FL/AC (decrease)	24–75%	44–93%
AFV increase	12–17%	92–98%
Ponderal index increase	13–15%	85–98%
High EFW increase	20–74%	93–96%
Growth score inc.	14%	91%
Macrosomia		
FL increase	24%	96%
AC increase	53%	94%
High EFW	11–65%	89–96%
BPD increase	29%	98%

- Renal/bladder abnormality: Any cause of reduction of urine formation as in renal (B/L) agenesis, ARPCKD or of obstruction to outlet of urine as in Prune-Belly syndrome, urethral atresia/stenosis, posterior urethral valve can lead to oligohydramnios (**Flowchart 20.13.1**). Look for signs of megacystis, i.e. UB >8 mm, hydronephrosis, i.e. pelvis >6 mm, abnormal renal parenchyma, dilated ureter and urethra.
- Polyhydramnios (**Flowchart 20.13.2**) occurs when either increased production or decreased fetal galloping of liquor is seen
- Cardiovascular decompensation:
  - Bradycardia - <100 bpm of >10 sec
  - Tachycardia - >180 bpm
  - PSVT   - 180–300 bpm with conduction rate 1:1
  - Flutter   - 300–400 bpm with conduction rate 2:1/4:1
  - Fibrillation - 400 bpm

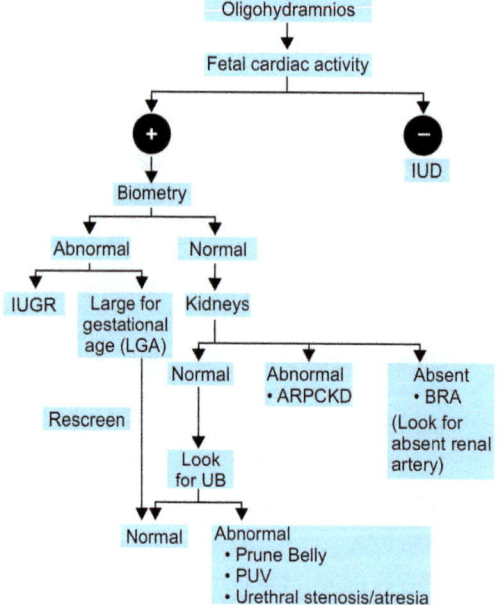

Flowchart 20.13.1: Oligohydramnios.

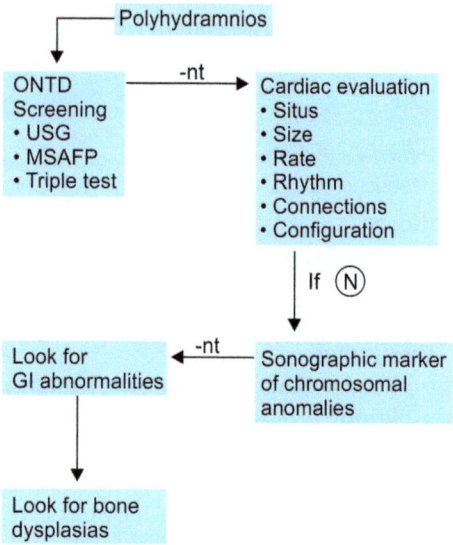

Flowchart 20.13.2: Polyhydramnios.

- *Diaphragmatic hernia*: Cystic areas in thorax with small abdomen. Absent fundic bubble, GB with portal vein pointing up
- Double bubble and triple bubble sign of duodenal and jejunal atresia should be looked for
- Skeletal dysplasia, chromosomal abnormalities detection have been described elsewhere.

20.14 INTRA-ABDOMINAL FETAL CALCIFICATION

Causes (Flowchart 20.14.1)

- *Peritoneal:*
  - Meconium peritonitis
  - Plastic peritonitis with hydrometrocolpos
- *Tumors:*
  - Hemangioma
  - Hemangioendothelioma
  - Hepatoblastoma
  - Metastatic neuroblastoma
  - Teratoma
- *Infections:*
  - Toxoplasma
  - Cytomegalovirus

Flowchart 20.14.1: Intra-abdominal fetal calcification.

```
                   Intra-abdominal fetal calcification
         ┌──────────────┬──────────────┬──────────────┐
      In liver       In spleen    Retroperitoneal/  In peritoneum
                     • CMV        gonadal           • Meconium
                     • Toxoplasma Teratoma,         • Peritonitis
                                  dermoid
      ┌──────┴──────┐
   Lumpy         Linear
   hepatoblastoma • Hemangio-
                   endothelioma/
                   hemangioma
```

- Results in abnormal large yolk sac (**Fig. 20.14.1**), abnormal G-sac (**Fig. 20.14.2**) or subchorionic hemorrhage (**Fig. 20.14.3**).

Salient Features

- *Meconium peritonitis:*
  - Occurs due to meconium exiting from the bowel lumen, due to perforation, causing sterile chemical peritonitis
  - Perforation occurs due to volvulus, jejunal/ileal atresia, meconium ileus
  - Immediately ascites occurs following which linear streaky or spotty calcification occurs
  - Pseudocyst formation may also occur
  - Calcified meconium balls in/out the lumen may also be seen
- Infections like *Toxoplasma* and CMV lead to calcifications in liver, spleen and also intracranial calcification
- Hemangiomas may occur at multiple sites in fetal body and may be associated with calcification
- *Hemangioendothelioma and hepatoblastomas:* Common fetal hepatic tumors which show areas of specky linear calcification associated with vascular spaces showing high velocity Doppler shifts

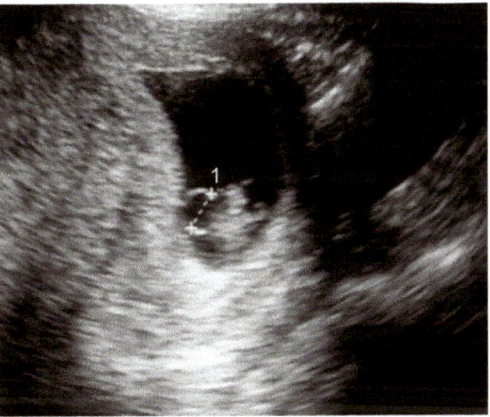

Fig. 20.14.1: Abnormally large yolk sac (calipers) in an early pregnancy.

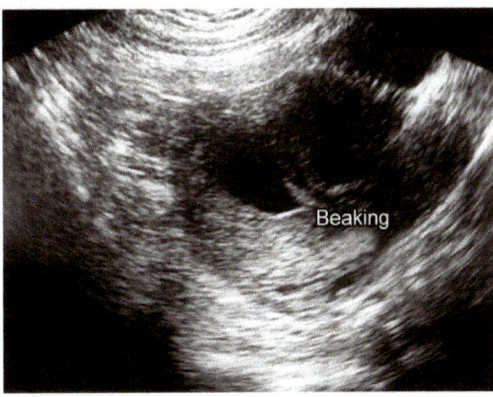

Fig. 20.14.2: Abnormal G-sac showing beaking.

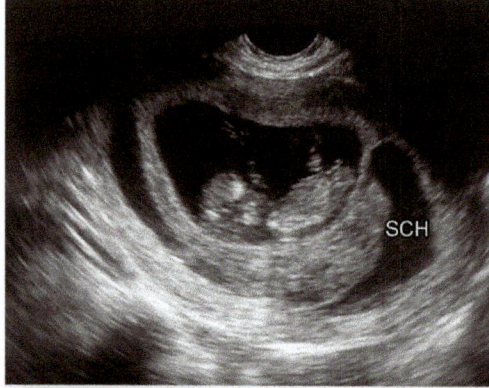

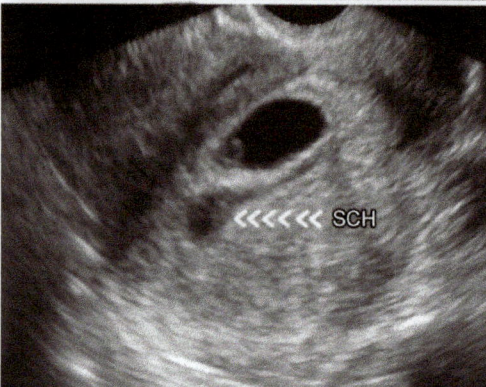

Fig. 20.14.3: Subchorionic hemorrhage (SCH) in two patients.

- Hepatoblastoma is the most common hepatic tumor (primary) in young and nearly all present before the age of five. Associated with hemihypertrophy, 11p13 chromosome and Beckwith-Wiedemann's syndrome. Serum AFP levels are almost always elevated. Shows lumpy calcification
- Neuroblastoma is the most common neonatal tumor usually occurring in the adrenal gland. It is an echogenic mass, heterogeneous in appearance. It commonly metastasizes to placenta, liver and subcutaneous tissues with the metastasis appearing echogenic calcified. Hydrops may commonly occur
- Teratomas and dermoids are common fetal tumors occurring in retroperitoneal and gonadal locations most commonly. These show solid and cystic areas with areas of calcification.

20.15 DIFFERENTIAL DIAGNOSIS OF FETAL THORACIC ABNORMALITIES

Causes

- Pleural effusion
- Congenital diaphragmatic hernias
- Pulmonary hypoplasia
- Pulmonary sequestration
- Pulmonary cystic adenomatoid malformation
- Congenital bronchogenic cyst
- Bronchial/laryngeal atresia
- Thymic enlargement
- Cystic hygroma
- Teratoma
- Enteric cysts
- Neuroblastoma.

Salient Features (Flowchart 20.15.1)

- *Pleural effusion:*
  - May be isolated or occurs as a result of generalized fetal hydrops
  - Fluid collects as a crescentic rim around lungs forming a 'Bat-wing-appearance' of lungs floating in fluid
  - U/L— congenital adenomatoid malformation (CAM), diaphragmatic hernia, sequestration, pulmonary hypoplasia
  - B/L—infections, CHF, Turner's, Down's, pulmonary lymphangiectasis
  - Long-lasting larger effusions may lead to pulmonary hypoplasia
  - May be treated by thoracocentesis.
- *Diaphragmatic hernias:*
  - *Bochdalek hernia:*
    - Posterolateral in location

Flowchart 20.15.1: Differential diagnosis of fetal thoracic abnormalities.

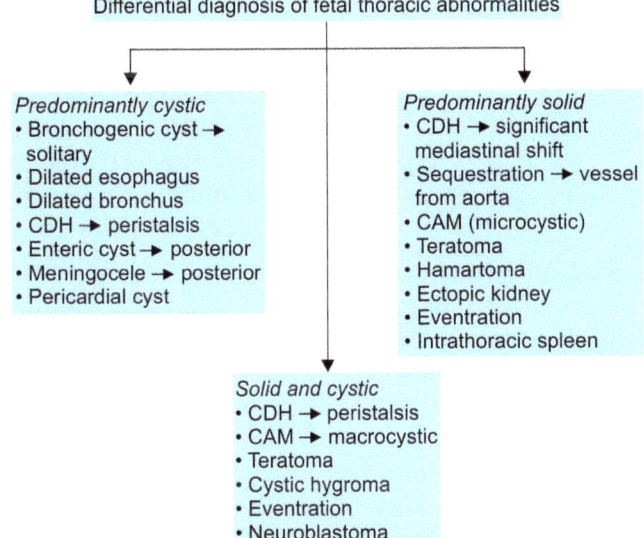

- Left >> right
- Small intestine (88%), stomach (60%), colon (56%), liver (51%), spleen (45%)
- Detected by sonography at 17 weeks
- Mediastinal deviation seen by change in position and axis of heart
- Hollow viscera may be seen with AC < 5th percentile and polyhydramnios
- Absence of GB in abdomen
- Umbilical vein displaced up.
- *Morgagni hernia:*
  - Anteriorly behind the sternum
  - Right>>> left
  - Omentum, colon, liver, stomach, small bowel
  - May be covered by peritoneum and pleura or only pleura or none at all. If pericardium is also absent, it lies in direct contact to heart.
- *Eventration of diaphragm:*
  - Due to absent muscle fibers in the diaphragm
  - U/L—asymptomatic
  - B/L—may cause pulmonary hypoplasia
  - B/L associated with trisomies 13 and 18, CMV infection, rubella infection and arthrogryposis multiplex congenital (AMC).
- *Pulmonary hypoplasia:*
  - U/L—rare, may be simulated by discordant rate of growth of both lungs. Due to thoracic masses
  - B/L—commoner, due to restricted chest cage as in thanatophoric dwarfism, Jeune's asphyxiating dystrophy, achondrogenesis and all causes of:

$$\frac{\text{Chest area} - \text{Heart area}}{\text{Chest area}} \times 100$$

  is an accurate (85% sensitive and specific) in diagnosis, as correlated to age.
- *Cystic adenomatoid malformation:*
  - Are hamartomas in lung divided by Adzich in macroscopic (cysts >5 mm) and microscopic (<5 mm) types
  - Macroscopic type has better prognosis and is less commonly associated with hydrops

- Size of the mass may decrease over the time
- Has to be d/d from diaphragmatic hernia, bronchial cyst, cystic dilatation of esophagus, pericardial teratoma.
- *Pulmonary sequestration:*
  - Is a segment or part of lung not communicating at the usually bronchovascular tree
  - Appears as solid echogenic masses inside (Intralobar sequestration) of the lung. Usually in basal parts
  - Extralobar may occur inside the diaphragm, pericardium, hila, mediastinum
  - In 50%, malformations of sternum and diaphragm are seen but no major anomaly is seen
  - D/D to diaphragmatic hernia, CAM and lobar emphysema
  - A supplying vessel from aorta is the most confirmatory sign.
- Up to 27 weeks, the thymus enlarges and appears as echogenic mass (from 14 weeks), after 27 weeks, it becomes hypoechoic
- Cystic hygroma (lymphangiomas) are cystic (predominantly) and solid dumbbell masses extending in the mediastinum
- Teratomas usually arise from pericardium and are surrounded by pericardial fluid (diagnostic point). Appearance is the same as in adults
- Neuroblastomas are echogenic masses with echolucent centers lying in paravertebral area
- Enteric cyst lined by GI mucosa are also seen in posterior mediastinum.

20.16 UNSUCCESSFUL FIRST TRIMESTER PREGNANCY

Abortion (Miscarriage)—termination of fetus before viability.

Type of embryonic/fetal loss:
- *Complete abortion*
  USG appearance
  Bulky uterus
  - Heterogeneous vascular myometrium
  - Thick heterogeneous endometrium
  - No products of conception seen
- *Incomplete abortion* **(Fig. 20.16.1):**
  - First three features are same as above
  - Minimal products of conception especial placenta is retained.
- *Septic:*
  - Apart from above features, some foreign body or signs of infection might be noted.
- *Inevitable/impending/imminent:*
  - Cervix dilated
  - Membranes protruding
  - Severe pain with uterine contractions
  - Low-placed GS, abnormal in shape.
- *Missed* **(Fig. 20.16.2):**
  - Whole of products of conception are retained inside for >2 months
  - Fetus is distorted
  - Normal components of conceptus may or may not be identifiable
  - Basically a heteroechoic mass is seen in a bulky uterus but vascularity is reduced.
- *Threatened abortion:*
  - A normal fetal pole with near-normal conceptus noted with the os closed
  - Basically diagnosed clinically.

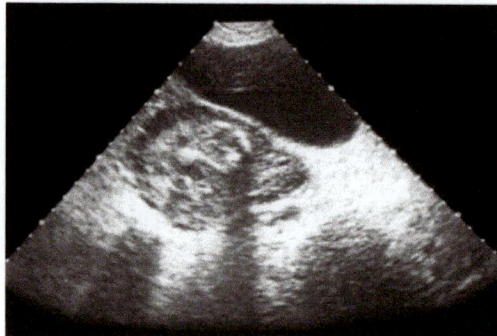

Fig. 20.16.1: Retained products of conception seen in the uterus in a case of incomplete abortion.

Gynecology and Obstetrics

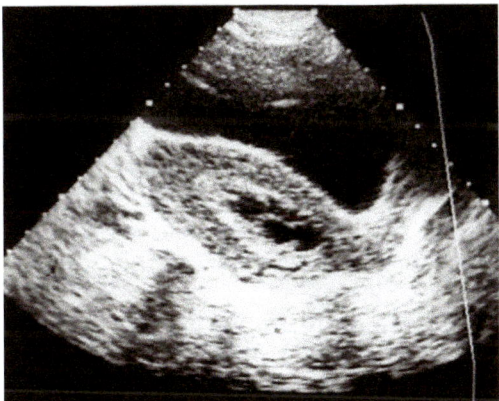

Fig. 20.16.2: Missed abortion—an irregular gestational ring with echoes inside it in normal-sized uterus.

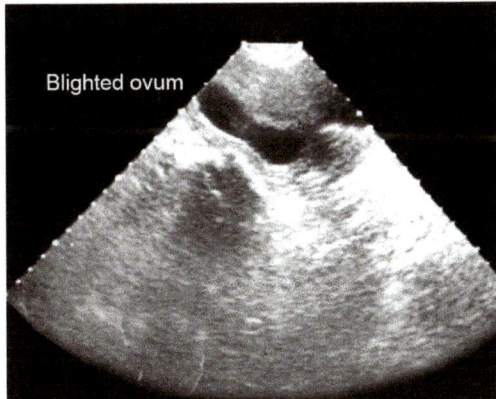

Fig. 20.17.1: Anembryonic gestational sac—no yolk sac is seen in the gestational sac.

Features of Abnormal Gestation Sac

- Abnormal/irregular shape
- Low position
- Abnormal sac size—most valuable [according to clinically judged age].
- Thin, weakly echogenic, incomplete trophoblastic reaction (<2 mm)
- Growth rate is reduced/absent growth on follow-up scans.

Abnormal Yolk Sac Features that Suggest Demise

- Threshold mean sac diameter—must see yolk sac.
  EVS = 8 mm
  TVS = 20 mm
- Yolk sac size >5.6 mm (5–10 weeks maternal = abnormal outcome age)
- Calcification in yolk sac.

20.17 FIRST TRIMESTER BLEEDING

- *With intrauterine conceptus identified:*
  - Blighted ovum
  - Vanishing twin syndrome
  - Implantation bleeding
  - Threatened abortion
  - Gestational trophoblastic disease
  - Ectopic pregnancy with a pseudo-gestation sac.
- *With empty uterus + beta hCG >1800 mIU/mL:*
  - Recent spontaneous abortion
  - Ectopic pregnancy.
- *With empty uterus + beta hCG <1800 mIU/mL:*
  - Early intrauterine pregnancy
  - Ectopic pregnancy.

Blighted Ovum

- Also known as anembryonic pregnancy/embryonic resorption **(Fig. 20.17.1)**
- Inner cell mass fails to grow further but the sac grows due to persistent trophoblastic function, though suboptimal
- *On USG:*
  - Large gestational sac without an embryo
  - Mean sac diameter >16 mm
    >25 mm without an embryo
  - Poor sac growth rate
  - Poor perisac trophoblastic reaction
  - Other features of an abnormal sac.

Ectopic Pregnancy (Figs. 20.17.2 to 20.17.4)

- *Specific features:* Live embryo in adnexa
- *Nonspecific features (need correlation to beta-hCG):*
  - Empty uterus with amenorrhea associated with recent spotting
  - Pseudogestation sac of ectopic pregnancy [created by decidual reaction and associated bleeding], no associated placenta seen.
  - Particulate ascites

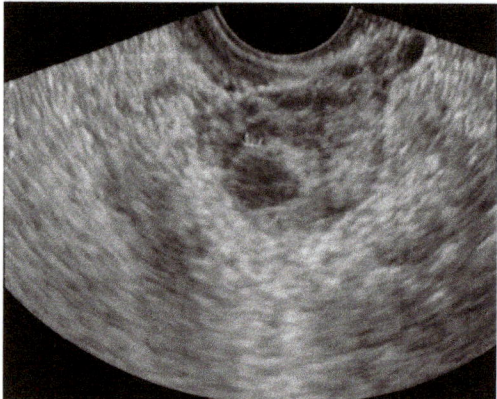

Fig. 20.17.2: Ectopic pregnancy—gray scale image showing a complex right adnexal mass.

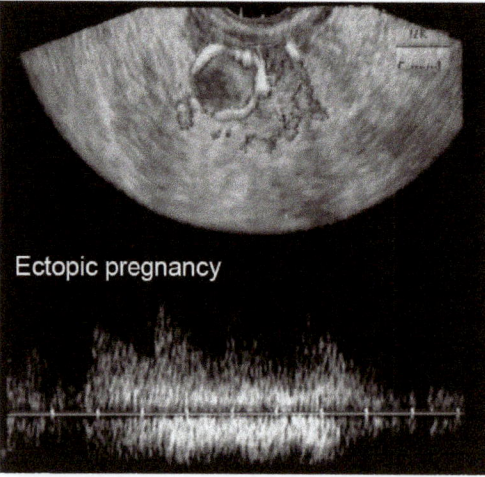

Fig. 20.17.3: Ectopic pregnancy—duplex Doppler demonstrates trophoblastic flow pattern.

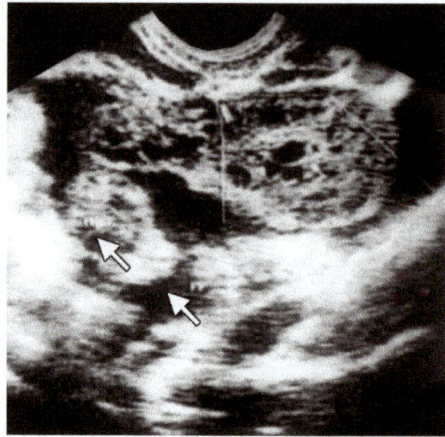

Fig. 20.17.4: Gray scale image showing small ectopic gestation (arrows).

  - Adnexal mass—heteroechoic
  - Ectopic tubal ring—concentric echogenic rim with increased vascularity circumferentially and central hypoechoic area
  - Adnexal tenderness
  - Interstitial line sign—thin echogenic line from endometrial canal to the ectopic sac.
- *Nonsupportive features:*
  - Live intrauterine pregnancy (as occurrence of heterotopic pregnancy is very rare)
  - Intradecidual sign and double decidual sign of early intrauterine pregnancy
  - Peritrophoblastic flow.

Gestational Trophoblastic Disease

- *Molar pregnancy:*
  - Complete mole (**Fig. 20.17.5**)
  - Partial mole (**Fig. 20.17.6**).
- *Persistent trophoblastic neoplasia (PTN):*
  - Invasive mole
  - Choriocarcinoma
  - Placental site trophoblastic tumor (PSTT).

Gynecology and Obstetrics

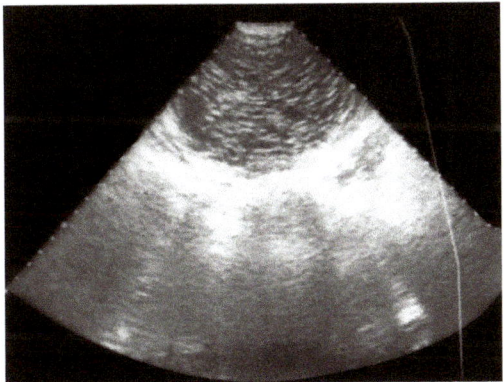

Fig. 20.17.5: Hydatidiform mole (complete). The entire uterus is filled with a heterogeneous mass with multiple anechoic cystic areas in a female with five-month amenorrhea.

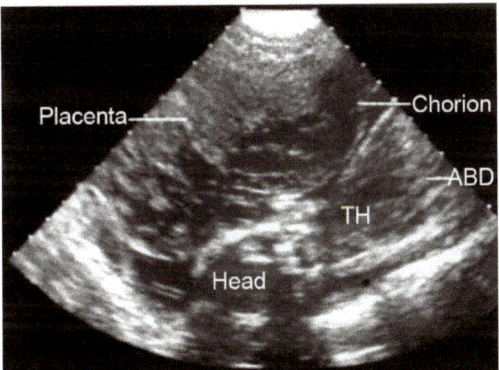

Fig. 20.17.6: Hydatidiform mole (partial)—multiple anechoic spaces in the region of placenta. Fetal parts are seen adjacent to it. (TH: thorax; ABD: abdomen)

On Ultrasonography

- *Echogenic soft tissue interspersed with multiple anechoic areas giving an overall appearance of a spongy mass:* Snow storm appearance
- Perilesional and intralesional vascularity increase in cases of invasive mole, choriocarcinoma, PSTT or any other complication (RI <0.5; PSV >50 cm/s)
- In partial mole, incompletely formed fetal porta may be seen
- In PTN, invasion of mass into myometrium is seen.

20.18 FETAL HYDROPS

- It is the abnormal accumulation of fluid in at least two body cavities
- It represents the terminal stage of a long list of conditions, majority of which are fetal in origin. It signifies fetal decompensation.

Sonographic Features

- Ascites (>2 mm) and hydrocele
- Pleural effusion
- Pericardial effusion (best over cardiac apex)
- Subcutaneous edema (>5 mm: Best over scalp)
- Arterial/venous Doppler abnormality
- Altered fetal wellbeing
- Placental edema (>4–5 cm in third trimester).

Hydrops immune	Nonimmune
• ABO incompatibility • Rh incompatibility • Any other blood group antigen involvement	• In West, most commonly due to infective, cardiovascular and chromosomal causes in east, thalassemia is most common

Immune Hydrops

- On USG:
  - Hyperdynamic fetal circulation
  - Enlarged liver and spleen
  - *Altered fetal blood parameters:*
    - Increasing antibody titer
    - Amniotic fluid spectrophotometry
    - Fetal blood sampling.

Nonimmune Hydrops

- *Fetal causes:*
  - *Cardiovascular:*
    - Malformations—cardiac tumors, myocarditis, cardiomyopathy, Ebstein anomaly, endomyocardial fibroelastosis, AV canal

- Arrhythmias—SVT, PAT, WPWS, complete heart block
- High output failure—Placental tumors, sacrococcygeal teratoma, vein of Galen aneurysm.

Neck/Thorax Abnormality

- Cystic hygroma
- Thoracic tumor
- Pulmonary sequestration
- Diaphragmatic hernia
- Congenital cystic adenomatoid malformation.

Gastrointestinal Abnormality

- Hepatic—cirrhosis; hepatitis; tumor
- Bowel—atresia; volvulus; meconium peritonitis **(Figs. 20.18.1A and B)**.

Urinary Tract Abnormality

Congenital nephrotic syndrome, Prune-Belly syndrome, polycystic kidney disease, upper/lower urinary tract obstruction **(Fig. 20.18.2)**.

Chromosomal Abnormalities

45 X, triploidy, trisomy 21, 18, 13.

Anemia

Alpha thalassemia (homozygous), HPV B19 infection, G6PD deficiency, fetomaternal hemorrhage, twin–twin transfusion (donor).

Infections

CMV, HPV, toxoplasma, syphilis, rubella.

Genetic Disorders

- Metabolic—Gaucher's, MPS
- Hypokinesis—AMC, Neu-Laxova, Pena-Shokeir syndrome, myotonic dystrophy
- Skeletal—achondroplasia, achondrogenesis, asphyxiating thoracic dystrophy, osteogenesis, thanatophoric dysplasia
    - Idiopathic (15-20%)
- *Maternal causes:*
    - Severe anemia
    - Severe hypoproteinemia
    - Severe diabetes.

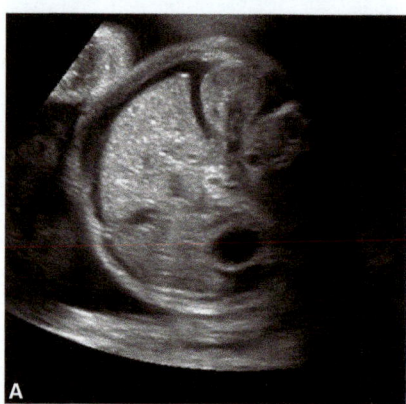
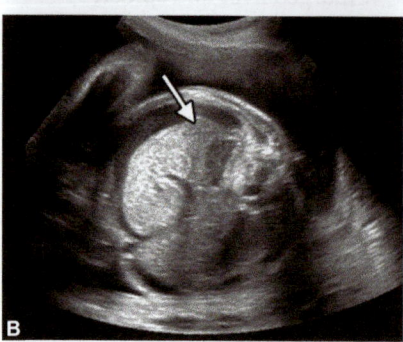

Figs. 20.18.1A and B: Transabdominal image showing fetal ascites and a focus of calcification at the liver surface suggesting meconium peritonitis.

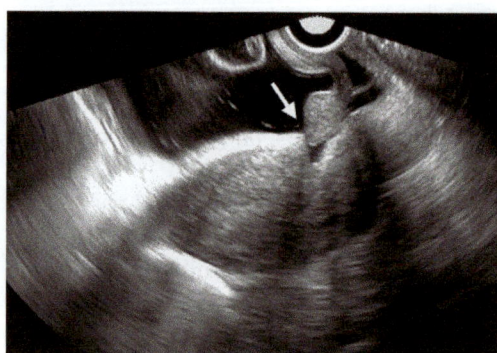

Fig. 20.18.2: TVS image showing vesicocervical fistula (arrow).

- *Placental:*
  - Chorioangioma
  - Venous thrombosis
  - *Cord torsion, knot, tumor:* USG features of above conditions are considered in detailed in relevant topics, in the following chapters.

20.19 TWIN PREGNANCY/ MULTIFETAL PREGNANCY

Aims of sonography in a clinically suspected case of multifetal pregnancy are **(Fig. 20.19.1)**:
- To confirm the diagnosis

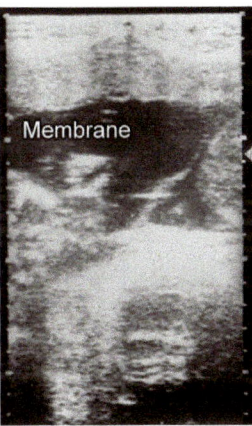

Fig. 20.19.1: A thin echogenic membrane is seen separating the two amniotic sacs in a case of twin pregnancy.

- To determine the chorionicity and amnionicity
- To determine the concordance/discordance in growth of fetuses
- To determine the complications, if any
- To follow up any such case till culminating in a successful outcome.

Sonographic determination of chorionicity and amnionicity:

Step 1: *Screen the placenta*
- Single placenta = Monochorionic or fused placenta
- >1 placenta = Dichorionic
- Diamniotic (DCDA) **(Figs. 20.19.2A and B)**

Step 2: *Screen for a membrane separating the fetuses*
- Membrane absent = Monochorionic
- Monoamniotic (MCMA)
- Membrane present = DCDA or MCDA

Step 3: *Determine the fetal sex*
- Similar sex = Zygosity cannot be inferred, either MC or DC
  Different sex = Dizygotic ... Dichorionic

Step 4: *Assess the presence of chorionic/twin peak sign*
  Present = DCDA
  Absent = Equivocal

Step 5: *Thickness of membrane in between*
  Thin = MCDA

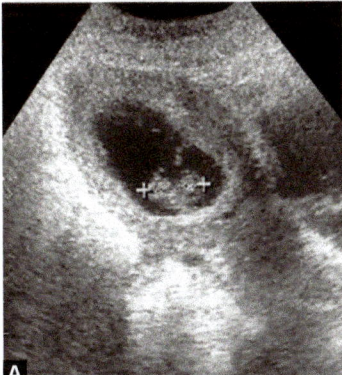 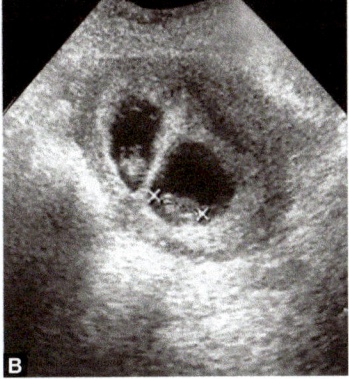

Figs. 20.19.2A and B: USG image showing echogenic septum between the two embryos suggesting dichorionic diamniotic twins.

Thick = DCDA before 22 weeks more reliable

Step 6: *Follow the cords from origin and at termination if reaching a common tangle = MCMA.*

Complications of Twin and Multifetal Pregnancy

- First trimester pregnancy loss
- *Monochorionic twin syndromes:*
  - Twin transfusion syndrome
  - Twin embolization syndrome
  - Acardiac parabiotic twin.
- *Problems specific to MCMA twins:*
  - Conjoined twins
  - Morbidity/mortality in nonconjoined twins, e.g. cord knotting, cord entanglement
  - Growth disparity among fetuses
  - Congenital anomalies in fetuses, e.g. CHD, VACTERL, congenital talipes equinovarus (CTEV), torticollis.

Sonographic Features

Twin Transfusion Syndrome (TTS)

- Arteriovenous or arterioarterial anastomosis in a single placental cotyledon loading to shunting of blood from 'donor' to 'recipient' twin
- Larger twin (recipient) is normal/macrosomic while donor is symmetrically growth retarded
- Recipient sac shows polyhydramnios while donor sac shows oligohydramnios
- Donor may even become a 'stuck twin'
- S/D ratio difference of two sides umbilical artery is >0.4.

Discordant growth
- 20–25% intrapair birth weight discrepancy
- Difference in AC of two of >18–20 mm
- Fetal weight disparity of >15%
- Second trimester BPD disparity >5 mm
- Umbilical artery S/D disparity >4.

Twin Embolization Syndrome (TES)

- Demise of co-twin leads to cerebral, hepatic and renal damage of the partner
- Due to exsanguination of live twin, due to embolization from dead twin of debris, clot or thromboplastin-rich blood.
- *On USG:*
  - Ventriculomegaly
  - Porencephaly
  - Brain atrophy
  - Microcephaly
  - Splenic/hepatic infarct
  - Gut atresias
  - Facial abnormality
  - Terminal limb abnormality
  - Renal cortical necrosis.

Acardiac Parabiotic Twins

- An arterioarterial or venovenous placental anastomosis leads to flow reversal in umbilical artery causing poorly oxygenated blood to reach the upper part of body of acardiac twin.
- *On USG:*
  - Anencephaly
  - Small rudimentary head with holoprosencephaly
  - Absent/hypoplastic upper tarso/limbs
  - Absent or anomalous two-chambered heart
  - Cystic hygroma
  - Severe oligohydramnios.

Conjoined Twins

On ultrasonography
- Continuous, fixed, abnormal/unusual complementary position of two twins
- Simultaneous movements
- Common/communicating organs
- Hyperextended head and neck.

20.20 DIFFERENTIAL DIAGNOSIS OF ECHOGENIC FETAL KIDNEYS

	Conditions	Renal size	Hydro-nephrosis	Liquor	Cyst	Cyst in parents	Family history	Associated features
1.	Infantile polycystic kidney	Large	No	Reduced	No	No	Yes in sibling	Hepatic fibrosis in later life
2.	Adult polycystic	Large	No	Normal	±	Yes, >20 years age	Yes in parents liver, spleen	Occasionally cysts in parents
3.	Obstructive cystic dysplasia	Small	Yes	Depends on degree of renal obstruction	Often	No	No	Hydronephrosis usually urethral obstruction
4.	Finnish type nephrotic syndrome	Large	No	Normal	No	No	Yes in sibling	Raised serum AFP
5.	Beckwith-Wiedemann syndrome	Large	No	Normal or increased	No	No	±	Macrosomia, Macroglossia, Hepatosplenomegaly, omphalocele
6.	Meckel-Gruber syndrome	Large	No	Reduced	±	No	Yes in sibling	Polydactyly, encephalocele
7.	Trisomy	Large	No	Normal	±	No	No	Microcephaly, hydrocephalus, Intracranial calcification, hydrops hepatosplenomegaly
8.	Cytomegalovirus infection	Large	No	Normal	No	No	No	Facial clefting, holoprosencephaly, polydactyly, cardiac defects
9.	Renal vein thrombosis	Large Usually U/L	No	Normal	No	No	No	Maternal diabetes, maternal pyelonephritis

20.21 DIFFERENTIAL DIAGNOSIS OF SYNDROMES ASSOCIATED WITH RENAL MALFORMATIONS

Name and chief renal findings	USG findings
• Renal agenesis	
– Fraser syndrome:	• Cryptophthalmos • Syndactyly of hand/feet • Large hyperechogenic lungs
• Cystic renal disease	
– Meckel-Gruber's syndrome:	• Large echogenic kidney • Polydactyly • Encephalocele
– Patau's syndrome (Trisomy 13):	• Large echogenic kidneys • Polydactyly • Holoprosencephaly • Facial clefting
– Beckwith-Wiedemann syndrome	• Large echogenic kidneys • Macrosomia • Hepatosplenomegaly • Macroglossia • Omphalocele
– Jeune's syndrome	• Echogenic kidney • Small thorax • Dwarfism/IUGR
– Short rib polydactyly syndrome (Majewski type)	• Large echogenic kidney • Polydactyly • Small thorax • Dwarfism/IUGR
– Laurence-Moon-Biedl syndrome (Bardet retinal dystrophy	• Renal cyst • Polydactyly • Mental deficiency • Hypogonadism
– Zellweger syndrome	• Cystic kidney • Hypotonicity • Limb contractures • Congenital cataract • Heterotopias • Hypoplastic corpus callosum

20.22 DIFFERENTIAL DIAGNOSIS OF FETAL HYDRONEPHROSIS

Causes (Figs. 20.22.1 to 20.22.9)

Unilateral	Bilateral
• Pelviureteric junction obstruction	• Pelviureteric junction obstruction
• Vesicoureteric junction obstruction	• Vesicoureteric reflux
• Duplex kidney with ureterocele obstruction	• Vesicoureteric junction
• Normal kidney with ureterocele	• Megacystis-megaureter syndrome
• Megaureter	• Posterior urethral valve
	• Urethral atresia
	• Obstructing ureterocele
	• Megacystis microcolon syndrome
	• Congenital megalourethra
	• Persistent cloaca
	• Hydrometrocolpos

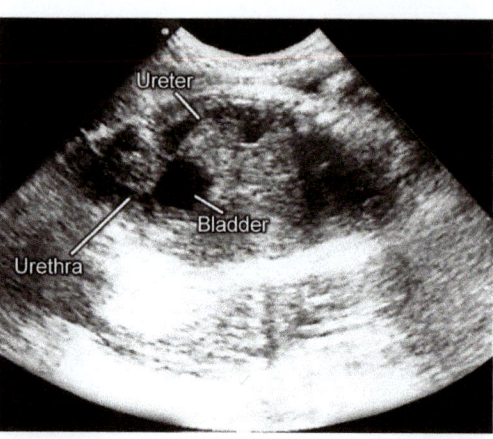

Fig. 20.22.1: Posturethral valve—a longitudinal scan showing dilated posterior urethra, urinary bladder, ureter and left kidney.

Genitourinary System

Dilatation at a median of 19 weeks (in mm) to label hydronephrosis and grading:

Gynecology and Obstetrics

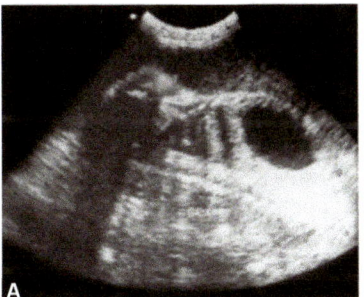 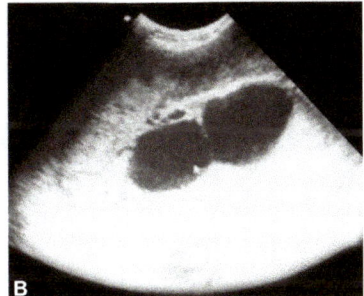

Figs. 20.22.2A and B: Pelviureteric junction obstruction.

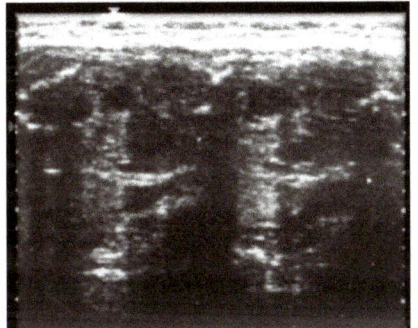

Fig. 20.22.3: Intrauterine hydronephrosis.

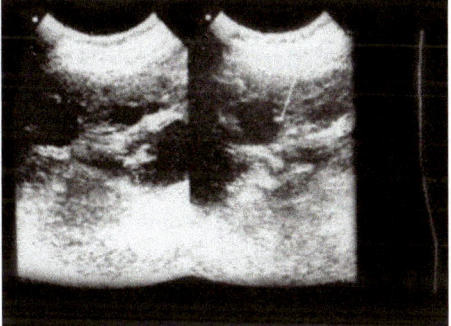

Fig. 20.22.5: Vesicoureteric (VU) reflux Jet.

- <4 mm—normal
- 5-9 mm—mild
- 10-15—moderate
- >15—severe.

Pelviureteric Junction Obstruction

- Most common cause
- Males > females
- About 90% unilateral

On Ultrasonography

- *Dilated PCS:* Normal ureter, bladder
- Renal parenchymal thinning
- Liquor volume normal/increased
- Perinephric urinoma
- Cystic renal dysplasia.

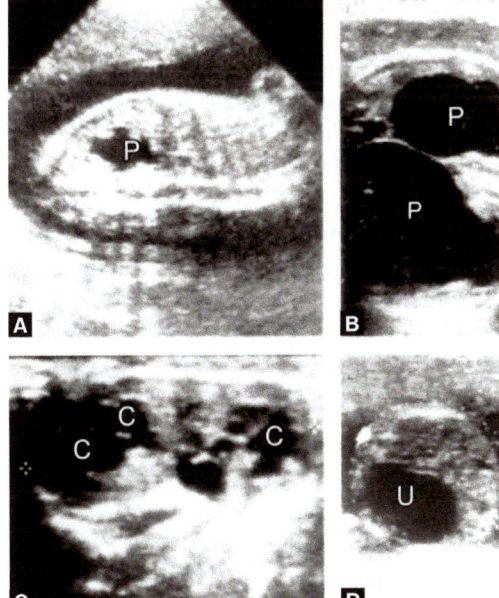

Figs. 20.22.4A to D: Pelviureteric junction (PUJ) obstruction: Obstruction with variable degree of obstruction P—pelvis, C—calyces, P-U—perinephric urinoma with rupture of calyceal system, seen as unilocular paraspinous cystic mass.

Vesicoureteric Junction Obstruction

- Also known as nonrefluxing megaureter
- Male > female
- About 10% cases of fetal hydronephrosis.

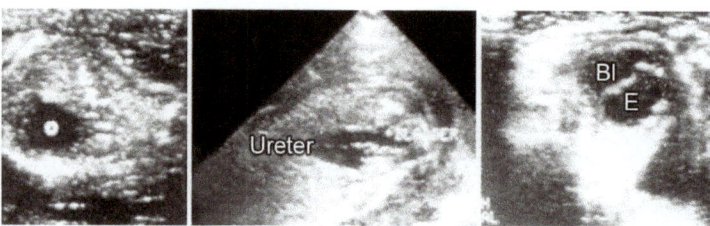

Fig. 20.22.6: Ectopic ureterocele: Ectopic ureterocele with ureterectasia to obstructed upper pole resembles a solitary cyst. It's thickened, displaced lower lobe parenchyma. (Bl: bladder; E: ectopic ureterocele)

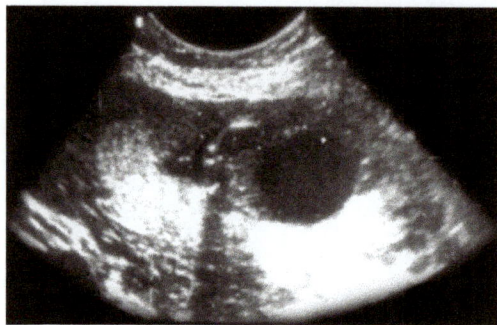

Fig. 20.22.7: Bladder outlet obstruction.

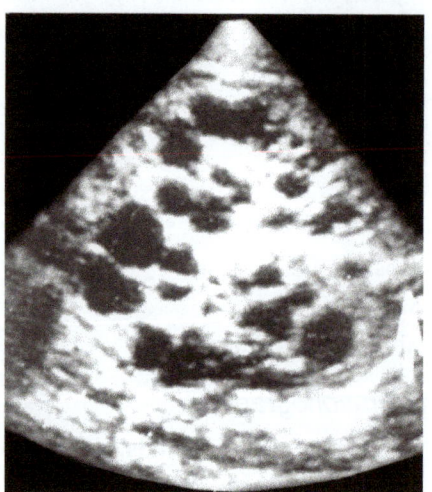

Fig. 20.22.8: Multicystic dysplastic kidney—multiple cysts seen with no communication.

On Ultrasonography

- Dilated ureter and PCS
- Bladder and liquor are normal
- No associated bladder outlet obstruction.

Vesicoureteric Reflux

- Female > male
- Associated with UTI postnatally
- Prenatal diagnosis more common in boys.

On Ultrasonography

Bilateral hydroureteronephrosis with normal liquor volume.

Ureterocele/Ectopic Ureter

- Are cystic dilatation of intravesicle segment of ureter
- Associated commonly with duplex collecting system, especially in girls. It usually collects the upper moiety
- In boys, it usually drains solitary PCS
- Ectopic ureter may be associated
- Insertions of ectopic ureter are inferomedial to normal opening at trigone, bladder neck, urethra, seminal vesicle, vas deferens, ejaculatory duct, vestibule, vagina, and uterus.

On Ultrasonography

- A large kidney is an indirect evidence of duplex PCS
- Hydroureteronephrosis so gross as to distort the definition of PCS and ureter
- Opposite UVJ may be obstructed by ureterocele
- *A ureterocele may prolapse and cause bladder outlet obstruction:* Other causes leading to lower urinary tract obstruction are discussed in next section.

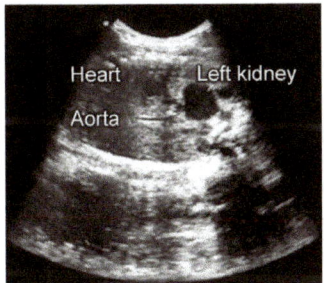
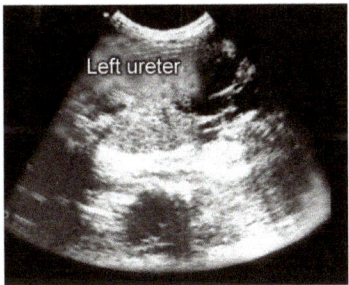

Fig. 20.22.9: Vesicoureteric reflux showing dilated pelvis and dilated ureter.

20.23 FETAL HEAD, NECK AND FACE

Over 150 different abnormalities of head and face have been described in literature. These can be classified according to the pathogenesis, location of anatomical defects and the structures involved **(Figs. 20.23.1A and B)**.

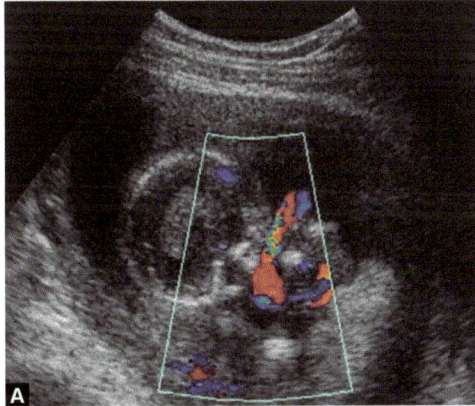
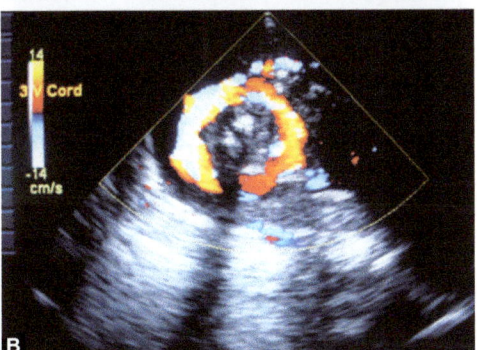

Figs. 20.23.1A and B: Cord around the neck in two patients.

Stewart's Classification

- Otocraniofacial syndromes, i.e. predominantly the ear and mandible involved: Treacher-Collins syndrome, Goldenhar syndrome
- Facial clefting
- *Midface syndromes:* Frontonasal dysplasia, holoprosencephalic malformation syndromes
- Craniosynostosis syndromes.

20.24 DIFFERENTIAL DIAGNOSIS OF MICROGNATHIA

- *Idiopathic:* Mild form
- *Chromosomal:* Trisomy 18, triploidy diseases
- *Skeletal dysplasias:*
  - Campomelic dysplasia
  - Diastrophic dysplasia
  - Achondrogenesis
  - Short rib polydactyly syndrome
- *Genetic syndrome:*
  - Treacher Collins syndrome
  - Goldenhar syndrome
  - Hemifacial microsomia
  - Pierre Robin syndrome
  - Pena-Shokeir syndrome
  - Seckel syndrome
  - DiGeorge syndrome
  - Hydrolethalus syndrome
  - Robert's syndrome
  - Mohr's syndrome
  - Miller's syndrome.

20.25 DIFFERENTIAL DIAGNOSIS OF SYNDROMES ASSOCIATED WITH HYPERTELORISM

- Frontonasal dysplasia
- Frontal encephalocele
- Craniosynostosis syndromes
- DiGeorge syndrome
- Hydrolethalus syndrome
- Coffin-Lowry syndrome
- Noonan's syndrome
- *Larsen syndrome:* 3, 4 and 5 of above are described in relevant sections.

Frontonasal Dysplasia (Median Cleft Syndrome)

A type of midfacial syndrome.

On Ultrasonography

- Marked hypertelorism
- Broad, frequently clefted nasal tip
- Median cleft lip.

Frontal Encephalocele

- East > West
- About 10% of all encephaloceles
- Better prognosis
- Brain tissue may herniate into the defect
- Associated agenesis of corpus callosum, hydrocephalus and microcephaly may be seen
- Anophthalmia may be seen.

Coffin-Lowry Syndrome

Associated with severe mental retardation.

On Ultrasonography

- Macroglossia
- Hypertelorism
- Persistently open mouth
- Cavum excavatum
- Thoracolumbar scoliosis.

Larsen Syndrome

May be diagnosed at 20 weeks I/U.

On Ultrasonography

- Multiple joint dislocation
- Talipes
- Abnormal broad thumb, short metacarpals
- Hemivertebra/butterfly vertebra
- Facial clefting
- *Cardiac defects:* A lethal variant leads to neonatal death due to laryngotracheomalacia and pulmonary hypoplasia. Abnormal palmar creases are seen.

20.26 DIFFERENTIAL DIAGNOSIS OF SYNDROMES ASSOCIATED WITH FRONTAL BOSSING

Skeletal Dysplasias

- Achondroplasia
- Achondrogenesis
- Thanatophoric dysplasia.

Craniosynostosis Syndromes

- Crouzon syndrome
- Pfeiffer syndrome
- Craniofrontonasal dysplasia.

Other Syndromes

- Russell Silver syndrome
- Robinson syndrome
- Hurler's syndrome
  Described in detail in relevant sections.

20.27 DIFFERENTIAL DIAGNOSIS OF SYNDROMES ASSOCIATED WITH CRANIOSYNOSTOSIS AND OTHER CAUSES (TABLE 20.27.1)

- Apert's syndrome
- Carpenter's syndrome

Table 20.27.1: Syndromes associated with craniosynostosis.

	Syndrome	Inheritance	Features	Intelligence
1.	Aperts	AD	• Hypertelorism, turricephaly • Prominent eyes • Syndactyly of toes and fingers (thumb rare)	• 50% mental retardation
2.	Carpenter	AR	• High forehead, flat facial • Midfacial hypoplasia profile • Polydactyly, preaxial—feet, Postaxial—hand	• Variable, can be N, IQ = 54–104
3.	Crouzon	AD	Proptosis, hypertelorism, Frontal boss, beak nose, Premature closure of coronal Sutures, ± clover leaf skull of coronal	Usually normal
4.	Pfeiffer	AD	Craniosynostosis of coronal, Neurological duplicate big toe, compromise is thumb, soft tissue syndactyly	Broad common Broad
5.	Saethre-Chotzen	AD	Hypertelorism, mid-face hypoplasia, high-flat forehead, small ears, craniosynostosis of coronal and lambdoid	Most normal
6.	CFN dysplasia	XLD	• Female > male, frontal bossing, hypertelorism, syndactyly of fingers and toes	Usually normal

(AD: autosomal dominant; AR: autosomal recessive; CFN: craniofrontonasal)

- Crouzon's syndrome
- Pfeiffer syndrome
- Saethre-Chotzen syndrome
- Craniofrontonasal dysplasia
- Isolated.

General Features

- Premature fusion of sutures with subsequent limitation of all related structures
- Secondary increase in ICT
- All sutures except metopic (18 months to 2 years) fuse after fourth decade of life
- Premature fusion of
  - Sagittal suture
  - Coronal suture

Name
Dolichocephaly
Brachycephaly
Acrocephaly
Turricephaly

- All sutures+ hydrocephalus   Clover leaf skull

20.28 DIFFERENTIAL DIAGNOSIS OF CLEFT LIP WITH/WITHOUT CLEFT PALATE

Chromosomal Defect

- Trisomy 18
- Trisomy 13
- Trisomy 21
- Triploidy.

Syndromes and Malformation

- Amniotic band syndrome
- Holoprosencephaly
- Ectodermal dysplasia syndrome

- Robert's syndrome
- Miller's syndrome
- Mohr syndrome
- Frontonasal dysplasia.

20.29 DIFFERENTIAL DIAGNOSIS OF CONDITIONS ASSOCIATED WITH FACIAL CLEFTING

- Facial clefting is the most common congenital anomalies
- Asians >> Black
- Males >> Females [except black boys]
- U/L >> B/L : Left >> Right
- Cleft lip and cleft palate are distinct entities and should not be considered as always one.
- *Four common combinations of facial clefting is noted:*
  1. U/L cleft lip
  2. U/L cleft lip and palate
  3. B/L cleft lip and palate
  4. Isolated cleft palate.
- It occurs due to failure of fusion of medial nasal swellings with the maxillary swelling. Ultrasound classification of facial clefts:

  Normal   Type 1
  Type 2   Type 3
  Type 4   Type 5

USG Appearance and Technique

- Antenatal diagnosis can be established in early second trimester but best is to scan at 18–20 weeks
- A vertical transonic median/paramedian area at upper lip in coronal scanning is noted. This extends to palate if cleft palate is associated
- Bilateral clefting is recognized by the presence of a central echodense mass in the region of upper lip known as premaxillary protrusion. This is best seen in sagittal and axial scanning. This represents abnormal alveolar and gingival tissue resulting from uninhibited growth of the premaxilla caused by lack of continuity of bony, gingival and lip structures.

Isolated Cleft Palate

- Flow of fluid both in mouth and nasopharynx on color Doppler during breathing
- Flow of fluid across the palate
- Polyhydramnios
- Small stomach bubble
- *Defect in posterior palate noted when the pharynx contains fluid:* Once diagnosed, always look for associated anomalies especially cardiac.

Amniotic band syndrome (and limb body wall complex).

- Early amnion rupture allows fetus to enter the chorionic cavity entrapping the fetal parts amongst the fibrous septa that traverse this cavity.

On USG

- Type 5 (usually) facial clefts
- Paramedian encephaloceles
- Gastropleuroschisis
- Limb amputation defects
- Spinal curvature abnormality.
  - Abdominal wall defect + spinal curvature defect—diagnostic.

Ectrodactyly—Ectodermal Dysplasia—Clefting Syndrome (EEC)

Autosomal dominant (AD).

On Ultrasonography

- Lobster claw deformity
- Hydronephrosis, VUR
- Cleft lip/palate.

Robert's Syndrome

Autosomal (lethal in neonates): Premature centromere separation (chromosome puffs) in centromeric staining is diagnostic.

On Ultrasonography

- Cleft lip with/without cleft palate
- Micrognathia
- Prominent premaxilla
- Prominent eyes
- Malformed ears
- Limb reduction defects (more severe in upper limb)
- Congenital heart disease
- Cystic dysplasia of kidneys.

Miller Syndrome (Acrofacial Dysostosis with Postaxial Defects)

Autosomal recessive (AR).

On USG

- Micrognathia
- Cleft lip
- Prominent eyes
- Absent fifth digit in all four limbs
- Ulnar/radial hypoplasia with incurving forearm.

Mohr Syndrome (Orofacial Digital Syndrome)

- Autosomal recessive
- Can be diagnosed as early as 20 weeks.

On USG

- Median cleft lip
- Micrognathia
- High/cleft palate
- Postaxial polydactyly in hand and feet and preaxial also in feet
- Severely hypoplastic tibia.

20.30 FETAL CENTRAL NERVOUS SYSTEM

- Central nervous system abnormalities are the most common cause of referral for prenatal diagnosis—ventriculomegaly and hydrocephalus
- Enlargement of ventricles is referred to as ventriculomegaly while above, when associated with increased intracranial tension and/or head enlargement, is known as hydrocephalus.

On USG

- Occipital horn >10 mm
- Distance of medial ventricular wall from medial border of choroid is >3 mm
- Total distance between lateral edges of the two anterior horns >20 mm (at GA <24 weeks and at BPD <6.5 mm)
- Ventricle to hemisphere ratio as correlated to gestational age from nomograms (35% at 25 weeks)
- Difference of >3 mm in the size of two atria
- Convex wall at anterior horns
- Asymmetry of choroids
- 'Droopy' or 'dangling' choroids
- Undulating septum pellucidum.

Acrania, Anencephaly and Exencephaly (Fig. 20.30.1)

- Acrania—absent cranial vault with a normal brain matter
- Anencephaly—acrania with absence of cerebral hemispheres and diencephalic structures which are replaced by an amorphous mass of neurovascular tissue known as area cerebrovasculosum orbits and face are normal.

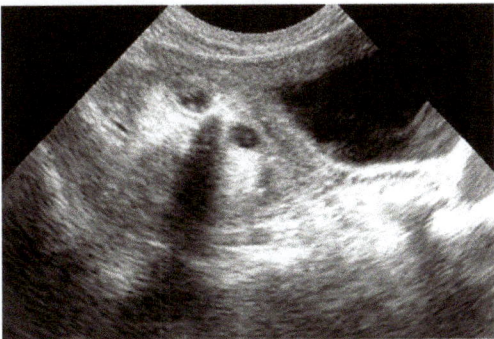

Fig. 20.30.1: US scan shows anencephaly.

- Exencephaly—the amorphous mass described above is identifiable with the normal brain matter
- Cranioschisis—dysraphic abnormality involves the head and entire spine.
    - Above abnormalities are associated with spinal **(Fig. 20.30.2)** non-CNS abnormalities and polyhydramnios
    - These should not be diagnosed with confidence until 11½ weeks when ossification of frontal bones is visible using TVS. The diagnosis is made with 100% confidence only after 14 weeks
    - D/D—amniotic band syndrome
    - Large encephaloceles.

Encephaloceles Including Cephaloceles and Myeloceles

- Are herniations of any part of neural tube through a defect in adjoining part of skull and spine **(Figs. 20.30.3 to 20.30.5)**
- Nomenclature depends on the exact site of defect and the part of neural tube protruding
- Seen as a cystic mass that may or may not contain echogenic internal contents
- *Meckel-Gruber's syndrome is a lethal autosomal recessive condition characterized by polydactyly postaxial (in 55% cases):*
    - Occipital cephalocele (60% to 85%). Polycystic kidneys (100%). Microcephaly may be an associated feature.
- *D/D-Cystic hygroma* **(Figs. 20.30.5A and B):**
    - Hemangioma
    - Teratoma
    - Branchial cleft cyst
    - Scalp edema.

Spina Bifida

Sonographic signs include:
- *Lemon sign—seen mostly <24 weeks:* Bifrontal indentations
- Ventriculomegaly
- Banana sign—obliterated cisterna magna with a smoothly convex posterior cerebellar margin without the bilobed configuration
- Spinal defect with cystic mass
- Slightly smaller fetal head measurement.

Iniencephaly

- Dysraphism involving the back of cranium and contiguous upper spine
- A short neck with star gazing position of child
- Associated anencephaly, Klippel-Feil syndrome may be seen.

Abnormal Cisterna Magna

- Normal size (anteroposterior) is 4–10 mm
- Small in Arnold-Chiari malformation.

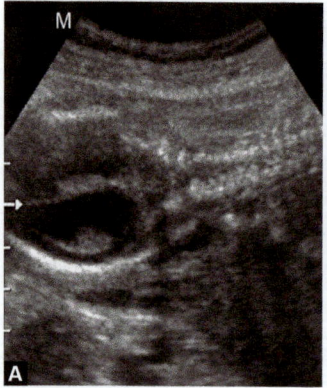
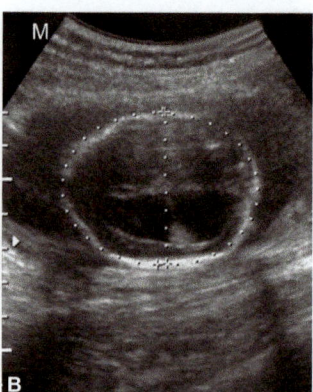

Figs. 20.30.2A and B: US scans show Chiari malformation. (M: mass)

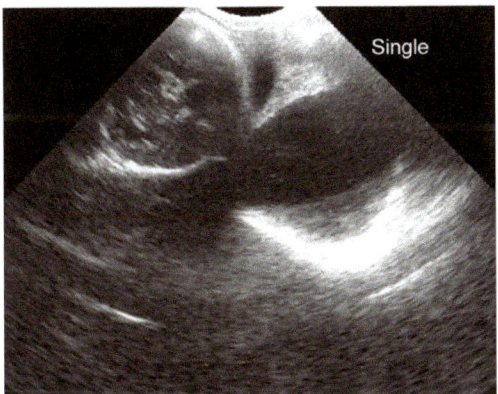

Fig. 20.30.3: US scan shows meningocele of head.

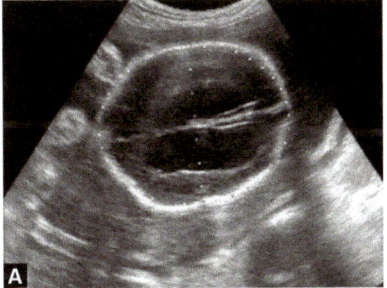

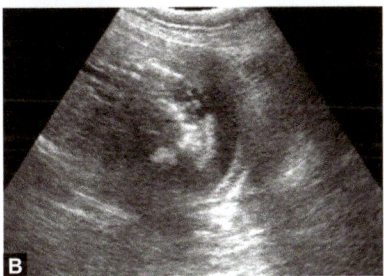

Figs. 20.30.5A and B: US scans show hydrocephalus and spina bifida with meningocele.

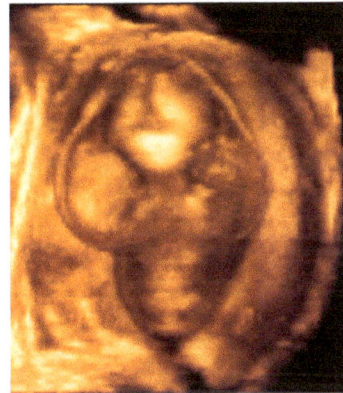

Fig. 20.30.4: 3D US scan shows cystic hygroma of neck.

- *Enlarged in—normal variant:*
  - Tonsillar/cerebellar hypoplasia
  - Communicating hydrocephalus
  - Arachnoid cyst

Dandy-Walker cyst (**Fig. 20.30.6**): Trisomy 18.

Holoprosencephaly

- Hypotelorism
- Midline maxillary cleft
- Cyclopia (Single eye with supraorbital proboscis)
- Ethmocephaly (hypotelorism with proboscis)
- Cebocephaly (hypotelorism with single nostril).

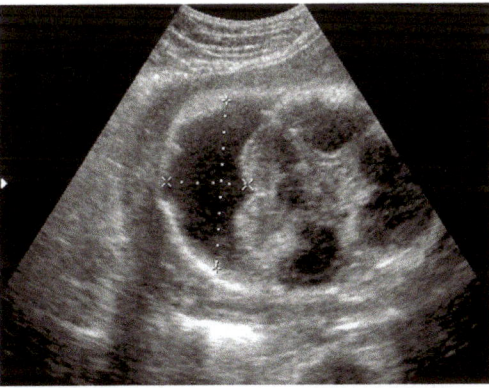

Fig. 20.30.6: US scan shows Dandy-Walker cyst.

- *Alobar type:*
  - Cup type—anterior cup-like cerebral mantle with a dorsal cyst
  - Pancake type—anterior small plate-like cerebrum with a large dorsal cyst
  - Ball type—single featureless
  - Monoventricle surrounded by a mantle of varying widths.
- *Semilobar type:*
  - Rudimentary occipital horns seen.

- *Lobar type:*
  - Absent cavum septum pellucidum
  - Fusion and squaring of frontal horns
  - Rudimentary, fused, abnormal-shaped fornices
  - *D/D—hydrocephalus:* Hydranencephaly.

Dandy-Walker Malformation

Diagnosed at >18 weeks:
- Vermian agenesis/hypoplasia
- Posterior fossa cyst communicating to fourth ventricle
- Elevated tentorium
- Ventriculomegaly
- Agenesis of corpus callosum
- Congenital heart disease
- Polydactyly
- *Genitourinary abnormality:* D/D-Arachnoid cyst—mega cisterna magna.

Hydranencephaly

- Supraclinoid carotid system not seen
- No cortical mantle seen
- Large fluid-filled cavities seen in head.
- *Head size commonly normal:*
  - *D/D—severe hydrocephalus:*
    - Alobar holoprosencephaly
    - Massive congenital subdural hygroma.

Schizencephaly

- On USG, clefts which may be bilateral and symmetrical are noted mainly in parietal and temporal areas
- Such clefts are smooth and lined by gray matter.

Lissencephaly (Agyria)

Diagnosed after 28 weeks:
- Mild ventriculomegaly
- Large, open Sylvian fissure
- Abnormal corpus callosum
- Gyri are absent or broad and flat, known as pachygyria.

Micro/Macrocephaly

- Head size (BPD) below or above 3 SD of normal for that particular age and sex
- *Also altered are:*
  - Head circumference
  - HC: AC
  - FL: HC
  - Frontal lobe size.

Agenesis of Corpus Callosum

- Disproportionately large occipital horns known as colpocephaly
- Lateral displacement of both medial and lateral ventricular wall
- Steer horn-shaped frontal horns
- Interhemispheric cyst/lipoma
- Sunray-like sulci and gyri radiating to ventricular margin
- Third ventricles is high placed and projects between lateral ventricles.

Aqueductal Stenosis

- Large lateral and third ventricles with thinned parenchyma
- Isolated, nonprogressive abnormality.

Space-occupying Lesions

- Arachnoid cyst
- Choroid plexus cyst **(Fig. 20.30.7)**
- Vein of Galen aneurysm
- Teratoma
- Glioblastoma
- Craniopharyngioma
- Neuroblastoma
- Subependymal hamartomas.
  No specific imaging features are noted, the location is the primary diagnostic feature.

Sacrococcygeal Teratoma

- Mass in rump/buttocks
- Solid/solid + cystic
- Calcification frequent

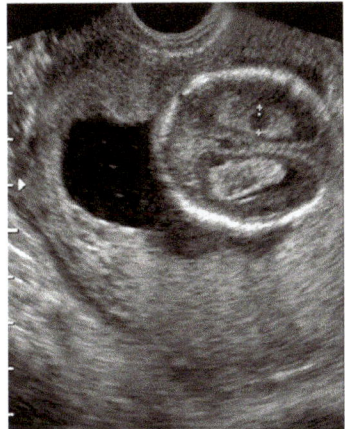

Fig. 20.30.7: US scan shows choroid plexus cyst.

- Displaced/distorted adjacent structures
- Hydronephrosis
- Fetal cardiac failure/hydrops
- *Size <4.5 cm—advise elective vaginal delivery*
  >4.5 cm—advise cesarean.
  - *Differential diagnosis:*
    - Chordoma
    - Anterior myelomeningocele
    - Neuroenteric cyst
    - Neuroblastoma
    - Bone tumor
    - Lymphoma
    - Rectal duplication
    - Lipoma
    - Sarcoma.

Caudal Regression Syndrome

- Ranging in severity from absence of sacrum (or only a part of it) to absence of whole lumbar spine
- Hypoplastic leg, oligohydramnios
- More common (25 times) in diabetic mothers
- Associated abnormalities are VACTERL, kyphoscoliosis, pelvic bone deformity, CTEV

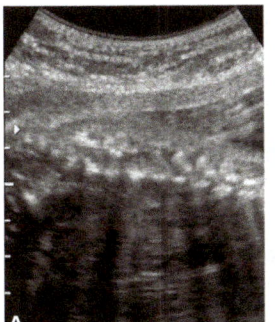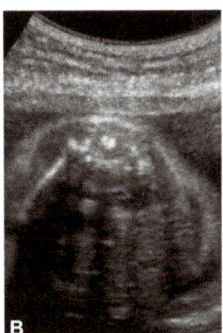

Figs. 20.30.8A and B: US scans show spina bifida with diastematomyelia.

- *Severest form if sirenomelia:*
  - Absent sacrum
  - Fused legs
  - Anorectal atresia
  - Renal agenesis/dysgenesis
  - Cardiac defects: This is also known as Mermaid syndrome.

Diastematomyelia (Figs. 20.30.8A and B)

- Sagittal cleft in spinal cord/conus/filum
- Hydromyelia
- Spina bifida
- Fibrous/bony sagittal septum.

Myelocystocele

- Dilated central canal
- Spina bifida may be absent
- Sac present posteriorly consists of skin, meninges and ependyma-lined hydromyelia sac.
  The overall appearance is known as the 'Cyst within Cyst'.

20.31 FETAL ABDOMINAL WALL DEFECTS

- Gastroschisis
- Omphalocele
- Pentalogy of Cantrell

- Limb-body wall complex known as body stalk abnormality
- Bladder and cloacal exstrophy.

Sonographic Features

Gastroschisis

- Full thickness abdominal wall defect
- Paraumbilical location (usually right) of the defect
- Small size (2–4 cm)
- Free-floating bowel loops in amniotic fluid
- No enveloping membrane.

Omphalocele

- Central anterior abdominal wall defect containing bowel/solid viscera
- Mass encompassed by umbilical cord
- Limiting membrane covering the defect.

Pentalogy of Cantrell

- Midline anterior wall defect usually involving the upper abdomen
- Ectopic heart
- Pericardial/pleural effusion
- Craniofacial abnormality
- Ascites
- Two-vessel-cord
- Omphalocele.

Limb-Body-Wall Complex

- Large ventral wall defect (usually left-sided) of the abdomen and thorax
- Craniofacial abnormality
- Marked scoliosis and/or spinal dysraphism
- Limb defects **(Fig. 20.31.1)**
- Short or absent umbilical cord
- Amniotic bands.

Cloacal Exstrophy (Table 20.31.1)

- Large infraumbilical anterior wall defect with irregular anterior wall mass
- Absent bladder
- Malformation of the genitalia
- May be neural tube defects.

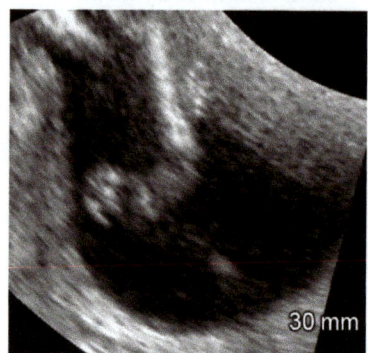

Fig. 20.31.1: 3D US scan shows clubfoot.

Table 20.31.1: Fetal limb body wall and cloacal defects.

		Gastroschisis	Omphalocele	Limb-body wall complex	Cloacal exstrophy
1.	Location	Right paraumbilical	Infraumbilical insertion site	Midline, at cord left	Lateral, usually
2.	Size of defect	Small (2–4 cm)	Variable (2–10 cm)	Large	Variable
3.	Membrane	—	+	+ (contiguous to placenta)	Variable
4.	Liver involvement	—	Common	+	+
5.	Ascites	—	Common	—	Variable
6.	Bowel thickening and dilatation	+	—	—	Variable (unless ruptured)

Contd...

Contd...

7.	Bowel complications	Common	—	—	—
8.	Cardiac abnormalities	Rare	Common (ASD, PDA) (complex)	Common	10–15%
9.	Chromosomal abnormalities	—	Common	—	Variable
10.	MS-AFP	+	+/–		
11.	Other abnormalities	Rare	Common	Always (scoliosis, cranial defect, limb defects)	Always genitourinary, spinal

20.32 NUCHAL FOLD AND TRANSLUCENCY

		Nuchal fold thickness	Translucency
1.	Measurement section	Axial; thalami, occipital bone and cerebellum seen	Sagittal; Midsagittal section of head
2.	From–to	Outer edge of bone to outer interface	Outer edge of bone to subcutaneous surface of skin
3.	Normal measurement with GA	14–18 weeks >5 mm—abnormal 4–5 mm—borderline <4 mm—normal 18–22 weeks >6 mm—abnormal 5–6 mm—borderline <5 mm—normal	10–14 weeks >3 mm is abnormal At 10–12 weeks 1.5 mm = 50th percentile 2.5 mm = 95th percentile At 12–14 weeks 2 mm = 50th percentile 3 mm = 95th percentile
4.	Indicate	• Trisomy 21	• Cardiac abnormality • Chromosomal abnormality (18,13,21) • Cystic hygroma

20.33 PRENATAL SONOGRAPHIC DIAGNOSIS OF CARDIAC ANOMALIES

Common indications for fetal echocardiogram:
- Abnormal four-chambered view on screening USG
- Fetal hydrops
- Polyhydramnios
- Fetal arrhythmias
- Chromosomal abnormalities
- Extracardiac abnormalities
- Family history of CHD/syndromes associated with CHD
- Maternal diseases as diabetes, phenylketonuria, collagen vascular diseases
- Teratogen exposure (Rubella, alcohol, and drugs)
- Monitoring response to intrauterine therapy
- Monitoring fetus at risk for decompensation in cases of hydrops, persistent tachyarrhythmias.

Best Timing for Echocardiography

- It is 18–22 weeks, as before 18 weeks, heart is very small; while after 22 weeks, bony

shadow, less liquor, awkward fetal position limit the examination
- With vaginal probe the procedure may be done as early as 12-13 weeks.

STRUCTURAL DEFECTS
Atrial Septal Defects
Arises after 4-6 weeks.

On Ultrasonography
- Difficult to distinguish small pathologic ASD from PFO
- A PFO is about 1 mm less than the aortic root diameter while ASD is larger than this
- The primum ASD is low placed in atrial septum near AV valve.

Ventricular Septal Defect
- Highest recurrence rate
- Most teratogen-associated defect.

On Ultrasonography
- An area of discontinuity in interventricular septum
- On color Doppler, bidirectional interventricular shunting with a systolic right to left and late diastolic left to right shunt
- Unidirectional shunting indicates additional abnormalities.

Atrioventricular Septal Defects
Occurs due to malformation in atrioventricular cushion.

On Ultrasonography
- Defect in atrial and/or ventricular septum
- Single abnormal A-V valve seen
- Demonstration of bridging leaflet is a confirmatory evidence of incomplete type AVSD
- Color Doppler shows a defect across endocardial cushion and abnormal A-V valve with valvular insufficiency
- A left ventricle to right atrial jet may be seen
- Holosystolic insufficiency on color Doppler is a late but ominous abnormality.

Ebstein Anomaly
- Inferior displacement of the tricuspid valve, frequently with leathered attachment of leaflets, tricuspid dysplasia and right ventricular dysplasia
- Most commonly associated with maternal lithium exposure.

On Ultrasonography
- Apical displacement of tricuspid valve in right ventricle
- Enlarged right atrium containing a part of atrialized right ventricle
- Reduction in size of atrialized right ventricle
- TR seen on color Doppler
- M-mode shows presence of arrhythmias, especially supraventricular tachycardias.

Hypoplastic Right/Left Heart Syndromes
Hypoplasia of ventricle due to inflow reduction (tricuspid/mitral atresia) or due to outflow reduction (pulmonary/aortic reduction).

On Ultrasonography
- Small respective ventricle with concentric hypertrophy
- Hypoplastic/atretic respective inflow and/or outflow channels
- On color Doppler, single area of flow at A-V valve level. A decreased flow is seen if only hypoplasia of channels is present
- Associated arrhythmias and CHF may be seen.

Univentricle Heart
Due to failure of development of interventricular septum, a single ventricle, having LV

morphology, but no outflow tract (type B) or common outflow tract (type A) is seen.

On Ultrasonography

- Single ventricle with absent interventricular septum
- Color Doppler is used to confirm or refute the presence of an outflow tract ... d/d between type A and B.

Tetralogy of Fallot

- Due to far anterior placement of conus septum, thus dividing the conus into smaller anterior right ventricular portion and a large posterior part. Closure of interventricular septum is thus incomplete leading to aortic over-riding
- Diagnosis can be made on or before 15 weeks using EVS probe.

On Ultrasonography

- Perimembranous VSD
- Dilated aorta.

Persistent Truncus Arteriosus

- A single large vessel arises from base of heart supplying coronary, systemic and arterial circulations
- VSD is almost always associated
- Truncal valve has two to six cusps and over-rides the ventricular septum.

On Ultrasonography

Around 15 weeks
- Above described defects seen
- Color Doppler is very helpful in localizing pulmonary arterial and estimating the presence of insufficiency.

Double Outlet Right Ventricle

More than 50% of both aorta and pulmonary artery arise from right ventricle.

On Ultrasonography

- Above defects are noted. Three types seen:
  - Aorta posterior and right to pulmonary artery
  - Both parallel with aorta to the right (Taussig-Bing syndrome)
  - Both parallel with the aorta anterior and to the left.

Transposition of Great Arteries

Two types:
1. *Complete or dextrotransposition (D-TGA):*
   - *Atrioventricular concordance with ventriculoarterial discordance:*
     - VSD present (30%)
     - VSD absent (70%)
2. *Congenitally corrected or levotransposition (L-TGA):*
   - Atrioventricular discordance with ventriculoarterial discordance
   - *On USG:*
     - Great vessels exit the heart parallel to each other rather than crossing
     - Color Doppler characterizes the flow.

Anomalous Pulmonary Venous Return

Due to failure of obliteration of normal embryological connections between the primitive pulmonary veins and the splanchnic, umbilical, vitelline and umbilical veins such that none or only few pulmonary veins drain into left atrium.

On Ultrasonography

- Mild prominence of right ventricle and pulmonary artery
- On duplex Doppler, a ratio of right to left flow of >2%
- Small left atrium.

Coarctation of Aorta

On Ultrasonography

- Right to left ventricle diameter ratio more than 2 SD above the normal
- Pulmonary artery to ascending aorta diameter ratio more than 2 SD than normal
- Presence of distal aortic arch hypoplasia.

Cardiosplenic Syndromes

Are defects of lateralization in which symmetric development of normally asymmetric organ/organ system occurs?

- *Asplenia (Bilateral right sidedness):*
    - Right atrial isomerism
    - Bilateral trilobed lung
    - Bilateral right bronchi
    - Bilateral right pulmonary arteries
    - Ipsilateral location of aorta and IVC
    - Absence of spleen
    - Midline horizontal liver
    - Bilateral superior vena cava
    - Severe and complex heart abnormalities.
- *Polysplenia (bilateral left sidedness):*
    - Interruption of IVC
    - Azygous continuation of IVC
    - Multiple spleens
    - Left atrial isomerism
    - Complete A-V block.

Cardiac Tumors

- 75%—Rhabdomyoma
- 19%—Teratoma
- 12%—Fibroma
- 2%—Cardiac hemangioma
- 2%—Mesothelioma of A-V node.

Rhabdomyoma

- Single/multiple
- Project in the cavity
- From interventricular septum
- 30–78% have tuberous sclerosis.

Teratoma

Solid + Cystic.

Ectopia Cordis

- Due to failure of fusion of the lateral body fold in the thoracic region
- Heart located out of thorax
- May be a part of pentalogy of Cantrell.

Arrhythmias (Diagnosed on M-Mode)

- Premature atrial/ventricular
- *Tachycardia:*
    - Heart rate >180 bpm
    - Mostly supraventricular
    - *Four types:*
        1. 180–300 bpm with conduction
        2. Rate 1:1 = PSVT
        3. 300–400 bpm + 2:1/4:1 = flutter
        4. >400 bpm atrial rate + ventricular rate 120–160 bpm = fibrillation
- *Bradycardia*: Prolonged heart rate <100 bpm for >10 seconds.

Index

Page numbers followed by *f* refer to figure.

A

Abdomen 37
Abdominal disease 8
Abdominal pathology 149, 151
Abdominal tuberculosis 105*f*, 142*f*
  case of 106*f*
Abdominal wall
  abscess 71*f*
  anterior 72
  defect 284
  masses 70
    common 70
    uncommon 71
Abortion 264
  complete 264
  incomplete 248, 248*f*, 264
  missed 265*f*
  threatened 264
Abscess 47, 49, 52*f*, 70, 92*f*, 110*f*, 156, 157, 206, 208
  amebic 51
  epididymal 157*f*
  hepatic 76
  iliopsoas 184*f*
  intraperitoneal 145
  mediastinal 10
  multiple 29*f*
  pyogenic 51, 84, 85
  renal 77
  scrotal 149*f*
  subperiosteal 206
  subphrenic 11, 78, 78*f*
Acalculus cholecystitis 68
Acardiac parabiotic twin 270
Acetabular roofline 181, 182*f*
Acetabulum labrum 181
Achalasia
  primary 98
  secondary 98
Achondrogenesis 268, 275, 276

Achondroplasia 276
Acinar cell tumor 93
Acquired immunodeficiency syndrome 41
Acrania 279
Actinomycosis 103
Acute respiratory distress syndrome 8
Addison's disease 140
Adenocarcinoma 93, 103, 131, 133, 137, 163
  colon 81*f*, 113
  colon, case of 88*f*
  mucinous 43
  of pyloric antrum 100*f*
  pancreatic 43
Adenofibrolipoma 175
Adenoid cystic tumor 206
Adenoma 14, 41, 93, 97, 121, 137
  adrenal 137, 137*f*
  nephrogenic 130
  papillary 63
  pleomorphic 28*f*, 200, 206
Adenomatous nodule 14, 16*f*
Adenomyomatosis 63, 63*f*, 64
Adenomyosis 236, 246
  focal 239*f*
Adenopathy
  hilar 1
  mesenteric 144*f*
Adenosis, sclerosing 169
Adhesions 254
Adnexal lesions, bilateral 237
Adnexal mass 230, 236, 250, 266
  cystic 232
Adnexal tenderness 266
Adrenal calcifications 140
Adrenal cortex, layers of 139
Adrenal gland 136, 139*f*
  bilateral large 136

Adrenal hyperplasia, congenital 136
Adrenal masses
  cystic 140
  large solid 139
  lesion 137*f*
  unilateral 137
Adrenocarcinomas 139
Agenesis 195
  renal 272
Agyria 282
Alkaptonuria 188
Alobar holoprosencephaly 210, 211, 214
Alpha thalassemia 268
Amebic abscess, large 52
Amniotic band 284
  syndrome 277, 278
Amniotic fluid assessment 259
Amniotic sacs 269*f*
Amorphous mass 280
Amyloid arthropathy 177
Amyloidosis 188
Amyotropic lateral sclerosis 11
Anaplastic carcinoma thyroid 21*f*
Anechoic retroperitoneal cyst 115*f*
Anemia 268
  maternal severe 255
  severe 268
Anencephaly 279
Aneurysm 176, 207
  dissecting 79*f*
Angioma, cutaneous 196
Angiomyolipoma 120, 121, 123
Angiosarcoma 86, 89, 168
Annular pancreas 102
Anomalous pulmonary venous return 287
Anophthalmia 195, 256
Anorectal malformation 228

Aorta
  aneurysm of 10
  coarctation of 258, 288
  ipsilateral location of 288
Apert's syndrome 207, 276
Appendiceal perforation 108
Appendicitis 106
  acute 80, 80f
  case of 110f, 111
  differential diagnosis of 108
Appendicolith 80, 111f
Appendicular lump 108, 111
Appendix, mucocele of 109f
Aqueductal stenosis 211, 282
  congenital 212
Arachnoid cyst 208, 215, 225f, 282
Arnold-Chiari malformation 212f, 280
Arrhythmias 288
Artefactual masses 74
Arterial bypass grafts, subcutaneous 73
Arterioarterial anastomosis 270
Arteriovascular malformations 207
Arteriovenous malformation 120, 201, 217
Artery
  sign, prominent feeding 112
  umbilical 256
Arthritis
  infective 178
  inflammatory 176
  pyogenic 179f
  septic 176, 177
Arthropathy
  crystal-induced 177
  hemophilic 177
Articular cartilage calcification, causes of 188
Ascaris lumbricoides 70
Ascending colon, thickening of 105f
Ascites 4, 11, 142f
  outlining bowel loops 143f
Asphyxia 219
Asphyxiating thoracic dystrophy 268

Asplenia 288
  syndrome 83
Asteroid hyalosis 197
Atherosclerotic plaque 33f
Atresia
  bronchial 262
  laryngeal 262
Atrial septal defects 286
Atrioventricular septal defects 256, 286
Atrophy 208
Autoimmune disorders 25
Autosomal dominant 120, 278
Avascular necrosis 176

B

Baker's cyst 176
Banana sign 280
Bardet retinal dystrophy 272
Baum's bumps 191
Beak sign 112
Bear's criteria 120
Beckwith-Wiedemann syndrome 272
Benign tumors 30, 47, 241
  cystadenoma 241
  cystic teratoma 241
  hemangioma 30
  lipoma 31
  nerve tumors 31
Bertin
  hypertrophied column of 117, 117f
  prominent septum of 117
Bile duct
  common 56f, 67f, 70f
  hamartoma 49, 50, 69
  malignancy 69
Biliary cyst
  adenoma 49, 54
  congenital 66
Biloma 49, 64, 70f
Bladder
  contour and caliber abnormality 133
  diverticulum 233
  masses 236
  mucosae herniate 233

  outlet obstruction 130, 132, 133, 164f, 274f
  case of 133f
  wall
    hypertrophy 133f
    thickening 130
Blighted ovum 265
Blood clot 123
Blunt abdominal trauma 55f
Bochdalek hernia 262
Bone
  cysts, aneurysmal 206
  dysplasias 258
  tumor 283
Bony fragments 176
Bowel
  and colon, small 102
  complications 285
  loops, adherent 242
  masses 236
  thickening 104f
Bowman's layer 189
Brachial cyst 28f
Brachycephaly 258
Bradycardia 260, 288
Brain
  abscess 216
  destructive lesions of 210
Branchial cyst 28
Breast 166
  abscess 167, 168f
    space-occupying lesion 168f
  anatomy 166f
  anechoic lesion 168f
  carcinoma 43, 174f
  chronic abscess 167f
  ductal ectasia in 170f
  fibroadenoma 173f
  fibrocystic disease of 172f
  lipoma in 171f
  metastatic 48f
  neoplasm, benign 169f
  parenchyma 166f
  prosthesis 171
  simple cyst in 167f
  ultrasound 166
Brenner tumor 236
Bromobenzyl cyanide 193
Brucellosis 45

Bruch's membrane 189, 196
Bulky lacrimal glands 205
Bull's eye 45, 47

C

Calcium pyrophosphate
    dehydrate deposition
    disease 188
Calculus
  cholecystitis, acute 62
  renal 123
Caliceal calculus, multiple 126f
Caliectasis, focal 125f
Campomelic dysplasia 275
Cancer, endometrial 247
Candida forming fungal balls 118
Candidiasis 41, 45, 87
Carcinoid 142
  fibrotic reaction of 142
Carcinoma 14
  adenosquamous 93
  anaplastic carcinoma thyroid 20
  cervix 245f
  colon 104f
  colorectal 43
  cortical 139
  endometrial 236, 246, 253, 254
  endometrioid 236
  esophageal 97
  follicular 19
  gastric 98
  intracystic 167, 172
  maxilla 206
  medullary thyroid 20
  mucoepidermoid 28
  pancreatic 70
  papillary 19, 24
  stomach, case of 99f
Carcinomatosis 145
Cardiac failure, congestive 41
Cardiosplenic syndromes 288
Caroli's disease 49, 50, 69
Caroticocavernous fistula 192, 193, 200, 207
Carotid artery, common 15, 26f
Carpenter's syndrome 276
Cartilage convexity,
    development of 182
Cataract 196
  case of 205
Caudal regression syndrome 223, 228, 283
Cavum
  excavatum 276
  septi pellucidi 216f
  septum pellucidum 216
  vergae 216, 216f
Cecum 103, 103f
Celiac artery 92
Cell implantation, malignant 9
Cellular lining 85
Central nervous system 218
Central retinal artery 192
  occlusion 192
Central retinal vein occlusion 192
Cephalocele 207, 280
Cerebellum 210
Cerebral
  edema 220
  hemorrhage 218
Cerebritis 220
Cerebrospinal fluid 210
  post-traumatic leakage of 223
Cerebrovascular complications 222
Cervical
  carcinoma 246, 254
  esophagus, tumor of 32
  fibroid 244f
  lymph nodes
    enlarged 19
    levels 33
    multiple enlarged 36
    posterior 34f
  lymphadenopathy 33
    features of 33
  phlegmon 29
  stenosis 254
Cesarean scar 72
Chemodectoma, malignant 32
Chest 1
  film, lateral 3
  wall 1
    cold abscess 188f
    muscle, worm in 187f
Chiari malformation 214, 280f
Chloroacetophenone 56f, 193
Cholangiocarcinoma, hilar 57f, 68
Cholangitis 46
  sclerosing 39, 113
Cholecystitis 45, 46
  acute 46f, 76
  chronic 60
  gangrenous 63, 64
  signs of chronic 61f
Choledochal cyst 66, 69
  types of 67f
Choledocholithiasis 70
Cholelithiasis 64f
Cholesterol
  crystals 85
  polyps 64
Chorioangioma 269
Choriocarcinoma 43, 159, 250, 266
Chorionic villi 251
Choristoma 196
Choroid
  detachment 204f
  disease of 199
  plexus
    cyst 208, 215, 282, 283
    enlarged 222
    papilloma 209, 220
    prominent 209
    tumor 222
Choroidal
  detachment 194
    differential diagnosis 199
  excavation 196
  hemangioma 192, 196
  melanoma 192, 196, 204f
  osteoma 196
Chromosomal abnormality 268, 285
  ultrasound signs of 256
Chromosomal defect 277
Ciliary artery occlusion 192
Cirrhosis 4, 37
  biliary 39
  case of 38f
  classified 38

etiology 38
portal vein wall 38f
sonographic findings of 39
Cisterna magna, abnormal 280
Classical hydatid cyst 53f
Claw sign 112
Cleft
　bilateral 215
　lip 256, 277, 279
　palate 256, 277, 278
　unilateral 215
Clinodactyly 256
Cloacal defects 284
Cloacal exstrophy 284
Clonorchis sinensis 70
Coat's disease 199
Coffin-Lowry syndrome 276
Colitis 76
Collagen vascular disease 8
Colloid goiter 17f, 35
Colpocephaly 208, 214
Conjoined twins 270
Connective tissue tumor 93
Cord
　atrophy 229
　laceration 229
Cornea 189
　layers of 191
Corpus callosum, agenesis of 215, 257, 282
Corpus luteal cyst 236
　ovary sign of 240f
Cortical sac 127f
Corticosteroids, endogenous 37
Craniopharyngioma 282
Cranioschisis 280
Craniosynostosis syndromes 275-277
Crohn's disease 104, 113
Crouzon's syndrome 207, 276, 277
Cryptophthalmos 195
Crystal deposition 176
Cubitus valgus 258
Cul-de-sac
　free fluid in 230
　posterior 230, 231
Curvilinear hyperechoic scar 175

Cyclophosphamide cystitis 130, 131
Cyclopia 256, 281
Cyst
　adrenal 140
　benign 156, 206
　bronchogenic 10
　congenital 10
　cortical 119
　epidermoid 83, 84, 154, 156, 157, 201f
　epididymal 160
　epithelial 140
　extrarenal 120
　filarial 168
　follicular 236
　functional 232
　hemorrhagic 230, 234, 236, 237f
　hepatic 49
　in testis 157
　infected 48f, 167
　interhemispheric 208
　leptomeningeal 208, 218
　mesenteric 145, 145f, 233
　neuroenteric 10, 283
　oil 167, 173
　peribiliary 49, 50, 69
　pericardial 10
　popliteal 176
　porencephalic 208, 210, 211
　post-traumatic 218
　renal 117
　　cortical 257
　retention 91, 162
　retroperitoneal 116
　subependymal 208, 215
　testicular 156f
　umbilical 72, 72f
　vitreous 206
　with debris 91
　with solid 91
Cystadenocarcinoma 49, 54, 56, 68, 236, 241f, 242
Cystadenoma 56, 58, 235, 236
　mucinous 243f
　serous 237f, 241f
Cystic adenomatoid malformation, pulmonary 262

Cystic degeneration 10, 16f
Cystic disease, uremia associated 120
Cystic dysplasia 154, 156, 157
　familial 118
　hereditary 118
Cystic lesion
　hypoechoic 145f
　infective 216
Cystic nephroma
　benign 121
　multilocular 119, 120, 121
Cystic pancreatic masses, differential diagnosis of 91
Cystic renal disease 272
　differential diagnosis of 118
Cystic teratoma, mature 10
Cysticercosis 198f, 206
Cysticercus 73f
　cyst 72
Cystitis
　cystica 132
　glandularis 132
Cytomegalovirus 136, 215, 220, 221

D

Dacryoadenitis 205
Dandy-Walker
　cyst 281, 281f
　malformation 208, 282
　syndrome 213f, 214
Daughter cysts, multiple 54
De Quervain's thyroiditis 19f
Debris 85
Dermal sinus 228
Dermoid 207, 240f
　cyst 238, 242f
　mesenteric 145
Descemet's membrane 189
Diabetes 37
　mellitus 154
　maternal 255, 285
Diabetic retinopathy 192, 200
Diaphragm
　bilateral 10
　eventration of 12, 263

part of 13
unilateral 11
Diaphragmatic hernias,
    congenital 262
Diastematomyelia 223, 225, 226f, 283
Diastrophic dysplasia 275
Dichorionic diamniotic twins 269f
Diffuse toxic goiter 19
    case of 18f
DiGeorge syndrome 275, 276
Dilated fluid-filled jejunal loops 102f
Dilated small bowel 102
    loop 106f
Distal small bowel obstruction 102
Distal ureters, dilated 233
Diverticular disease 106
Diverticulitis 76, 142
Dorsal dermal sinus 223, 225
Dorsal interhemispheric cyst 215
Double outlet right ventricle 256, 287
Down's syndrome 101
Dromedary hump 117
Duct
    ectasia 170
    dilated 170
Ductal carcinoma
    in situ 170
    invasive 170, 173
Ductal dilatation 170
Ductal ectasia, mucinous 92
Dumb-bell masses, solid 264
Duodenal atresia 256
Duodenum 101
    dilatation of 101
    mechanical obstruction 101
Dysgerminoma 243
Dysostosis, acrofacial 279
Dysplasia
    craniofrontonasal 276, 277
    fibrous 206
    frontal 276, 278
    renal 256

    cystic 118
    thanatophoric 268, 276
Dysraphic defect, large 225f

E

Ears, malformed 279
Ebstein anomaly 286
Echinococcal cyst 140
Echinococcus granulosus 43, 51
Echogenic fetal kidneys,
    differential diagnosis of 271
Ectodermal dysplasia syndrome 277
Ectopia cordis 288
Ectopia lentis 196
Edema
    placental 267
    subcutaneous 186f, 267
    subserosal 68
Egg shell-like calcification 22
Ejaculatory duct
    calculi 154
    cyst 163
    dilatation, bilateral 163f
    obstruction 162
    prominent 164
Embedded organ sign 112
Emboli, pulmonary 8
Embryonal cell carcinoma 153, 158
Empyema 3, 208, 217, 222
    subdural 209f
Encephalocele
    frontal 276
    paramedian 278
Encephalomalacia, cystic 208, 211
Endodermal sinus 158
    tumor 153, 158, 243
Endometrial cavity 253f
Endometrial hyperplasia 236, 247, 251
    causes 251
    ultrasound 251
Endometrial polyp 247, 251, 251f-253f
    feeding vessel sign of 253f

Endometrioma 72, 234, 236, 237, 238f
Endometriosis 132, 254f
Endometritis 254
Endometrium 80
    hyperplastic 230f
    thickened 247
Endophthalmitis 192, 197
Entamoeba histolytica 51
Enteric cyst 264
Ependymoma 220
Epididymal tubules, dilated 160
Epididymis 156
    chronic 150f
    cystic lesion in head of 150f
    enlargement of 161
    region of head of 160f
Epididymitis 149, 160f
    chronic 151, 161
    thickened 150
Epigastrium
    differential diagnosis for 75
    transverse scan of 92f
Episcleritis 202
Epithelioma, bronchial 32
Epithelium 189
Escherichia coli 222
Esophageal duplication cyst 10
Esophagus 97
Ethyl iodoacetate 193
Extracapsular nodal spread 33
Extraocular muscles, lesions of 202
Exudative pleural effusion,
    causes of 6
Eye, vertical section of 191f
Eyeball 189
    evaluation of 191
    lesions of 202
    vascular layer of 189

F

Fallopian tube 231f
    carcinoma of 236, 240
    dilated 255f
Fasciola hepatica 70
Fat
    fluid levels 113
    necrosis 169, 173

Fatty infiltration 37
  focal 38f, 41
Fatty metamorphosis 43
Femur head 182, 183f
Fetal
  abdominal wall defects 283
  anemia 255
  arrhythmias 285
  calcification, intra-
    abdominal 260, 261
  cardiac failure 283
  central nervous system 279
  echocardiogram, indications
    for 285
  head, neck and face 275
  hydronephrosis 272
  hydrops 255, 285
  limb body wall 284
  lobulations 117
  thoracic abnormalities,
    differential diagnosis
    of 262, 263
Fibrillation 260
Fibrin balls 8, 9
Fibroadenolipomas 171
Fibroadenoma 169, 169f, 172,
    172f
  juvenile 169, 173
Fibroid 236
  uterus 243f
Fibroma 13, 98, 288
  nonossifying 206
  pleural 8, 9
Fibromatosis 142
Fibrosis 41
  retroperitoneal 113
  scar 175
  secondary 99
Fibrous histiocytoma
  benign 193
  malignant 86, 113
Fibrous septae 222
Fine-needle aspiration cytology
    18f, 74f, 82f, 169f, 174,
    201f
Floating aorta sign 82
Fluid
  debris level 146f, 235f
  distended bowel 233
  endometrial 254
  filled bowel, wall of 97

Follicular adenoma 24f
  case of 20f
Fraser syndrome 272
Fuchs spots 196
Fungal infection 118

G

Galactocele 168
Galen aneurysm, vein of 282
Galen malformation, vein of
    208, 211, 217
Gallbladder 39f
  adenomyomatosis of 63f
  anterior wall of 65f
  carcinoma 62-64
  dilatation 62
  mass 64f
  neck mass 58f, 64f
  perforation 61f, 62, 68
  polyp, evidence of 65
  thickening 40
    focal 63
  tumefactive sludge in 66f
  wall
    posterior 61
    thickened 68f
    varices 63
Gallstone 46
  with acoustic shadowing 65f
  with intrahepatic dilatation
    69f
Gamna-Gandy nodules 89, 90
Ganglion cysts 176
Ganglioneuroma 31, 139, 140
Gartner duct cyst 255
Gastric
  dilatation 99, 101
    gas in stomach wall 100
    mechanical obstruction
      99
    paralytic ileus 100
  diverticulum 140
  emphysema, interstitial 100
  fundus 140
  lymphoma 98
  wall
    hypertrophic 101f
    thickening of 98
Gastrinoma 93, 95
Gastritis

  emphysematous 100
  granulomatous 99
Gastrocnemio-
    semimembranosus
    bursa 176
Gastroesophageal junction 98f
Gastrointestinal
  abnormality 268
  tract 97, 196
    ultrasound differential
    diagnosis of 97
Gastropleuroschisis 278
Gastroschisis 283, 284
Gaucher's disease 86, 87
Genetic
  disorders 268
  syndrome 275
Genital tract
  calcification, extratesticular
    male 154
  obstructed 232
Genitalia, malformation of 284
Genitourinary
  abnormality 282
  system 272
Germ cell
  origin, benign tumors of 157
  tumors 113, 151, 153, 158,
    236
  differentiating features of
    159
  malignant 243
  mixed 159
  necrotic 235
Germinal matrix hemorrhage
    218, 218f
Gestation
  ectopic 233
  sac 265
Gestational sac, anembryonic
    265f
Gestational trophoblastic
  disease 248, 265, 266
  neoplasia 258
Ghost artifact 74
Giant fibroadenoma 169, 173
  large mass 169f
Gland, adrenal 138
Glandular enlargement, diffuse
    17
Gliding sign 8

Glioblastoma 282
Glioma 200, 202
Gliotic white matter 210
Glomerulonephritis, acute 4
Glucogenoma 93
Glycogen storage disease 37
Goldenhar syndrome 275
Gonadal stromal tumor 153
Gout 188
Granuloma 89, 206
  healed 44f
Granulosa cell tumor 154
Graves' disease 19, 192, 201, 202, 206
Great arteries, transposition of 287
Gut atresias 256
Gynecomastia 172

H

Haemophilus influenzae 222
Hair tufts 223
Halo, absence of 16
Hamartoma 86, 168, 171, 175
  subependymal 282
Hamartomatous lesions 140
Hansemann's giant cells 118
Harada's disease 199
Hashimoto's thyroiditis 19
  case of 19
Head
  complete dislocation of 183f
  femur development of 178
  meningocele of 281f
Heart
  disease, congenital 279, 282
  univentricle 286
Hemangioendothelioma 260, 261
Hemangioma 41, 42, 55, 86, 92, 98, 131, 132, 139, 141, 168, 187f, 205, 206, 260
  capillary 200, 201
  cardiac 288
  cavernous 42, 47, 49, 92, 200
  giant cavernous 55
  retinal capillary 192
  tip of nose 187f
Hemangiothelioma 31f

Hematocolpos 232f
Hematohydrocolpos 244
Hematoma 49, 70, 84, 151, 175, 202, 206, 230, 233
  acute 175
  chronic 218
  intraparenchymal 84
  perisplenic 84f
Hematometra 232f, 255f
Hematometrocolpos 244f
Hematopoiesis, extramedullary 116
Hematosalpinx 255f
Hemifacial microsomia 275
Hemochromatosis 39, 188
Hemorrhage
  adrenal 77, 136
  intracranial 209, 209f, 218
  intraocular 192
  intraparenchymal 219
  intraventricular 209, 210f, 219, 222
  placental 257f
  splenic 80
  subarachnoid 219
  subchorionic 262
  subependymal 218, 219
  subhyaloid 197, 198
  vitreous 194, 198, 200, 201f
Hemothorax 3
Henoch-Schönlein purpura 149, 151
Hepatic adenoma 47, 56
  presence of 42f
Hepatic dysfunction 62
Hepatic hematoma 42f
Hepatic laceration 55f
Hepatic metastasis 3f
  patterns of 58
Hepatic parenchyma 38f
Hepatitis 37, 39
  acute 40f, 76
  alcoholic 37, 39
  chronic 37, 39
  granulomatous 37, 39
Hepatobiliary system 37
Hepatoblastoma 260-262
Hepatocellular carcinoma 48, 49, 55, 56, 58, 58f
Hepatoduodenal ligament, echogenic fat in 66

Hepatoma 41, 42, 45
Hepatorenal pouch 142
Hernia 71
  diaphragmatic 12, 12f, 268
  evidence of 72f
  type of 71
Herniated sac 225f
Herpes simplex 221
Heterogeneous echotexture 122f
  lesion of 43
Heterogeneous mass 139f, 229
  solid 138f
Hilar lip 117
Hilum, splenic 96
Hip
  abnormal 179, 182
  congenital dislocation of 180
  coronal sonography 182f
  dysplasia, classification of 181
  joint 185f
  pediatric 178
Hippel-Lindau disease 199
Histiocytoma, fibrous 141
Hodgkin's disease 10
Hodgkin's lymphoma 49, 88, 202
Holoprosencephaly 208, 214, 214f, 256, 277, 281
Homozygous alpha thalassemia 255
Horseshoe kidney 116, 258
Human chorionic gonadotropin 159, 248
Hurler's syndrome 276
Hyaloid artery, persistent 206
Hydatid 175, 206
  cyst 49, 53f, 118f, 167
  parenchyma like 1
  disease 51
  infected 53f
  sand 85f
  splenic 85
Hydatidiform mole 248
  complete 267
  early 250f
  partial 267f
Hydranencephaly 208, 210, 211, 282

Hydrocele 149f, 155f, 160f
  acute 149
  gross 155f
Hydrocephalus 208, 210, 211, 215f, 219, 222
  causes of 211, 213
  diagnosis of 212
  imaging after development of 219
Hydrolethalus syndrome 275, 276
Hydromyelia 223, 224f, 227
Hydronephrosis 126f, 283
  intrauterine 273
  moderate 124f
Hydropneumothorax 4, 7f
Hydrops
  fetal 267
  immune 267
  nonimmune 256, 258, 267
Hydrosalpinx 81, 236, 239
Hydrothorax 256
Hydroureteronephrosis 274
Hygroma, cystic 28, 256, 258, 262, 264, 268, 270, 281f
Hyperechoic
  lesion 168, 249f
  metastasis 59, 59f
  nodule 22
  renal nodules, differential diagnosis of 123
  splenic lesion 89
Hyperlipidemia 37
Hyperparathyroidism 188
Hyperplasia 136
  cystic endometrial 249f
Hyperplastic
  adenomatous nodule 14
  nodule 15f
Hypertelorism 276
  syndromes with 276
Hypertrophy
  compensatory 117
  iliopsoas 133, 135
Hypervascular masses 112
Hyphema 193
Hypochondrium, differential diagnosis for 75
Hypoechogenicity, periportal 46

Hypoechoic
  deposits, multiple 48
  lesions 30f, 48, 150, 163
    multiple 30f, 88f
    solid 114f
  nodular lesions, multiple 82f
  renal sinus, differential diagnosis of 123
  solid mass 74, 107f
    lesion 7f
  space occupying lesion 4f, 12f
Hypogastrium, differential diagnosis in 76
Hypoplasia 282
  pulmonary 262, 263
Hypoproteinemia, severe 268

I

Iliac artery aneurysm 133
Iliac fossa 108, 114f
  transverse scans of 108
Iliac line 182
Iliac region, differential diagnosis in 76
Iliac vein varices 133
Infarct, cystic degeneration of 83
Infarction, pulmonary 8
Inflammatory mass
  chronic 96f
  in ovary 236f
Inguinal canal 73f, 154f
Inguinal hernia, case of 155f
Iniencephaly 280
Injury, spinal trauma mode of 229
Insulinoma 93, 95
Interbowel loop fluid 106f, 143f
Interstitial line sign 266
Interventricular septum 286, 287
Intrahepatic bile ducts, dilated 68f
Intrahepatic biliary
  calculi 69
  dilatation, differential diagnosis of 68

radicals 38f
  dilated 70f
Intrahepatic neoplasm 68
Intranodal blood flow pattern 14
Intraocular
  structures, evaluation of 190
  tumors, evaluation of 191
Intraorbital
  calcification, differential diagnosis of 207
  fat 206
Intrauterine
  growth restriction 256
  infections 255
Intussusception 77
  evidence of 107f
Iridocyclitis 192
Iris 189
Ischemia 220
Islet cell tumor 91
  nonfunctioning 96
Isoechoic nodule 23

J

Jeune's syndrome 272
Joint
  capsule 178, 181
  effusion 178
  neuropathic 176
Juxtaportal intrahepatic mass 69

K

Kaposi's sarcoma 43, 45
Keratoconjunctivitis sicca 25
Kidney
  cystic dysplasia of 279
  medullary sponge 119, 120
  multicystic dysplastic 118, 120
  multilocular nephroma of 120
Klatskin tumor 68
Klippel-Trenaunay-Weber syndrome 86

Knee
  joint 185
    effusion 184f
    synovitis of 185
Koch's abdomen, case of 144f

L

Lacrimal gland
  carcinoma 207
  lesions of 205
Lamina propria 131
Larsen syndrome 276
Laurence-Moon-Biedl
    syndrome 272
Legg-Calvé Perthes disease 179, 180
Leiomyomatosis peritonealis
    disseminated 147
Leiomyosarcoma 104, 113, 141, 246
Lemon sign 280
Lens 190
  disease of 196
  dislocation 197
Leptomyelolipoma 226, 227, 228
Lesions
  anechoic 208
  appendiceal 108
  cystic 13f, 98, 167, 208
  malignant 173
  sclerosing 171
  solid 209
Lesser sac posterior 147
Leukemia 45, 121
Leukomalacia
  periventricular 211, 219, 220
  subcortical 220
Leydig cell tumor 153
Limb
  amputation defects 278
  body wall complex 284
  defects 284
  reduction defects 279
Limbus 189
Linitis plastica, case of 99f
Lipodystrophy 142
Lipoleiomyoma 244
Lipoma 41, 141, 171, 283

intradural 226f, 227
intraspinal 227, 228
Lipomatosis, diffuse infiltrative 142, 148
Lipomeningocele 228
Lipomyelocele 226
Lipomyelomeningocele 223, 224
Lipomyeloschisis 228
Liposarcoma 32, 142
Lissencephaly 282
Listeria 222
Liver 47, 52f
  abscess
    amebic 12f
    information 47f
    multiple 51
  cyst 50f
  cystic lesions of 49
  echogenicity of 37
  focal hypoechoic lesions 47
  focal nodular hyperplasia
    lesion in 41f
  generalized decrease in
    echogenicity of 40
  hematoma 55
  in transverse scan 11f
  left lobe of 147
  lesions, differential diagnosis
    of 37
  mass 12
    isoechoic 49, 58f
    multiple hydatid cysts in 54f
    right lobe of 42f, 45f, 48f, 59f
    shadowing lesions of 43
    subcostal scan of 53f
    target lesion of 45
    transabdominal scan of 57f, 64f
Lobar holoprosencephaly,
    sonographic findings
    in 214
Lumbar quadrants, differential
    diagnosis for 75
Lumbosacral
  region 228f
  spine 224
  vertebrae 224f
Lung
  abscess 4f

carcinoma 43
collapse 1
hydatid 2f
lesions 13
normal 1
parenchyma 1
right lower lobe of 2f
scan, pleural 7f
tumor 1
  primary 11
Lymph nodes 73, 82f, 99f, 104
  intramammary 169
  lymphomatous 82
  mass, conglomerate 113f
  metastasis to 10
  metastatic 34f
  multiple matted 29f
  necrotic mesenteric 143f
  submental 33
Lymphadenopathy 112
  abdominal 81
  mediastinal 9
  retroperitoneal 140
Lymphangioma 10, 86, 92, 98, 116, 200, 201, 206, 264
  cystic 29f
Lymphatic
  obstruction, malignant 46
  periportal 46
Lymphocele 146, 116, 168, 233
Lymphoma 9, 14, 43, 45, 91, 103, 104, 112, 133, 135-137, 141, 142, 146, 170, 174, 200, 206, 283
  case of 113f

M

Macroglossia 276
Macronodular cirrhosis 39
Malakoplakia 130, 132
  renal 118
Malformations, congenital and
    developmental 214
Malignant disease 8
Malignant infiltration, diffuse 40
Malignant ovarian
    lesions, ultrasound features
    of 242

mass 242f
neoplasm 242
Mammilopontine distance 211
Mandible, radicular cyst of 186
Masses
  cystic 280
  hypoechoic 82f
  pleural 3, 8
  pulmonary 3f
  renal 120
Mastitis 171, 171f
Matted bowel loop 102f
Meckel-Gruber's syndrome 280
Meconium peritonitis 144, 146, 148f, 151, 260, 261, 268
Median cleft syndrome 276
Mediastinum 1
  anterior 1
  cystic mass of 10
  vascular lesions of 10
Mediterranean fever, familial 149
Medullary carcinoma 21f, 170
  case of 21f
Medullary granulomatous masses 118
Megacisterna magna 208, 215, 256
Megaureter 272
Melanoma 202
  malignant 86
Ménétrier's disease 99
Meningioma 202, 207
Meningitis 222
Meningocele
  herniation, posterior 225f
  lateral 10
  posterior 223
  simple posterior 225
Mesenteric artery
  superior 80, 81f, 93
  syndrome, superior 102
Mesenteric dermoid tumors 146
Mesenteric lymph nodes
  enlarged 143f
    isolated 147
    multiple enlarged 148, 148f

Mesenteric masses 141
Mesenteric thickening 141f
  ascites 104
Mesenteric vein, superior 80f, 102
Mesoblastic nephroma 120, 121
Mesothelioma 145, 146
  cystic 144, 146
  malignant 8
  peritoneal 142
  pleural 9
Metastasis 8, 43, 45, 88, 103, 104, 136, 147, 170, 174, 202
  cystic 55, 59
  echopoor 58, 59f
  hypoechoic mass 137f
Metastatic lesions 54f
  cystic 60f
  different types of 58
Michaelis-Gutmann inclusion bodies 118
Microabscess 84
Microcalcification, presence of 16
Micrognathia 257, 279
  differential diagnosis of 275
Microlithiasis, isolated 152
Midface syndromes 275
Miliary tuberculosis 85, 86, 88
Miller's syndrome 275, 278, 279
Mirizzi's syndrome 69
Mohr's syndrome 275, 278, 279
Molar placenta 257
Mondor's disease 171
Monochorionic twin syndromes 270
Morgagni hernia 263
Mucocele 206
Mucoepidermoid tumor 206
Müllerian cyst 162
Multicystic dysplastic kidney 274f
Multinodular parenchymal pattern, heterogeneous 21f
Mural nodule 242
Musculoskeletal system 176
Mustard gas 193

Myasthenia gravis 11
Mycobacterium
  avium intracellulare 85
  tuberculosis 85
Myelocele 224, 280
Myelocystocele 223, 224, 283
Myelofibrosis 90
Myelolipoma 137, 139
  adrenal 139
Myelomeningocele 223, 224, 257
  anterior 283
Myotonic dystrophy 268

N

Neck
  abnormality 268
  lesions 14
Neonatal
  and infant brain 208
  spinal canal, indications for ultrasound of 223
Neoplasm 12
  cystic 84
Neoplastic lesions 233
Nephrocalcinosis 124
Nephrotic syndrome 4
  congenital 268
Nerve root tumors 10
Neural arches 224f
Neural tissue, part of 224
Neural tumors 141
Neurilemmoma 176
  malignant 193
Neurinomas 31
Neuroblastoma 138, 138f, 139, 262, 264, 282, 283
  metastatic 260
Neurocysticercosis, intraocular 206
Neurofibroma 31, 206
Neurofibromatosis 207
Neurogenic bladder 130, 132
Neuromuscular disorders 11
Nodal disease, criteria for assessing 81
Nodular
  goiter 18f
  hyperplasia, focal 41

Nodule
  benign 22
  hypoechoic 22
  metastatic 63, 64
  pleural 3
Non-Hodgkin's lymphoma 74, 88
Nonskin covered back mass 223
Noonan's syndrome 276
Nuchal
  fold 285
  thickening 256
  translucency 256, 285

O

Obesity 11
Obstruction, intrahepatic 70
Obstructive uropathy, signs of 126f
Ocular inflammatory diseases 199
Ocular tumors, common 195
Oligohydramnios 258, 259, 260
Omental
  cyst 147, 233
  infarction 78
  sarcoma, evidence of 143f
Omentum, thickened 103f
Omphalocele 256, 283, 284
Oncocytoma 121, 123
Oophoritis 236
Ophthalmic vein, superior 201f
Optic nerve 190
  avulsion 192, 194
  head, disease of 200
  lesions of 202
Ora serrata 189
Orbit 189, 190
  vertical section of 191f
Orbital
  cellulitis 206
  color Doppler 192
  cyst 195
  cysticercosis 195, 202f
  diseases, sonological features of 193
  hemorrhage 195
  lesions, sonographic classification of 200
  muscle enlargement, differential diagnosis of 201
  pathology 200
  trauma 192
  sonoanatomy and technique 190
  indications 190
  systematic evaluation 191
  ultrasound technique 191
  trauma 192, 193
Orchitis 149
Ormond's disease 113
Orofacial digital syndrome 279
Osteochondromatosis, synovial 177
Osteomyelitis 185f
Otocraniofacial syndromes 275
Ovarian
  carcinoma 43
  cyst 233
    adenoma 233
    functional 239f
    hemorrhagic 238f
    large 240
  dermoid 235f, 242f
  enlargement 232
  lesions 234
  malignancy 242f
  mass, cystic 236
  stimulation, case of 238
  torsion 236, 239
  tumors 236
    benign 241
    malignant 241
Ovary
  cystadenocarcinoma of 243f
  endometriotic cyst in 239f
  massive edema of 238

P

Pancreas 91
  cystic
    mass 96f
    tumors of 91
  diffuse fatty, infiltration of 95f
  enlargement of 78
  head of 94, 95f
Pancreatic masses, inflammatory 93, 95
Pancreaticoblastoma 93
Pancreatitis 78, 142
Panuveitis 192
Papillary carcinoma, case of 20f
Papillary tumors, intraductal 91
Papilloma 97, 173
  intracystic 167
Paraganglioma 131, 132
Paralysis, diaphragmatic 11
Paralytic ileus 102, 103
Paranasal sinus malignancy 200
Paraovarian cyst 232, 236, 238
Parasites, biliary 70
Parasitic
  cyst 84, 85
  infection 118
  infestation 72
Paratubal cyst 238
Parenchyma
  homogeneous 15f
  hyperplasia of 117
  pulmonary 7f
Parotid gland 28f
  enlarged 30f
Paroxysmal nocturnal hemoglobinuria 41
Patau's syndrome 272
Peak systolic velocities 192
Pediatric
  neoplasm, solid 93
  testicular masses 157
Pelvic
  abscess 145f, 146f, 230, 231, 234f
  hematoma 133, 135, 235f
  inflammatory disease 80, 230
    case of 78f
  lipomatosis 133
  malignancies 131
  masses
    cystic 232
    solid 236
  nodes 135
  tumors 112

Pelvicalyceal system, dilatation of 126f
Pelvis 123, 141f, 142f
  renal 127f
  transverse scan of 232f, 243f
Pelviureteric junction obstruction 125f, 272, 273, 273f
Pena-Shokeir syndrome 268, 275
Pericholecystic fluid 62, 68
  differential diagnosis of 68
Pericholecystic inflammation, signs of 66
Perichondrium unite 181
Perinodal blood flow 14
Periovarian inflammation 81, 231
Peripancreatic collaterals 92f
Peripheral nerve sheath 192
Peritoneal
  cavity 145f
    duplication cyst 107f
    with internal septae 144f
  dialysis 4
  inclusion cyst 148, 233
  lesions, solid 145
  masses 141
Perthes' disease 180f
Pfeiffer syndrome 276, 277
Phantom sign 112
Pheochromocytoma 136, 137, 138, 138f, 139, 140
  large 139f
Phleboliths 207
Phrenic nerve paralysis 11
Phthisis bulbi 194
Phylloides tumor 173
Pierre Robin syndrome 275
Placental cotyledon, single 270
Placode 224
Pleural disease, drug-related 8
Pleural effusion 3f, 4, 6f, 8f, 262, 267
  and ascites outlining diaphragm 5f
  and collapsed lung 6f
  superior to diaphragm 5f
Plexiform neurofibroma 201
Pneumobilia echogenic foci 46f

Pneumocystis 123
  carinii infection 84, 85
Pneumothoraces 4
Polycystic
  kidney disease 69, 119, 119f, 120, 240f, 268
    infantile autosomal recessive 120
  liver 50f
  ovarian disease 239
  renal disease 50
Polydactyly 257, 282
Polyhydramnios 258, 260, 285
Polypoidal mass 130f
Polysplenia 288
  syndrome 83
Popliteal fossa, cystic mass in 176
Portal hypertension, noncirrhotic 46
Postmeningitis hydrocephalus 222f
Post-vasectomy changes 161
Pott's spine 116
Pouch of Douglas 230f
Pregnancy
  and lactation, late 175
  anembryonic 265
  ectopic 230, 230f, 231f, 234, 248, 250f, 258, 265, 266, 266f
  first trimester 264
  intrauterine 244, 247, 248, 248f, 258
  loss, first trimester 270
  molar 266
  multifetal 269
  ruptured ectopic 230
  test 258
Prephthitic eyeball 194
Pressure, intra-articular 179
Primitive gonadal stroma, tumor of 154
Proliferative disease 248
Prostastitis, chronic 154
Prostate 162
  abscess 164
  acute 165
  advanced carcinoma of 164f
  calcification 165, 165f
  carcinoma 163f, 164f
  chronic 165
  cyst
    differential diagnosis of 162
    simple 165
  dysplasia 165
  midline cyst in 162f
  retention cysts cluster of 164
  tissue, normal 164
Prostatic hyperplasia, benign 164
Prostatic hypertrophy, benign 162, 162f
Prostatitis, granulomatous 163, 165
Protruding tongue 256
Prune-Belly syndrome 260, 268
Pseudoachalasia 98
Pseudoaneurysm 73, 92
Pseudoangiomatous stromal hyperplasia 169, 173
Pseudocyst 92, 140
  pancreatic 10, 84, 86, 92f, 116, 147
  paracardiac 144
Pseudogestation sac 266
Pseudokidney sign 103, 104f
Pseudolithiasis, drug-induced 63f
Pseudomasses
  adrenal 140
  differential diagnosis of 116
Pseudomembranous colitis 106
Pseudomyxoma peritonei 144, 147
Pseudostaphyloma 200
Pseudotumor 117, 202
  inflammatory 86
  pleural 8
  renal 117
Psoas abscess 114f, 115f, 116
Ptotic kidney 116
Pulsatile proptosis, differential diagnosis of 207
Pyelonephritis
  acute 125f
  case of 127f
  xanthogranulomatous 118

Pyloric stenosis
    hypertrophic 101f
    infantile hypertrophic 100f
Pyogenic cholangitis, recurrent 45, 46
Pyometra 244
Pyonephrosis
    secondary 127f
    stone 123
Pyosalpinx 81

Q

Quadrants, division of 75f

R

Radial scar 169
Radiation cystitis 130, 132
Rectal endosonography, role of 111
Rectus abdominis muscles 71f
Reflux nephropathy 117
Renal cell carcinoma 43, 118f, 119, 121, 122, 123f
    mass 122f
    presence of 122f
Rendu-Osler-Weber syndrome 217
Reninoma 120
Retina 190
    disease of 198
Retinal detachment 194, 203, 204
Retinoblastoma 195, 202, 203, 203f
Retractile mesenteritis 142
Retroperitoneum 112
Retrotumoral attenuation 170
Rhabdomyoma 288
Rhabdomyosarcoma 32, 131, 201
Rhadomyoma 205
Rhesus isoimmunization 255
Rheumatoid arthritis 8, 177, 188
Rib
    fracture 8
    with distal shadowing 1f
Riedel's lobe 37f

Riedel's struma 113
Robert's syndrome 275, 278
Robinson syndrome 276
Rocker bottom feet 256
Rotator cuff 177f
Roundness index 33
Rubella 220, 221
    clinical features 221
    ultrasonography 221
Russell silver syndrome 276

S

Sacral meningocele, anterior 223, 227
Saethre-Chotzen syndrome 277
Salivary gland, enlargement of 25
Sandwich sign 81f
Sarcoidosis 9, 86, 87, 152, 154, 188, 206
Sarcoma 91, 170, 175, 205
    botryoides 131
    osteogenic 13
    retroperitoneal 114f
Scalp edema 280
Scar granuloma 169, 175
Schistosomiasis 45, 130, 131, 151
Schizencephaly 208, 214, 282
Schwannomas 31
Sclera 189
Scleral injury 194
Scleritis 202
Sclerocornea, disease of 199
Scoliosis, thoracolumbar 276
Scrotal
    calcification, differential diagnosis of 151
    edema, idiopathic 149, 150
    fat necrosis 149
    gas, differential diagnosis of 152
    masses, differential diagnosis of 153
    pearls 151, 152
    sac 153f, 155f
        calcification in 152f
        tubercular collection in 151

Scrotolith 151f
Scrotum 149
    differential diagnosis of 149
Sebaceous cysts 167
Seckel syndrome 275
Semilobar holoprosencephaly 208
    sonographic findings in 214
Seminal vesicles
    absent 163f
    cyst 133, 163
    normal 163f
Seminiferous tubules 150
Seminoma 158
    testis 154f
    tumors 159
Sepsis 63
Septate uterus 245f
Septic emboli 45
Seroma 71
Serpentine sonolucencies transgress 63
Serpiginous tortuous hypoechoic vascular structures 207
Sertoli's cell tumor 151, 153
Sex cord tumors 236
Short rib polydactyly syndrome 272
Shoulder joint cavity 184f
Sialadenitis
    acute 25
    chronic 25
Sialolithiasis 26
Sickle cell anemia 199
Sigmoid colon 76
Silhouette sign 82
Silicon granulomas 175
Simple cyst 156
Sinonasal malignancies 206
Sinus of Valsalva, aneurysm of 10
Sinusoidal dilatation 43
Situs inversus 80
Sjögren's syndrome 25
Skeletal dysplasias 275, 276
Skin covered back mass 223
Soft splenic calcification 90f

Soft tissue
  nodule causes of 188
  sarcomas 121
  tumors 236
Solid masses, differential diagnosis of 112
Solitary thyroid nodule 15f
Somatostatinoma 96
Sonopathology 192
Space-occupying lesion 92f, 93f, 282
Sperm granuloma 160
Spermatocele 160, 160f
Sphenoid wing dysplasia 207
Spill meconium 146
Spina bifida 280, 283
  aperta 223, 224
  cystica 223, 224
  with meningocele 227f, 281f
Spinal childhood tumors 229
Spinal cord, area of clefting 226f
Spinal defect 280
Spinal dysraphism 223, 227, 284
  occult 223, 225, 228
  overt 223
Spinal lipoma 223, 226
Spinal trauma 223, 229
  etiology 229
Spleen 83
  abscess 79
  absence of 288
  cystic, lesion of 83
    cystic neoplasm 86
    epidermoid cyst 84
    infection or inflammation 85
    post-traumatic 85
    vascular 84
  multiple hydatid cysts in 85f
  star-sky 89
  traumatic fragmentation of 83
Splenic
  abscess, case of 84
  infarction 86, 87
  laceration 83, 84
  lesion, solid 86
  parenchyma, abscess in 84
  vein 85
Splenoma 86

Splenomegaly 85, 87, 90
Split notochord 227
  syndrome 223
Squamous cell carcinoma 121, 130, 133
Squamous tumors, small 97
Staghorn calculus 127f
Staphyloma 199
  posterior 205f
Stenosis 260
Sternocleidomastoid muscle 28
Stewart's classification 275
Stomach 98
Stroma 189
Stromal tumors 159
Sturge-Weber syndrome 196
Subarachnoid space 217
Subcutaneous fat 225f
Submandibular gland, transverse scan of 25f
Submucosa, disease of 131
Submucosal fibroid 244f
Subretinal fluid 194, 199
Sunray spiculation 44
Supraspinatus tendon 187f
Swelling, diffuse 220
Synovitis, proliferative 185f
Systemic lupus erythematosus 8

T

Tachycardia 260
Taenia solium 72
Target lesion 104f
Target sign 103
Taussig-Bing syndrome 287
Teeth, apical cyst of 186f
Tendinitis, signs of 177
Tendo-Achiles chronic, partial rupture of 184f
Tendon tears 177
Tenosynovitis 185f
Teratocarcinoma 156
  gonadoblastoma 151
Teratogen exposure 285
Teratoma 113, 151, 158, 260, 262, 282, 288
  cystic 91, 236
  sacrococcygeal 282

Testicular
  appendages, torsion of 149
  calcification 151, 152f
  lesions, cystic 156
  malignancy 153f
  metastasis 159
  microlithiasis 151
  torsion 149
  trauma 149, 150
Testis 150, 156
Tethered cord 228
  causes of 228
  risk factors for 228
Tetralogy of Fallot 287
Thalamus 210
Theca cell tumor 154
Theca lutein cyst 232, 237, 250
Thickened placenta 255, 255f
  differential diagnosis of 255
Thoracic meningocele, lateral 223, 227
Thoracic tumor 268
Thorax abnormality 268
Thymic cyst 10
Thymic enlargement 262
Thyroglossal cyst 28
Thyroid 14
  calcification 22
  colloid nodule of 23f
  disease, diffuse 17
  function tests, abnormal 206
  gland, heteroechoic enlarged 19f
  inferno 19
  isthmus of 15f
  left lobe of 23f
  multinodular goiter, nodule in 22f
  nodule
    benign 16, 17
    cystic 23
    degeneration in 24f
    differential diagnosis on 22
    malignant 16, 17
    with internal calcification 24f
Tissue inhomogeneity 193
Tortuous brachiocephalic artery 10

Index

Toxocara infection 195
Toxoplasma 261
Toxoplasmosis 136, 220, 221
Transabdominal
  scan 57*f*
  sonography 248
Transient uterine contraction 244
Transitional cell
  carcinoma 121, 121*f*, 128*f*, 130, 130*f*, 133
  papilloma 130
Transudative pleural effusion, causes of 4
Transvaginal sonography 248
Traumatic cystic lesions 218
Treacher-Collins syndrome 275
Trilobed lung, bilateral 288
Triploidy 255, 257
Triradiate cartilage 183*f*
Trophoblastic
  disease 247
    invasive 246
  neoplasia, persistent 266
  tumor, placental site 251, 266
Truncus arteriosus, persistent 287
Tubal lesions 232
Tubercular
  abdomen 105*f*
  abscess, multiple 29*f*
  arthritis, right hip 179*f*
  epididymitis 161*f*
  epididymo-orchitis 150*f*
  lymphadenopathy 82*f*
  peritonitis 106*f*
    case of 143*f*
    thickened omentum 144*f*
  tubo-ovarian mass 232*f*
Tuberculosis 9, 103, 131, 142
  peritoneal 144, 147
  renal 129
Tuberculous pleural effusion 7*f*
Tubo-ovarian
  abscess 81, 81*f*, 231, 235, 235*f*, 238
  complex 231
  mass 231*f*
Tubular ectasia 154, 156, 157

Tubular structures, multiple 69*f*
Tumefactive sludge 63, 65
Tumors 74, 220, 229
  benign submandibular 26*f*
  cardiac 288
  cystic
    change in 162
    spindle-shaped 144
  desmoid 74, 141, 142, 145
  endometrioid 243
  epithelial 93, 97
  esophageal 97
  extradural 229
  lipomas 74
  malignant 32, 47
  metastasis 74
  metastatic 243
  neuroendocrine 43
  neurofibromas 74
  neuromas 74
  occult primary 159
  pancreatic 140
  pleural 8
  renal 117
  retroperitoneal 112
  sacrococcygeal 229
  thrombus in portal vein 49*f*
Tunica albuginea cyst 154, 156, 157
Turner's syndrome 258
Twin
  and multifetal pregnancy, complications of 270
  embolization syndrome 270
  peak sign 269
  pregnancy 257*f*, 269
    case of 269
  transfusion syndrome 270
Typhlitis, amebic 103

U

Umbilical region, differential diagnosis for 76
Undescended testicles 72
Unilocular cystic lesion 238
Urachal cyst 72, 134*f*
Ureter, ectopic 274
Ureterocele, ectopic 274*f*
Urethra, dilated posterior 272*f*

Urethral atresia 260
Urethral diverticulae 255
Urethral valve, posterior 260
Uric acid, calcium precipitates 176
Urinary bladder 130, 146*f*, 237*f*
  clot in 130*f*
  hemangiomatous lesion 131*f*
  multifocal carcinoma 131
  polypoidal mass from
    anterior wall 132*f*
    posterior wall of 130*f*, 134, 234*f*
  transitional cell carcinoma of 131*f*
  walls of 130*f*
Urinary tract
  abnormality 268
  obstruction 4
Urinoma 116, 119*f*, 233
Uterine
  cavity 253*f*, 255*f*
  endometrium 247*f*
  enlargement, diffuse 246
  fibroids 243, 244*f*
  fundus 238
  lesions 234
  masses 243
    adenomyosis 246
    benign 243
    cervical carcinoma 246
    focal myometrial contraction 246
    leiomyoma 246
    leiomyosarcoma 246
    lipoleiomyoma 246
    malignant 246
    rudimentary horn of bicornuate uterus 246
  synechia 254*f*
Uterus
  adenomyoma of 245
  foreign body in 254*f*
  obstructed 232
  peritoneal surfaces of 148
  small lipoma of 245*f*
Utricle cyst 162
Uveal melanoma 196
Uveal tract 189
Uveitis 202

V

Vaginal lesions detected on
    ultrasound 255
Vanishing twin syndrome 265
Varicocele 73, 152f
Vascular
    abnormalities 171
    aneurysms 92
    disease 192
    extratesticular mass 150f
    lesions 217
    malformations and
        aneurysm 118
    masses 73
Vein of Galen, aneurysm of 217f
Vena cava
    bilateral superior 288
    inferior 12f, 115f
    superior 4
Venous thrombosis 269
Venovenous placental
    anastomosis 270
Ventral wall defect, large 284
Ventricular septal defect 286
Ventriculoarterial discordance 287
Ventriculomegaly 208, 211
Vermian agenesis 282
Vertebral body 228f
Vesical calculus 134f
Vesicocervical fistula 268f
Vesicoureteric junction 272
    obstruction 272, 273
Vesicoureteric reflux 272, 274, 275f
    jet 273f
Vessel
    encasement 14
    tear, cause of 198
Villous hyperplasia 63
Vipoma 96
Viral hepatitis 39f, 46
Vitreous humor, evaluation of 191
Volvulus 99
    malrotation with 102
von Hippel-Lindau disease 91
von Meyenburg complex 49, 50

W

Wall-echo-shadow sign 61
Wandering spleen 83
Wegener's granulomatosis 201
Wharton's duct 26f
Wilms' tumor 13, 119, 121–123
Wilson's disease 39, 188
Wolman's disease 137
Wyburn-Mason syndrome 217

X

Xerostomia 25

Y

Yolk sac 265, 265f
    tumor 153, 156, 158

Z

Zellweger syndrome 215, 272

EU GSPR Authorised Reprsentative
Logos Europe, 9 rue Nicolas Poussin
1700, La Rochelle, France
Phone: +33 (0) 6 67 93 73 78
E-mail: contact@logoseurope.eu

www.ingramcontent.com/pod-product-compliance
Ingram Content Group UK Ltd.
Pitfield, Milton Keynes, MK11 3LW, UK
UKHW050429150426

5217IPUK00019B/1306